ALLE ZEIT WACH
1842

R. Felix M. Langer (Eds.)

Advances in CT

II

2nd European Scientific User Conference
SOMATOM PLUS
Berlin, March 1992

With 147 Figures
in 266 Separate Illustrations
and 29 Tables

Springer-Verlag
Berlin Heidelberg New York
London Paris Tokyo
Hong Kong Barcelona
Budapest

Professor Dr. R. Felix
Professor Dr. M. Langer

Freie Universität Berlin
Universitätsklinikum Rudolf Virchow
Strahlenklinik und Poliklinik
Augustenburger Platz 1
W-1000 Berlin 65, FRG

ISBN-13:978-3-642-77465-2 e-ISBN-13:978-3-642-77463-8
DOI: 10.1007/978-3-642-77463-8

Softcover reprint of the hardcover 1st edition 1992

21/3145–5 4 3 2 1 0 – Printed on acid-free paper

Preface

Computed tomography with a continuously rotating X-ray tube and the capacity to perform subsecond CT scans was introduced into clinical routine nearly 4 years ago. At the first European Scientific User Conference – Somatom Plus, organized by the Radiological Department of the University of Zürich, Professor Fuchs demonstrated its great value and its potentional in clinical applications. The 2nd European Scientific User Conference, held here in Berlin, showed that further significant developments, featured by the Siemens Somatom Plus, have opened new fields for diagnostic imaging in computed tomography.

Spiral CT with a continuously rotating X-ray tube and synchronous table increments for up to 60 cm in less than half a minute make radiological diagnosis more accurate. Blind gaps, due to different depths of inspiration, will no longer pose a problem, and all structures, especially in the lungs, can be identified and diagnosed. This fact is of increasing relevance in the staging and follow-up of tumor patients.

Dynamic CT, angio CT, and the cine display of incremental CT of the abdomen and dental-CT will open new dimensions in diagnostic imaging by probably simultanously increasing the sensitivity and the specificity of computed tomography.

The value of two- and three-dimensional multiplanar reconstructions will increase in the future. Their value for therapy planning has already been established, and the increasing preciseness and resolution of the images will increase their diagnostic value even further.

The organizers of the 2nd European Scientific User Conference – Somatom Plus hope that publishing these proceedings will illustrate the state of the art and future perspectives of subsecond computed tomography. We would like to thank all authors for their efforts in preparing their papers and for their understanding regarding the tight deadlines, which were necessary to achieve rapid publication.

We would like to thank all our colleagues at the Strahlenklinik, Universitätsklinikum Rudolf Virchow, for their help in preparing the conference and during the symposium itself.

We want to express our special thanks to Siemens for generously sponsoring the 2nd European Scientific User Conference – Somatom Plus and to Springer-Verlag for marvellously organizing the symposium and publishing these proceedings.

Berlin, March 1992 *Roland Felix and Mathias Langer*

Contents

Thoracic CT and Pediatric Applications
Chairmen: W. A. Fuchs, A. L. Baert, and R. Felix

Clinical Application I
Chairmen: J. Lissner, U. Mödder, and K. J. Wolf

Spiral CT
Chairmen: E. Zeitler and M. Galanski

Chairmen

Prof. A. L. Baert
Universitaire Ziekenhuizen Leuven, Gasthuisberg, Heerestraat 49,
B-3000 Leuven

Prof. C. D. Claussen
Eberhard-Karls-Universität, Radiologische Universitätsklinik,
Abt. Radiologische Diagnostik, Hoppe-Seyler-Straße 3, W-7400 Tübingen,
FRG

Prof. R. Felix
Universitätsklinikum Rudolf Virchow, Strahlenklinik und Poliklinik,
Augustenburger Platz 1, W-1000 Berlin 65, FRG

Prof. W. A. Fuchs
Institut für Radiologie, Universitätsspital Zürich, Rämistraße 100,
CH-8091 Zürich

Prof. M. Galanski
Medizinische Hochschule Hannover, Abt. Diagnostische Radiologie,
Konstanty-Gutschow-Straße 8, W-3000 Hannover 61, FRG

Prof. K. Lackner
Radiologisches Institut und Poliklinik der Universität Köln,
Joseph-Stelzmann-Straße 9, W-5000 Köln 41, FRG

Prof. M. Langer
Universitätsklinikum Rudolf Virchow, Strahlenklinik und Poliklinik,
Augustenburger Platz 1, W-1000 Berlin 65, FRG

Prof. J. Lissner
Radiologische Universitätsklinik, Klinikum Großhadern,
Marchioninistraße 15, W-8000 München 70, FRG

Prof. U. Mödder
Institut für Diagnostische Radiologie, Heinrich-Heine-Univ. Düsseldorf,
Moorenstraße 5, W-4000 Düsseldorf, FRG

Prof. H. E. Riemann
Klinikum der Joh.-Wolf.-Goethe-Universität, Theodor-Stern-Kai 7,
W-6000 Frankfurt 70, FRG

Prof. P. Vock
Institut für Diagnostische Radiologie, Inselspital, Universität Bern,
CH-3010 Bern

Prof. K. J. Wolf
Radiologische Universitätsklinik, Klinikum Steglitz, Hindenburgdamm 30,
W-1000 Berlin 45, FRG

Prof. E. Zeitler
Klinikum Nürnberg Nord, Radiologisches Zentrum, Flurstraße 17,
W-8500 Nürnberg 1, FRG

Prof. D. zur Nedden
Medizinische Universitätsklinik, Anichstraße 35, A-6020 Innsbruck

Speakers

A. Adam, M. D.
Hammersmith Hospital, Department Radiology, Du Cane Road,
GB-London W12 ONN

Dr. T. Bareiter
Klinikum Nürnberg, Radiologisches Zentrum, Abteilung Diagnostik,
Flurstraße 17, W-8500 Nürnberg, FRG

PD Dr. W. Bautz
Technische Universität München, Institut für Röntgendiagnostik,
Klinikum rechts der Isar, Ismaninger Straße 22, W-8000 München 80, FRG

Dr. R. Braunschweig
Eberhard-Karls-Universität Tübingen, Radiologische Universitätsklinik,
Abt. Radiologische Diagnostik, Hoppe-Seyler-Straße 3, W-7400 Tübingen,
FRG

Dr. P. Brennan
Universitätsspital Zürich, Röntgendiagnostisches Zentralinstitut,
Rämistraße 100, CH-8091 Zürich

Dr. A. Dickschas
Bezirkskrankenhaus Erlangen, Abteilung Neurologie, Am Europakanal 71,
W-8500 Nürnberg, FRG

Dr. R. Dore
Policlinico S. Matteo, Istituto di Radiologia, I-Pavia

Dr. K. Engelhard
Krankenhaus Martha-Maria-Nürnberg, Abteilung Radiologie,
Stadenstraße 58, W-8500 Nürnberg, FRG

Dr. Th. Fleiter
Eberhard-Karls-Universität Tübingen, Radiologische Diagnostik,
Hoppe-Seyler-Straße 3, W-7400 Tübingen, FRG

PD Dr. R. Frahm
Klinikum der Stadt, Institut für Radiologie, Röntgenstraße 20,
W-7730 VS-Schwenningen, FRG

Dr. J. Gaa
Institut für Klinische Radiologie, Klinikum Mannheim
der Universität Heidelberg, Theodor-Kutzer-Ufer, W-6800 Mannheim 1, FRG

P. A. Gevenois, M. D.
Université Libre de Bruxelles, Hôpital Erasme, Departments of Radiology,
Route de Lennik 808, B-1070 Bruxelles

J. C. Hacking, M. D.
University of Cambridge, Department of Radiology,
Addenbrooke's Hospital, Hills Road, GB-Cambridge CB2 2QQ

M. Hayball, M. D.
Department of Nuclear Medicine, Addenbrooke's Hospital, Hills Road,
GB-Cambridge CB2 2QQ

Prof. Dr. M. Herbst
Universität Regensburg, Klinik für Strahlenkunde und Nuklearmedizin,
Franz-Josef-Strauß-Allee 1, W-8400 Regensburg, FRG

Dr. K. G. Hering
Abteilung Radiologie, Knappschaftskrankenhaus Dortmund,
Wieckesweg 27, W-4600 Dortmund, FRG

PD. Dr. H. Hirschfelder
Orthopädische Universitätsklinik und Poliklinik,
Waldkrankenhaus St. Marien, Rathsberger Straße 57, W-8520 Erlangen, FRG

Dr. R. Hupke
Siemens Medical Systems, 186 Wood Avenue South, USA-Iselin, NY 08830

Dr. P. E. Huppert
Eberhard-Karls-Universität Tübingen, Radiologische Universitätsklinik,
Abt. Radiologische Diagnostik, Hoppe-Seyler-Straße 3, W-7400 Tübingen,
FRG

Dr. habil. W. Kalender
Siemens AG, Medizinische Technik, Henkestraße 127, W-8520 Erlangen,
FRG

Dr. U. Keske
Universitätsklinikum Rudolf Virchow, Strahlenklinik und Poliklinik,
Augustenburger Platz 1, W-1000 Berlin 65, FRG

PD Dr. M. Lenz
Technische Universität München, Institut für Röntgendiagnostik,
Klinikum rechts der Isar, Ismaninger Straße 22, W-8000 München 80, FRG

Dr. S. Lieberenz
Universität Leipzig, Abt. Radiologie, Liebigstraße 20, O-7010 Leipzig, FRG

Dr. U. Lörcher
Universitätsklinik, Zentrum Radiologie, Theodor-Stern-Kai 7,
W-6000 Frankfurt 70, FRG

Prof. G. Marchal
Katholieke Universiteit Leuven, Herestraat 49, B-3000 Leuven

Prim. Dr. F. Mieß
A.Ö. Krankenhaus der Elisabethinen, Zentralröntgen, Fadingerstraße 1,
A-4010 Linz

Dr. Oberhauser
Medizinische Universitätsklinik, Anichstraße 35, A-6020 Innsbruck

Dr. M. Oldendorf
Klinikum Nürnberg, Abteilung Diagnostik, Radiologisches Zentrum,
Flurstraße 17, W-8500 Nürnberg, FRG

Dr. M. Oudkerk
Dr. Daniel Den Hoedklinik, Groene Hilledijk 301, NL-3075 EA Rotterdam

Dr. M. Prokop
Medizinische Hochschule Hannover, Diagnostische Radiologie I,
Konstanty-Gutschow-Straße 8, W-3000 Hannover 61, FRG

Dr. A. Rieber
Eberhard-Karls-Universität Tübingen, Radiologische Universitätsklinik,
Abt. Radiologische Diagnostik, Hoppe-Seyler-Straße 3, W-7400 Tübingen,
FRG

Prof. Dr. R. Rienmüller
Klinikum Großhadern, Radiologische Klinik und Poliklinik,
Marchioninistraße 15, W-8000 München 70, FRG

Dr. K. Rosenkranz
Universitätsklinikum Rudolf Virchow, Strahlenklinik und Poliklinik,
Augustenburger Platz 1, W-1000 Berlin 65, FRG

Dr. C. Schaefer
Medizinische Hochschule Hannover, Diagnostische Radiologie I,
Konstanty-Gutschow-Straße 8, W-3000 Hannover 61, FRG

Dr. M. Soucek
Abteilung Diagnostische Radiologie, Universität Bern, Inselspital, Freiburgstraße, CH-3010 Bern

Dr. H. Steinkamp
Universitätsklinikum Rudolf Virchow, Strahlenklinik und Poliklinik, Augustenburger Platz 1, W-1000 Berlin 65, FRG

Dipl.-Phys. Ch. Süss
Siemens AG, Medizinische Technik, Henkestraße 127, W-8520 Erlangen, FRG

Dr. M. O. Tanyü
Universitätsklinikum Freiburg, Radiologische Abteilung, Hugstetter Straße 55, W-7800 Freiburg, FRG

Dr. J.-P. Wakat
Eberhard-Karls-Universität Tübingen, Radiologische Universitätsklinik, Abt. Radiologische Diagnostik, Hoppe-Seyler-Straße 3, W-7400 Tübingen, FRG

PD. Dr. C. Zwicker
Universitätsklinikum Rudolf Virchow, Strahlenklinik und Poliklinik, Augustenburger Platz 1, W-1000 Berlin 65, FRG

Thoracic CT and Pediatric Applications

Chairmen: W. A. Fuchs, A. L. Baert, and R. Felix

CT Quantification of Pulmonary Emphysema – Correlation with Pulmonary Function Tests: Preliminary Results on 15 Patients*

P. A. Gevenois, P. De Vuyst, M. Littani, J. Zanen, P. de Franquen, J. C. Yernault, and J. Struyven

Introduction

Pulmonary emphysema has been redefined as "a condition of the lung characterized by abnormal, permanent enlargement of the airspaces distal to the terminal bronchioles, accompanied by destruction of their walls, without obvious fibrosis"[1]. This diagnosis can theoretically only be established either at autopsy or by examination of surgically resected lobes or lungs. Emphysema is difficult to diagnose accurately during life and almost impossible to quantify. In the 48 autopsy lungs available from the 228 patients who died during the NIH trial of intermittent positive-pressure breathing involving 935 non-hypoxemic patients, Nagai showed that there were no significant relationships between clinical or physiologic variables and either the interalveolar wall thickness or the alveolar surface area, as calculated from measurements of the mean linear intercept [2].

The increase of airspace volume with destruction of the airspace walls will reduce the physical density of the lung, which can be measured by computed tomography (CT). On CT, emphysema is characterized by the presence of areas of abnormally low attenuation. This technique has been shown to be sensitive in evaluating the presence and the severity of emphysema [3–11]. Recently, Kalender et al. presented semiautomatic evaluation procedures for quantitative CT of the lung ("pulmo-CT") [12]. Using this technique, we quantitated the relative area in both lungs with an attenuation of less than – 950 HU and less than – 900 HU. In this preliminary report, we present the correlation of the results obtained with this program with pulmonary function tests in 15 patients.

Material and Methods

Computed tomography scans and pulmonary function tests were performed on 15 patients scheduled for thoracotomies for lung tumors (n = 15) and for lung transplantation because of end-stage lymphangioleiomyomatosis (n = 1). The age of the patients ranged from 29 to 69 years (mean 55). There were 12 men and 3 women. All but two were smokers. The CT scans were obtained on a Somatom Plus (Siemens AG, Erlangen, Germany) at 1-cm intervals, from the apex to the diaphragm at both

* Supported by the Fondation Erasme

full inspiration and maximal expiration using 1-mm collimation. The scan parameters were 1 s scan time, 250 mA tube current, 137 kVp voltage. Patients were positioned supine on the CT couch. No contrast medium was used. Quantification with "pulmo-CT" program was subsequently performed. After tracing the lung contours, the image background, i.e., everything but the lung parenchyma, is erased [12]. Histograms were determined for the left, the right, and both lungs. In their analysis, mean values, standard deviations, and arbitrary percentiles of the histograms are calculated [12]. We have evaluated the relative area of lung for which the attenuation values range from −900 to −1024 HU and from −950 to −1024 HU, at maximal inspiration and expiration, respectively. All these results are calculated for each section and for the entire pulmonary volume. The pulmonary function tests measured by body plethysmography selected for comparison with quantification by CT were (a) forced vital capacity (FVC, % predicted); (b) 1-s forced expiratory volume (FEV1, % predicted); (c) 1-s forced expiratory volume/forced vital capacity (FEV1/FVC, %); (d) total lung capacity (TLC, % predicted); (e) residual volume (RV, % predicted); (f) residual volume/total lung capacity (RV/TLC, %); (g) single breath diffusing capacity for carbon monoxide (DLCO, % predicted); (h) diffusing capacity for carbon monoxide/alveolar volume (DLCO/AV, % predicted). The results of quantitative CT were compared with the functional measurements using linear regression analysis. Significance was set at the level of 5%.

Results

The statistical results are summarized in Table 1 and most significant correlations are illustrated in Figs. 1–4.

Table 1. Significance of the correlation between respiratory function tests and "pulmo-CT" in full inspiration and maximal expiration for attenuation values less than −950 HU and less than −900 HU

	[−950, −1024]		[−900, −1024]	
	Inspiration	Expiration	Inspiration	Expiration
RV	<0.01	<0.01	NS	<0.05
FEV_1	<0.01	<0.01	NS	<0.01
FRC	<0.1	<0.01	NS	<0.05
TLC	NS	<0.1	NS	NS
RV/TLC	<0.01	<0.01	NS	<0.01
FEV_1/FVC	<0.05	<0.01	NS	<0.02
DLCO	NS	NS	NS	NS
DLCO/VA	NS	NS	NS	NS

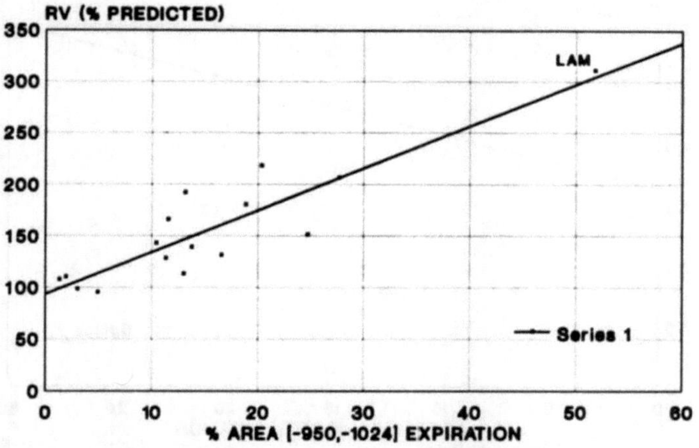

Fig. 1. Relationship between relative area (%) of attenuation values less than −950 HU and RV (% predicted). There was a significant correlation between the two ($P < 0.01$). *LAM*, lymphangioleiomyomatosis

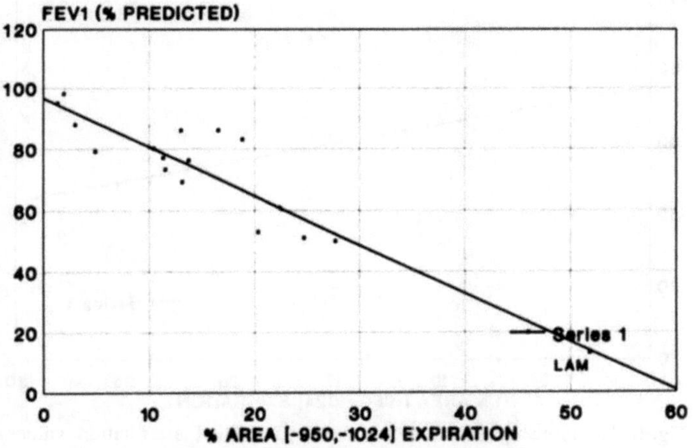

Fig. 2. Relationship between relative area (%) of attenuation values less than −950 HU and FEV_1 (% predicted). There was a significant correlation between the two ($P < 0.01$). *LAM*, lymphangioleiomyomatosis

Discussion

Introduction of treatment that could modify the course of emphysema [13] would make necessary more precise quantification of the disease than the data available with pulmonary function studies. To evaluate the accuracy of CT for the quantification of emphysema, pathologic and functional correlations must be performed. We used the semiautomatic evaluation procedure [12] to quantitate areas with attenuation values less than −900 and −950 HU, which were taken to represent areas of

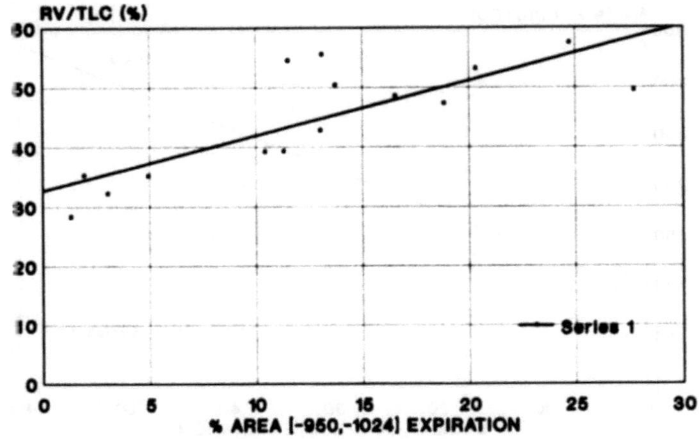

Fig. 3. Relationship between relative area (%) of attenuation values less than −950 HU and RV/TLC (%). There was a significant correlation between the two ($P < 0.01$)

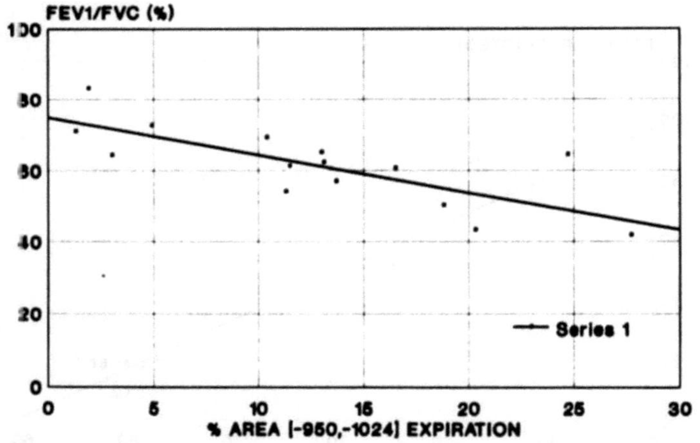

Fig. 4. Relationship between relative area (%) of attenuation values less than −950 HU and FEV_1/FVC (%). There was a significant correlation between the two ($P < 0.01$)

emphysema, and to provide an overall percentage of lung involvement by this disease. Our results showed that attenuation values of less than −950 HU are more discriminant than attenuation values of less than −900 HU. In other studies, several authors have considered −900 or −910 HU and observed significant correlations [10, 11]. R. J. Knudson recently suggested that expiratory CT can reveal the abnormal permanent enlargement of airspaces which defines emphysema and provides a method of assessing lung morphology [11]. Our preliminary results confirm these conclusions; except for the FVC, all correlations are more significant in expiration than in inspiration.

In this small number of patients, we did not find any correlation with DLCO and DLCO/VA. Kinsella and coworkers [10] examined the correlation of CT evaluation of emphysema using the "density mask" method of Müller and associates [9] with spirometric and diffusing capacity measurements in 85 patients. These authors performed CT of the entire chest with 10-mm thick slices and defined "emphysema" as pixels with attenuation values less than −910 HU. They found that DLCO/VA correlated well with what they term the extent of emphysema. By using 8-mm sections at two levels, Knudson and colleagues found a significant correlation, too.

While these results must be confirmed by a larger number of patients, by using a spirometric gating [14], and by pathologic correlations, CT appears to be an accurate method for the quantification of emphysema.

References

1. Snider GL, Kleinerman J, Thurlbeck WM, Bengali ZH (1985) The definition of emphysema. Report of a National Heart, Lung and Blood Institute, Division of Lung Diseases workshop. Am Rev Respir Dis 132: 182–185
2. Nagai A, West WW, Thurlbeck WM (1985) The National Institute of Health intermittent positive-pressure breathing trial: pathology studies. II. Correlation between morphologic findings, clinical findings, and evidence of expiratory air-flow obstruction. Am Rev Respir Dis 132: 946–953
3. Hayhurst MD, Flenley DC, McLean A, Wightman AJA, MacNee W, Wright D, Lamb D, Best J (1984) Diagnosis of pulmonary emphysema by computerised tomography. Lancet 2: 320–322
4. Bergin CJ, Müller NL, Miller RR (1986) CT in the quantitative assessment of emphysema. J Thorac Imag 1: 94–103
5. Bergin C, Müller NL, Nichols DM, Lillington G, Hogg JC, Mullen B, Grymalosky MR, Osborne S, Pare PD (1986) The diagnosis of emphysema: a computed tomographic-pathologic correlation. Am Rev Respir Dis 133: 541–546
6. Foster WL Jr, Pratt PC, Roggli VL, Godwin JD, Halvorsen RA Jr, Putman CE (1986) Centrilobular emphysema: CT-pathologic correlation. Radiology 159: 27–32
7. Hruban RH, Meziane MA, Zerhouni EA, Khouri NF, Fishman EK, Wheeler PS, Dumler S, Hutchins GM (1987) High resolution computed tomography of inflation-fixed lungs: pathologic-radiologic correlation of centrilobular emphysema. Am Rev Respir Dis 136: 935–940
8. Gould GA, Macnee W, McLean A, Warren PM, Redpath A, Best JJK, Lamb D, Flenley DC (1988) CT measurements of lung density in life can quantitate distal airspace enlargement – an essential defining feature of human emphysema. Am Rev Respir Dis 137: 380–392
9. Müller NL, Staples CA, Miller RR, Abboud RT (1988) "Density mask": an objective method to quantitate emphysema using computed tomography. Chest 94: 782–787
10. Kinsella M, Müller NL, Abboud RT, Morrison NJ, DyBuncio A (1990) Quantification of emphysema by computed tomography using a "density mask" program and correlation with pulmonary function tests. Chest 97: 315–321
11. Knudson RJ, Standen JR, Kaltenborn WT, Knudson DE, Rehm K, Habib MP, Newell JD (1991) Expiratory computed tomography for assessment of suspected pulmonary emphysema. Chest 99: 1357–1366
12. Kalender WA, Fichte H, Bautz W, Skalej M (1991) Semiautomatic evaluation procedures for quantitative CT of the lung. J Comput Assist Tomogr 15: 248–255
13. Snider GL, Stone PJ, Lucey EC (1990) The specific treatment of emphysema. Eur Respir J 3: 23s–28s
14. Kalender WA, Rienmüller R, Seissler W, Behr J, Welke M, Fichte H (1990) Measurement of pulmonary parenchymal attenuation: use of spirometric gating with quantitative CT. Radiology 175: 265–268

Medium-Sized Slice Thickness, High-Resolution Reconstruction Algorithm, and Wide-Ranged Window Settings: Optimal Parameters in CT of the Lung

U. Lörcher, J. Peters, M. Gossmann, and H. E. Riemann

Introduction

Initially, the technique for computed tomography (CT) examination of the lung parenchyma was the same as that for other parenchymal organs like the liver or kidney. In contrast to those organs, the structure of lung parenchyma shows extremely high density gradients, and very small anatomic and pathologic structures are of great diagnostic importance. Therefore, a different technical approach than that used in examing parenchymal organs is needed to optimize CT examination of the lung.

Slice Thickness

In order to optimize slice thickness with regard to anatomical structures and spatial resolution, the following study was performed. In 100 patients three scans were taken at five different levels with slice thicknesses of 10, 5, and 1 mm. They were reconstructed using a high-frequency algorithm and a zoom-factor of 2.3. Five radiologists determined the number of vessels in the subpleural region and the number of bronchi that could be identified in the ventral portion of the right and the left lung.

We found that there is a great difference in the visibility of anatomical structures between different slice thicknesses. Using a 10 mm slice thickness, 45 vessels can be identified in the lung parenchyma. Using a slice thickness of 5 mm, 41 vessels can be seen. If the slice thickness is reduced to 1 mm, only 16 elements can be identified as vessels.

In the lung parenchyma, the extremely high density gradients increase the importance of the partial volume effect: A structure of high density (vessel) surrounded by low density parenchyma can be identified even if it is considerably smaller than the slice thickness. Blood vessels can be differentiated from septal lines and nodules because of their characteristic dichotomous pattern.

As the slice thickness is reduced, the partial volume effect is reduced also. As a result, vessels are seen as round or oval structures only, and their dichotomous pattern disappears. Therefore, it is often impossible to differentiate those elements from pathologic structures like nodules or fibrotic lines.

For the bronchi, we obtained the following results: Using 10-mm collimation only 1 bronchus is seen, whereas with 5-mm collimation, 3 and with 1-mm collimation, 6 bronchi can be identified.

With thin collimation, the bronchi can be identified by their ring-shaped appearance. It is difficult to define normal bronchial walls on 10-mm scans. They may appear as linear structures accompanying vessels.

The vascular anatomy and structure form the road map for lung anatomy. Vessels are best seen using thick collimation (10 mm). There is no significant loss of detectability of vessels in thinner sections down to 5 mm, while fine details and small structures especially in the subpleural region are better defined on thinner slices (5 mm).

Very thin slices (1 mm) show the best spatial resolution, and very small lines and points can be seen. However, reduction of the partial volume effect leads to a reduction of visibility of the pulmonary vascular anatomy. Therefore, there is a loss of diagnostic reliability.

Another disadvantage of very low slice thickness is the concomitant high radiation dose and/or increasing noise.

As a result of our study we found a slice thickness of 5 mm to be the best for CT examination of diffuse lung disease.

Image Reconstruction Algorithm

Comparing different reconstruction algorithms, we found that the effects on image quality and diagnostic certainty depend on slice thickness. A high-frequency reconstruction algorithm (Siemens 041) leads to an improvement of the detectability of details to a greater extent in images with 10-mm collimation than in those with 1-mm collimation. With 10-mm collimation, 97 % of images reconstructed using a high-frequency algorithm were classified as being better than those reconstructed with a standard (033) algorithm. With 5-mm collimation, in 80 % of images the high-frequency reconstruction algorithm showed a higher quality, and in 6 % of images the standard reconstruction algorithm gave superior results. With 1-mm collimation, in only 52 % of cases was the high frequency reconstruction algorithm superior to the standard algorithm, and in 17 % the standard algorithm seemed to be better than the high-frequency reconstruction algorithm.

Using the results of our study with regard to slice thickness and type of algorithm, we conclude that 5-mm collimation and a high-frequency reconstruction algorithm will yield the best results and may be called high resolution CT.

Window Settings

Lung tissue itself shows a wide range of density. Free air has by definition a density value of – 1000 HU.

Emphysematous or hyperinflated lung tissue shows densities of about – 850 HU, normal lung tissue has a density of about – 800 HU, and hilar structures up to 50 HU. Density values of parenchymal organs range from – 150 HU (fat) to 50 HU (muscle) or 100 HU (thyroid gland).

In order to differentiate the various pulmonary structures, the lower limit of window values must include densities of −950 HU. Mediastinal structures and structures of the thoracic wall may be distinguished if the upper window limit includes the value of 100 HU. This means that a window width of less than 1000 HU cannot present all the diagnostically important information.

In order to find optimal window parameters, different (normal and abnormal) CT scans were presented to 12 radiologists. CT scans were documented in a set of differ-

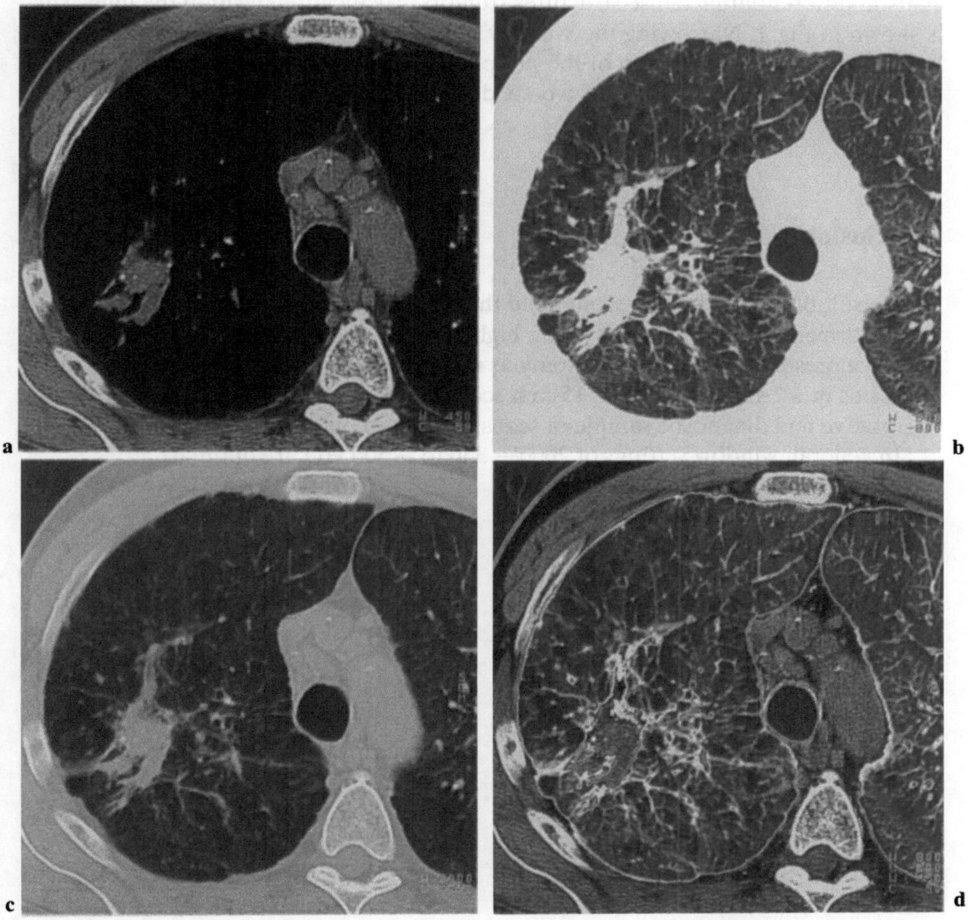

Fig. 1. CT scan showing a silicotic mass within an emphysematous lung is displayed with different window settings. Mediastinal window setting (450/50 HU) *(upper left)* shows best mediastinal lymph nodes and calcification within the silicotic mass. Lung window setting (800/ − 800 HU) *(upper right)* demonstrates emphysematous lung structure. Diagnostic evaluation of pleura, mass, and mediastinum is impossible. Double window setting *(lower right)*, a combination of mediastinal and lung window, leads to artificial frontier lines between aerated and solid structures which are easily misinterpreted as an anatomical structure (pleura). Interface between lung and silicotic mass cannot be analyzed. Thoracic window setting (2000/ − 500 HU) *(lower left)* demonstrates emphysematous lung structure and pleural junction, mediastinal structures and lymph nodes, as well as calcification within the silicotic mass

ent window settings, widths ranging from 800 to 2500 HU and centers from −100 to −800 HU. This study group found a window width of 1800–2000 HU and levels between −350 to −500 HU to be the optimal setting.

The presentation of two different images, one optimized to lung structures (800/−800 HU) and the other to mediastinum (450/50 HU), was found to be of less diagnostic quality. A single image presentation with wide-ranged window settings was preferred by all of the examiners. The presentation of two different images of the same scan with lung and mediastinal settings leads to diagnostic difficulties, especially in differentiating dense structures (tumors, calcifications) within the lung. This is shown in Fig. 1. Narrowing the window improves the visibility of lucencies in the lung parenchyma. Evaluation of the peripleural region and demonstration of bronchial changes, however, becomes worse, due to a loss of visibility of partial volume effects.

Conclusion

As a result of our study, we recommend that CT examination of diffuse lung disease be performed with 5-mm scans using high resolution algorithm. These parameters lead to a presentation of lung anatomy as in a 10-mm scan with a resolution of small details as in a 1-mm scan. Also, 15-mm scan intervals are sufficient to obtain a representative and diagnostic sample of scans for diffuse pulmonary disease.

In general, window settings of 2000/−350 to −500 HU are optimal.

Quantitative Analysis of CT Value Changes of the Lung with Different Respiratory Volumes

R. Rienmüller, H. Schulz, T. Beinert, F. Mehnert, P. Heilmann, A. Hillebrecht, J. Behr, and P. Brand

Introduction

In a preliminary experimental study to characterize the influence of air pollution on the behaviour of the airways and lung parenchyma, high resolution computed tomography (CT) studies of the lungs of beagle dogs were performed. The purpose of this study was to establish the exact relationship between CT values of the lungs at different levels of respiratory volumes.

Material and Methods

Seven beagle dogs with an average body weight of 15.7 ± 1.8 kg and mean age of 24.3 ± 14.8 months were examined. Their lung function parameters were as followed: total lung capacity (TLC) 1.4 ± 0.1 l, a compliance 0.1 ± 0.02 l, dead space 0.13 ± 0.005 l. High resolution CT studies were performed in supine anaesthesized (Surital) and intubated animals at 5 standardized lung volumes, defined by an intratracheal pressure of zero (FRC), + 10 cmH_2O, + 15 cmH_2O, + 20 cmH_2O and + 25 cmH_2O (TLC). The scans were performed at the tracheal carina as well as 4 cm above and below. A fast contour tracing algorithm was used to isolate the lung parenchyma, followed by determination of CT mean values and by a quantitative histogram analysis of the frequency distribution of CT values, including the full width at half-maximum (FWHM) [1–4].

The analysis contains the separate evaluation of all slices from each side of both lungs. Additional ventrodorsal CT value gradients (CTG) were determined for each of both sides of the lungs at various lung volumes.

Table 1. CT mean values (HU), full width at half-maximum (FWHM) and ventrodorsal CT mean value gradient (CTG) of the lungs of beagle dogs (n = 7), determined at the level of the tracheal carina and at 4 cm above and below, and total lung capacity (TLC) at defined intratracheal pressures

Intratracheal pressure (cmH_2O)	HU ($\bar{x} \pm SD$)	FWHM ($\bar{x} \pm SD$)	CTG ($\bar{x} \pm SD$)	TLC (%)
0	−748 ± 24	251 ± 15	2.01 ± 0.71	42
10	−848 ± 21	122 ± 14	0.7 ± 0.39	73
15	−872 ± 14	93 ± 5	0.35 ± 0.22	83
20	−883 ± 12	85 ± 4	0.28 ± 0.18	92
25	−889 ± 11	81 ± 3	0.25 ± 0.14	100

Results

The CT mean values, FWHM and CTG decrease with increasing lung volume (Table 1, Figs. 1–5). The largest changes of CT mean values were observed between 42% and 73% of TLC (−748 ± 24 HU vs. −848 ± 21 HU). Differences of CT mean values minimized between lung volumes of 73% and 100% of TLC (−872 ±

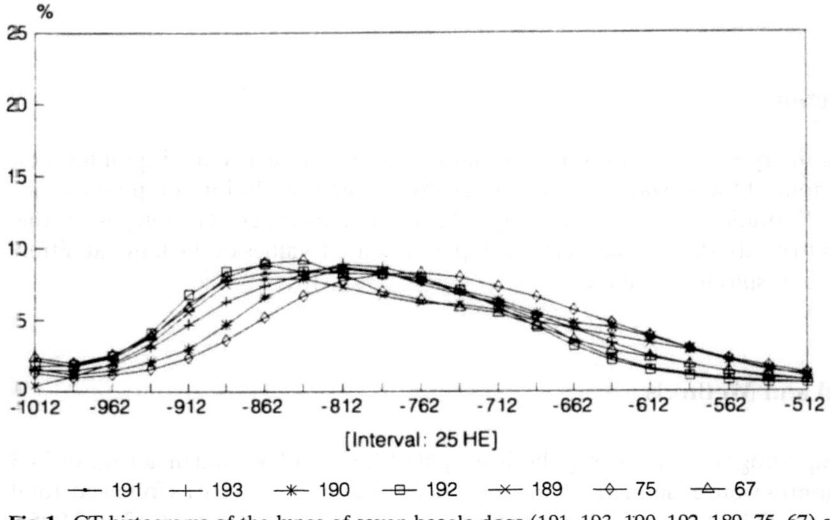

Fig. 1. CT histograms of the lungs of seven beagle dogs (191, 193, 190, 192, 189, 75, 67) at an intratracheal pressure of 0 cmH_2O

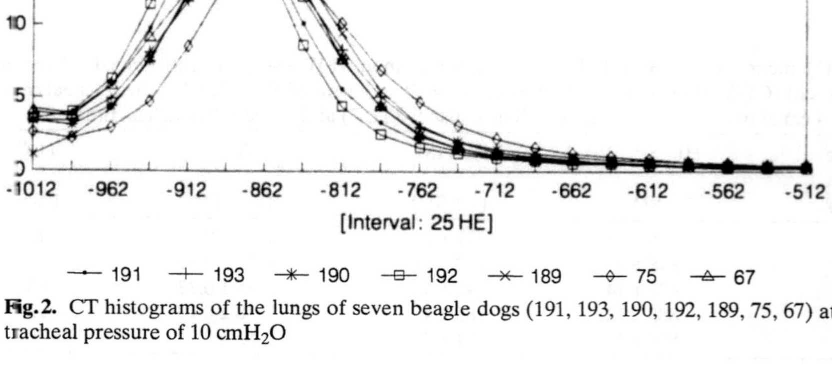

Fig. 2. CT histograms of the lungs of seven beagle dogs (191, 193, 190, 192, 189, 75, 67) at an intratracheal pressure of 10 cmH_2O

14 HU vs. − 889 ± 11 HU). The variance of standard deviations of CT mean values, of FWHM and of CTG was found to decrease with increasing TLC by a factor of 2 or 5 (Table 1). The histogram analysis revealed a constant frequency distribution of CT values at the HU interval between − 1024 and − 999 HU at 83%–100% of TLC (Figs. 1–5). In contrast to these findings between 43% and 83% of TLC, the frequency distribution of CT values in the same interval increased two fold.

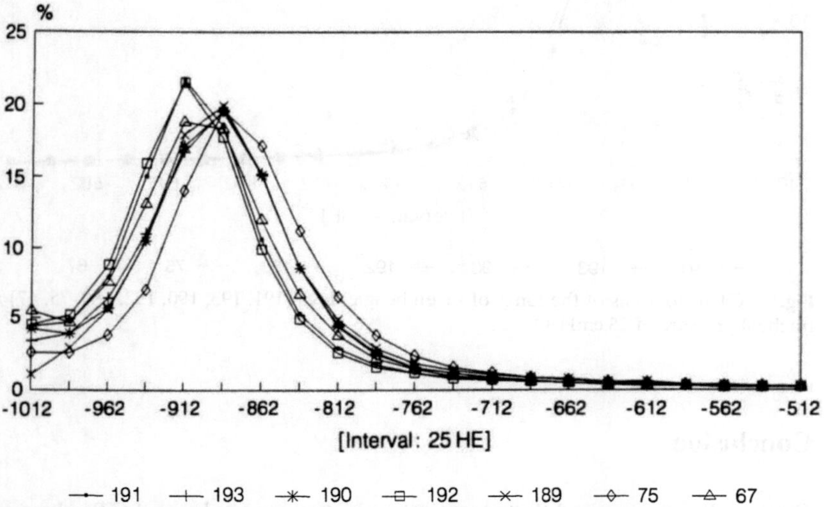

Fig. 3. CT histograms of the lungs of seven beagle dogs (191, 193, 190, 192, 189, 75, 67) at an intratracheal pressure of 15 cmH_2O

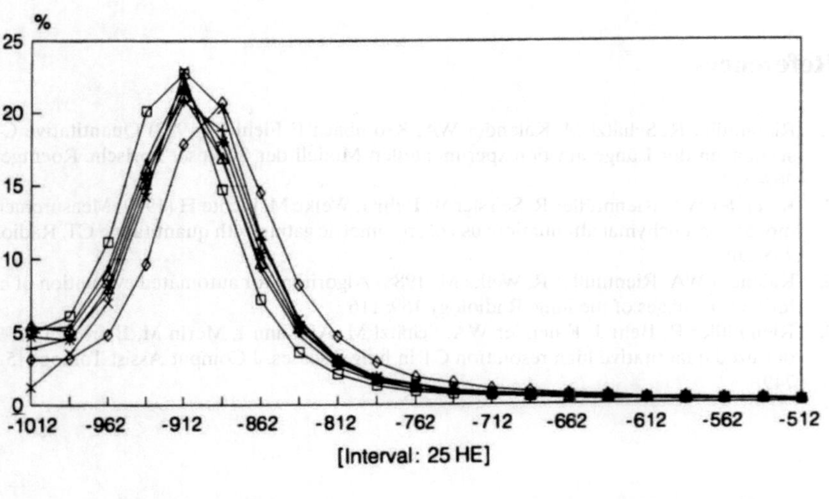

Fig. 4. CT histograms of the lungs of seven beagle dogs (191, 193, 190, 192, 189, 75, 67) at an intratracheal pressure of 20 cmH_2O

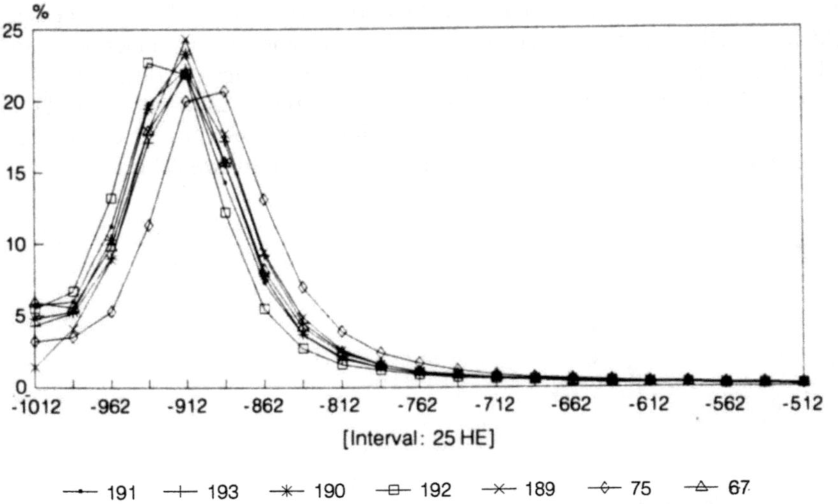

Fig. 5. CT histograms of the lungs of seven beagle dogs (191, 193, 190, 192, 189, 75, 67) at an intratracheal pressure of 25 cmH_2O

Conclusion

Our results recommend that quantitative histogram analysis of CT values of the lung in beagle dogs should be performed at constant lung volumes above 75% TLC to minimize interindividual differences of CT mean values.

References

1. Rienmüller R, Schätzl M, Kalender WA, Krombach F, Fiehl E (1988) Quantitative CT-Untersuchungen der Lunge am tierexperimentellen Modell der Silikose. Fortschr Roentgenstr 148: 367–373
2. Kalender WA, Rienmüller R, Seissler W, Behr J, Welke M, Fichte H (1990) Measurement of pulmonary parenchymal attenuation: use of spirometric gating with quantitative CT. Radiology 175: 265–268
3. Kalender WA, Rienmüller R, Welke M (1988) Algorithm for automated evaluation of high resolution CT images of the lung. Radiology 169: 116
4. Rienmüller R, Behr J, Kalender WA, Schätzl M, Altmann I, Merin M, Beinert T (1991) Standardized quantitative high resolution CT in lung diseases. J Comput Assist Tomogr 15 (5): 742–749

Evaluation of CT Histograms Determined by Spirometrically Standardized High Resolution CT Studies of the Lung in Man

R. Rienmüller, J. Behr, T. Beinert, F. Mehnert, and W. Kalender

Introduction

In diffuse pulmonary diseases it has been shown [1] that histogram analysis of frequencies of values determined by spirometrically standardized high resolution computed tomography (HRCT) provides objective quantitative data that reflect changes of pulmonary structures corresponding to lung function impairments.

For a wider clinical application, however, it is necessary to determine the variance of the frequency distribution of CT values in healthy subjects and in patients with defined diseases.

Material and Methods

The group studied consisted of 26 healthy adults. In all of them, lung function tests were performed including the following: vital capacity (VC), specific resistance (SR), total lung capacity (TLC), intrathoracic gas volume (IGV), residual volume (RV), forced expiratory volume in 1 s (FEV_1) and peak expiratory flow (PEF).

In all individuals of lung function results of TLC, IGV, RV, FEV_1 and PEF were "normal" as defined by European Community for Coal and Steel (ECCS) [2]. The results of VC were ≥ 80 (% predicted) and of SR ≤ 1.0 (kPa × s).

In addition to this group of 26 healthy adults with normal lung function data, patients with well-defined pulmonary diseases were studied. In these patients the results of functional tests were expressed as predicted values [2]. As a measure of the diffusing capacity (DCO), the carbon monoxide transfer factor was obtained by a single breath method using a gas mixture containing 0.15% CO and 4% helium.

The HRCT studies of the lung were performed using thin section HR CT at 50% of the actual VC and controlled spirometrically during each exposure. In all patients the CT scan was performed in inspiration at 50% of the actual VC to determine the level of the carina. There and 5 cm below and above this level, three 1-mm HRCT scans of the lungs were done. Each of these three HRCT slices was obtained again after spirometrical determination and maintenance of an inspiration level of 50% of actual VC. Using our CT machine (Somatom Plus, Siemens, Erlangen, Germany) for HRCT slices of 1 mm thickness, scanning parameters of 137 kV, 260 mA and 1-s exposure time were available. The lungs were isolated by means of a fast contour tracing algorithm, and the CT values were evaluated as mean values and by quantitative histogram analysis. The threshold value for the contour finder was optimal at −200 HU [3–6].

Theoretical Remarks

As most CT voxels consist of various amounts of air, lung tissue, blood, lung fluid and sediments, the measured CT value of any voxel does not represent an arithmetic mean value but an "effective" value (Fig. 1). The size of this CT effective value is mainly determined by its air/lung tissue relationship. This is the reason why in the histograms of the lungs no positive CT value exists. Comparative evaluation of CT values and lung function data reveals that it is not sufficient to determine only the mean values and the standard deviation, it is also necessary to determine the distribution frequency of CT values at defined intervals (Table 1). We call these intervals A, B, C and D. The CT value interval A shows the highest correlation with the IGV and SR. Both of these determine the extent of emphysema or bronchial obstruction. Thus, the greater the proportion of CT values present in interval A, the more extensive the present emphysema and/or bronchial obstruction is and vice versa. The intervals B and D show the highest positive or negative correlation with the VC, DCO capacity and exercise PaO_2, these being the functional parameters. Thus, the greater

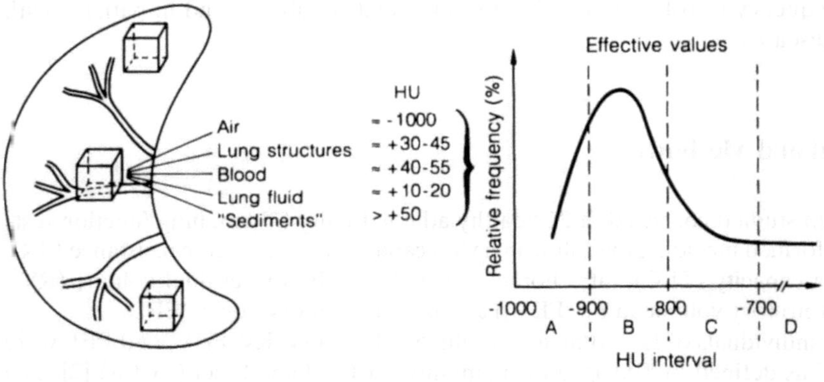

Fig. 1. Relationship between CT values and CT histogram of the lung

Table 1. Correlation of lung function data with mean CT values and with the frequencies of CT values at defined intervals: A, B, C and D ($n = 63$)

	VC (% pred.)	DCO (% pred.)	Exercise PaO_2 (mmHg)	IGV (% pred.)	SR (kPa·s)
Mean CT value (HU)	r = −0.57	−0.34	−0.44	−0.54	n.s.
Frequency (%) of CT values at Interval					
A ...< 900 HU	r = n.s.	n.s.	n.s.	0.73	0.48
B −899... −800 HU	r = 0.69	0.63	0.68	n.s.	n.s.
C −799... −700 HU	r = −0.26	n.s.	−0.34	−0.39	n.s.
D > −699... HU	r = −0.56	−0.40	−0.47	−0.43	n.s.

$P \leq 0.05$–$P \leq 0.001$

the proportion of CT values present in interval B, the better the lung function is, and similarly for interval D, the lower the lung function is and vice versa [1].

On the basis of these theoretical considerations and of our practical clinical experience, we have been using instead of the four above-mentioned CT intervals, only three: E for emphysema index, L for lung parenchyma index and F for fibrosis index. Hereby, the interval E reaches up to −925 HU, the interval L from −924 to −800 HU and the interval F above −799 HU.

The intervals E, L and F correlate only slightly less with the above-mentioned lung function data than the former intervals A, B and D, yet being easier to work with they are more suitable for the daily clinical diagnosis.

Results

By averaging the frequency of all CT values ($\bar{x} \pm SD$) of the lung in the group of 26 healthy normals, a new "normal CT histogram curve" and its CT value range for defined indexes of emphysema, lung parenchyma and fibrosis (Fig. 2) for all three levels together and for each level separately (Fig. 3) were determined. These results of healthy normals serve as control data in the clinical evaluation of patients with known or suspected pulmonary disease, as shown in the following examples.

1. The results of lung function tests of a 71-year-old woman with idiopathic fibrosis were as follows: VC = 95 (%pred.), IGV = 78 (%pred.), FEV = 92 (%pred.), RV = 81 (%pred.), TLC = 83 (%pred.), DCO = 59 (%pred.), SR = 0.31 (kPa × s). The histogram analysis reveals a global decrease of the lung parenchyma index to 53.5 % and an increase of the fibrosis index to 42.2 % (Table 2) accompanied by a normal emphysema index of 4.1 %. The additional analysis of the regional frequency distribution of the CT values demonstrates (Table 3) that fibrosis is mainly localized at the right lung and at the level of carina and at both sides of the lungs at the level of 5 cm below the carina (Fig. 4), whereas both sides at levels

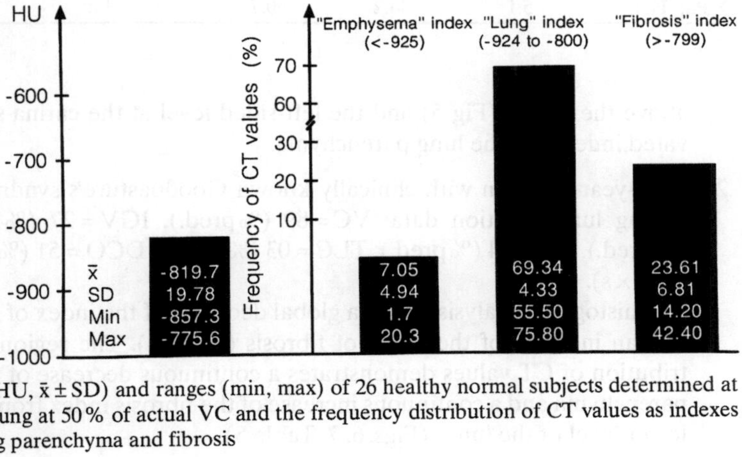

Fig. 2. CT values (HU, $\bar{x} \pm SD$) and ranges (min, max) of 26 healthy normal subjects determined at three levels of the lung at 50 % of actual VC and the frequency distribution of CT values as indexes of emphysema, lung parenchyma and fibrosis

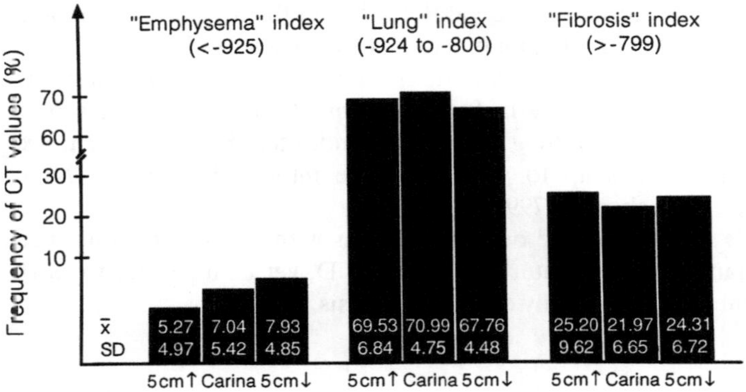

Fig. 3. Frequency distribution of CT values as indexes of emphysema, lung parenchyma and fibrosis at the level of the carina and 5 cm below and above

Table 2. Normal range and median of the indexes of emphysema (E), lung parenchyma (L) and fibrosis (F) in 26 healthy normal subjects and in the patient with idiopathic fibrosis

	E	L	F
Normal range (95%)	<14%	>62%	<35%
Median	6.6%	70.2%	23.2%
Actual data Pat. H. I.	4.1%	53.5%	42.2%

Table 3. Regional frequency distribution (%) of CT values at defined HU intervals as indexes of emphysema (E), lung parenchyma (L) and fibrosis (F) in the patient with idiopathic fibrosis

Index / Level	Right lung			Left lung		
	E	L	F	E	L	F
5 cm ↑	6.3	74.1	19.6	4.3	78.9	16.8
Carina	2.3	43.2	45.5	3.4	63.6	33.0
5 cm ↓	6.8	36.2	57.0	2.4	54.3	43.3
Σ Pat. H. I.	5.1	44.2	50.7	3.2	62.8	34.0

above the carina (Fig. 5) and the left-sided level at the carina show slightly elevated indexes of the lung parenchyma.

2. A 24-year-old man with clinically known Goodpasture's syndrome had the following lung function data: VC = 89 (%pred.), IGV = 27 (%pred.), FEV = 84 (%pred.), RV = 54 (%pred.), TLC = 03 (%pred.), DCO = 51 (%pred.), SR = 0.87 (kPa × s).
The histogram analysis shows a global decrease of the index of lung parenchyma and an increase of the index of fibrosis (Table 4). The regional frequency distribution of CT values demonstrates a continuous decrease of the index of lung parenchyma and a continuous increase of the fibrosis index from the upper to the lower level of the lungs (Figs. 6, 7, Table 5).

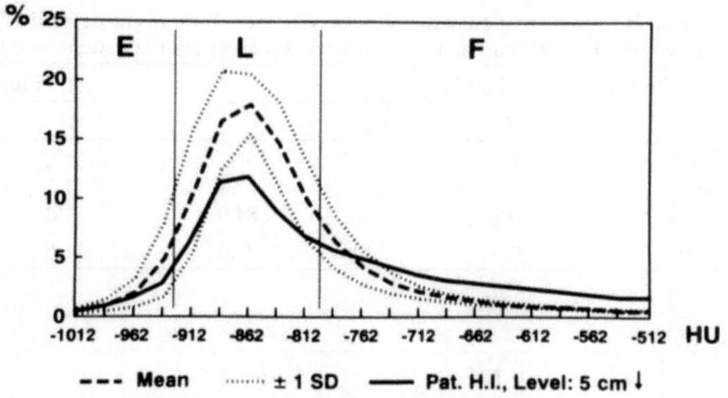

Fig. 4. CT histogram of 26 healthy normal subjects (mean ± SD) and of the patient with idiopathic fibrosis 5 cm below the carina

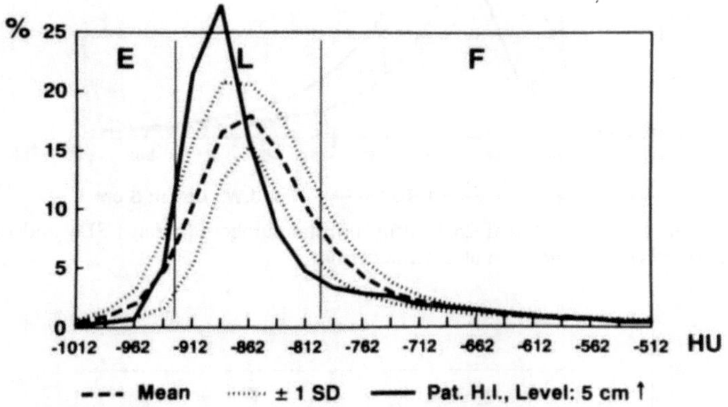

Fig. 5. CT histogram of 26 healthy normal subjects (mean ± SD) and of the patient with idiopathic fibrosis 5 cm above the carina

Table 4. Normal range and median of the indexes of emphysema (E), lung parenchyma (L) and fibrosis (F) in 26 healthy normal subjects and in the patient with Goodpasture's syndrome

	E	L	F
Normal range (95%)	< 14%	> 62%	< 35%
Median	6.6%	70.2%	23.2%
Actual data Pat. J. W.	1.1%	32.6%	66.3%

3. A 47-year-old woman with a homozygous α_1-PID (proteinase inhibitor deficiency) had these lung function data: VC = 49 (%pred.), IGV = 18 (%pred.), FEV = 28 (%pred.), RV = 89 (%pred.), TLC = 30 (%pred.), SR = 7.13 (kPa × s). The histogram analysis demonstrates a global increase of the emphysema index to 48.8% and a decrease of the lung parenchyma index to 34.7% with a very low fibrosis index of 16.5% (Fig. 8, Tables 6, 7).

Table 5. Regional frequency distribution (%) of CT values at defined HU intervals as indexes of emphysema (E), lung parenchyma (L), and fibrosis (F) in the patient with Goodpasture's syndrome

Level \ Index	Right lung			Left lung		
	E	L	F	E	L	F
5 cm ↑	1.1	47.7	51.2	1.2	57.3	41.5
Carina	1.2	31.5	67.3	2.3	44.4	53.3
5 cm ↓	0.5	14.6	84.9	1.0	19.0	80.0
Σ Pat. J.W.	0.9	28.1	71.0	1.6	37.4	61.0

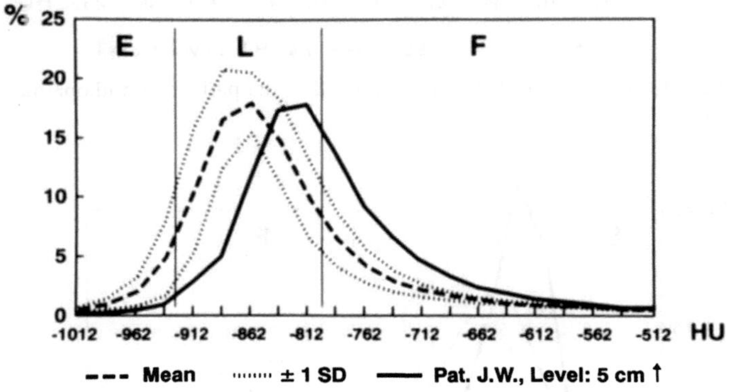

Fig. 6. CT histogram of 26 healthy normal subjects (mean ± SD) and of the patient with Goodpasture's syndrome 5 cm above the carina

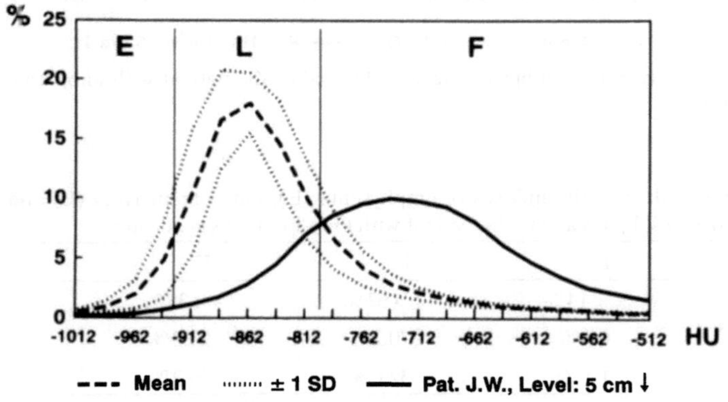

Fig. 7. CT histogram of 26 healthy normal subjects (mean ± SD) and of the patient with Goodpasture's syndrome 5 cm below the carina

The analysis of the regional frequency distribution of CT values shows a somewhat higher increase of the emphysema index of the right lung than of the left lung. In contrast, the index of lung parenchyma is somewhat higher in the left than in the right lung.

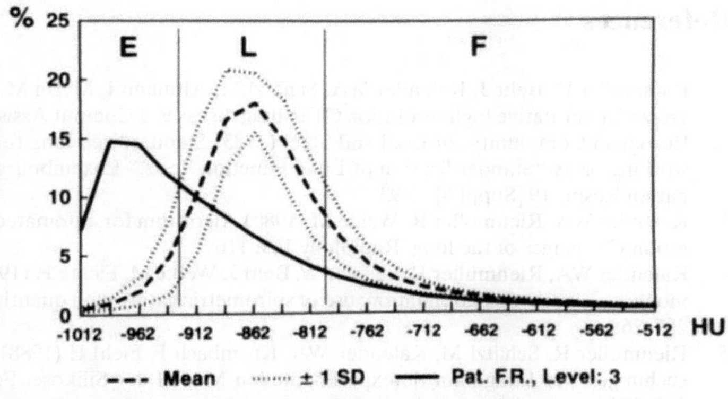

Fig. 8. CT histogram of 26 healthy normal subjects (mean ± SD) and of the patient with emphysema of α_1-PID type of all three levels

Table 6. Normal range and median of the indexes of emphysema (E), lung parenchyma (L) and fibrosis (F) in 26 healthy normal subjects and in the patient with emphysema of α_1-PID type

	E	L	F
Normal range (95%)	<14%	>62%	<35%
Median	6.6%	70.2%	23.2%
Actual data Pat. F.R.	48.8%	34.7%	16.5%

Table 7. Regional frequency distribution (%) of CT values at defined HU intervals as indexes of emphysema (E), lung parenchyma (L) and fibrosis (F) in the patient with emphysema of α_1-PID type

Index / Level	Right lung			Left lung		
	E	L	F	E	L	F
5 cm ↑	51.0	34.4	14.6	44.6	39.4	16.0
Carina	54.0	31.2	14.8	39.7	40.6	19.7
5 cm ↓	57.7	26.3	16.0	43.0	39.6	17.4
Σ Pat. F.R.	55.1	29.8	15.1	42.1	40.0	17.9

Conclusion

The CT values and CT histogram curves of the healthy normal subjects may serve as control data for the clinical evaluation of pulmonary diseases. However, for clinical and epidemiological studies it is necessary to increase the number of healthy normal subjects studied to determine more precisely the normal ranges of pulmonary CT values for each decade of human life. Therefore, a protocol was developed to start an interinstitutional European cooperation study for the evaluation of the CT data of the healthy normal subject as was previously done in the evaluation of the normal values for the CT densitometry of bones. Any research group is cordially invited to participate in this exciting project.

References

1. Rienmüller R, Behr J, Kalender WA, Schätzl M, Altmann I, Merin M, Beinert T (1991) Standardized quantitative high resolution CT in lung diseases. J Comput Assist Tomogr 15 (5): 742–749
2. European Community for Coal and Steel (1983) Standardized lung function testing. Report of working party "Standardization of Lung Function Tests." Luxembourg, 1983. Bull Eur Physiopathol Respir 19 [Suppl 5]: 7–93
3. Kalender WA, Rienmüller R, Welke M (1988) Algorithm for automated evaluation of high resolution CT images of the lung. Radiology 169: 116
4. Kalender WA, Rienmüller R, Seissler W, Behr J, Welke M, Fichte H (1990) Measurement of pulmonary parenchymal attenuation: use of spirometric gating with quantitative CT. Radiology 175: 265–268
5. Rienmüller R, Schätzl M, Kalender WA, Krombach F, Fiehl E (1988) Quantitative CT-Untersuchungen der Lunge am tierexperimentellen Modell der Silikose. Fortschr Roentgenstr 148: 367–373
6. Rienmüller R, Altmann I, Behr J, Krombach F, Kalender WA (1990) Spirometrically standardized quantitative high resolution CT of interstitial lung diseases. In: Fuchs WA (ed) Advances in CT. Springer, Berlin Heidelberg New York, pp 102–108

Single-Breath-Hold Spiral Volumetric CT of the Lung

A. Rieber, T. Fleiter, P. Wakat, H.-J. Brambs, and C. D. Claussen

Introduction

A variety of computed tomography (CT) techniques have been described in the detection and assessment of small pulmonary nodules [3, 4]. However, the problem of reproducing consistent inspiratory levels for successive scans to obtain an anatomically continuous study persists [3]. The introduction of spiral volumetric CT has added a new dimension to the assessment of lung nodules and seems to be a solution of this problem. We describe the use of spiral volumetric CT (SVCT) of the lung in comparison with standard CT. The aim was to evaluate the advantages and disadvantages of SVCT.

Material and Methods

Forty patients were examined prospectively. Eleven patients had known lung metastases, in 10 patients lung metastases were to be excluded, 18 patients had one or multiple suspected pulmonary nodules which should be assessed, and in 1 patient with artificial respiration ARDS was suspected.

Using a standard CT scanner (Siemens, Somatom Plus) allowing up to 24 continuous 1-s rotations, we synchronized data acquisition with longitudinal patient motion. A table feed of 10 mm/s was used, covering a distance of 120 mm with a single, 12-s-long breath hold. To examine the complete volume of the lung, a second SVCT was performed coupled onto the last scan of the first SVCT. Additionally, 39 patients were scanned with conventional CT techniques with 10-mm section thickness at 10-mm intervals from the lung apices to the bases. The number, size, and location of nodules were recorded for both the conventional and SVCT examinations. In the patient with artificial respiration we performed only the SVCT, during which the artificial respiration was interrupted. A conventional CT scan was not implemented because SVCT showed an ARDS, and so further confirmation was unnecessary.

Results

In nine patients, SVCT detected all lung metastases noted on conventional CT. The sizes of nodules detected with SVCT did not differ in comparison with these on conventional CT.

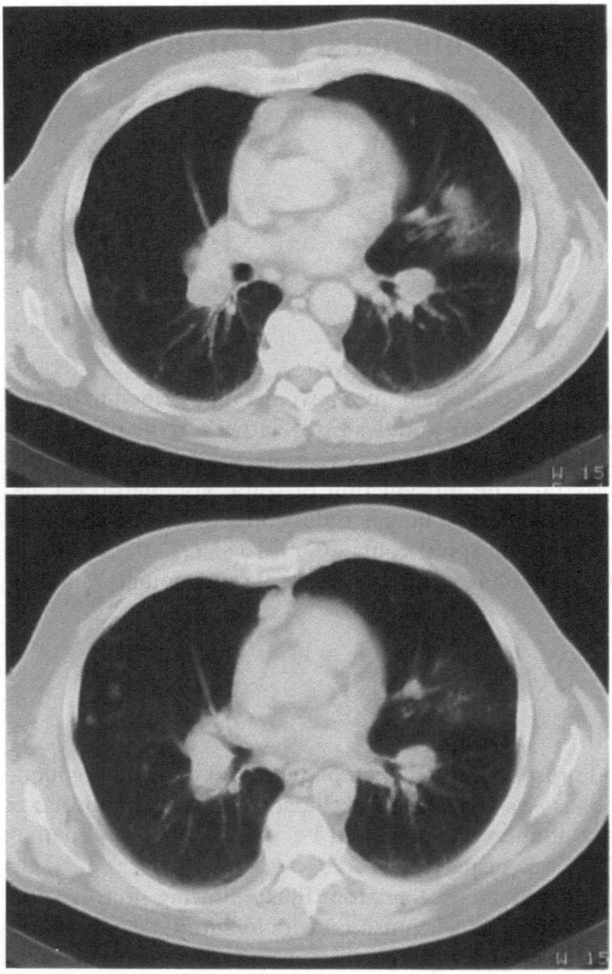

a

b

Fig. 1 a. Patient with known lung metastases. **a** Conventional CT, only a few metastases are detected. **b** Spiral volumetric CT at the same table position, multiple metastases are detected, omitted on conventional CT

Five single nodules that were missed on conventional CT were detected with SVCT in two patients (Fig. 1). Ten patients had no nodules either on conventional CT or on SVCT.

In 18 patients, SVCT helped to differentiate suspected nodules. Eight patients had specific changes of tuberculosis. SVCT detected the pleural reference or calcifications in these nodules better than conventional CT.

In four patients with one pulmonary suspected nodule, SVCT demonstrated that the suspected nodule was only a fibrous scar. In six patients, the tentative diagnosis of bronchogenic carcinoma was confirmed with SVCT. This suspicion was verified at operation in these six patients. In one patient, SVCT detected an ARDS, so that confirmation by conventional CT became unnecessary (Fig. 2).

Radiation-induced fibrosis became blurred on SVCT in two patients (Fig. 3). Hypostasis and the pleural membrane were missed on SVCT in two patients.

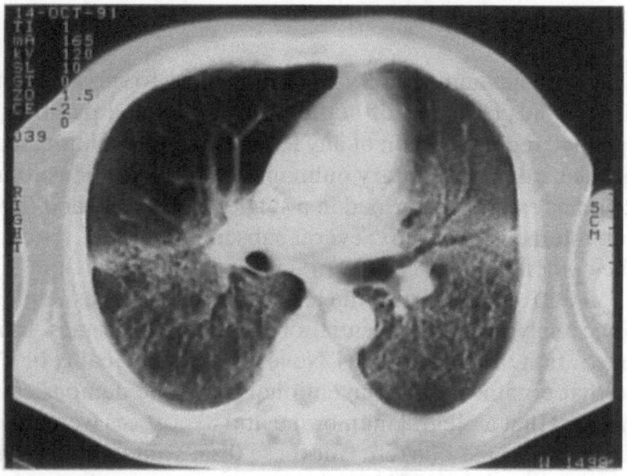

Fig. 2. Spiral CT of patient with ARDS: typical ground glass opacity

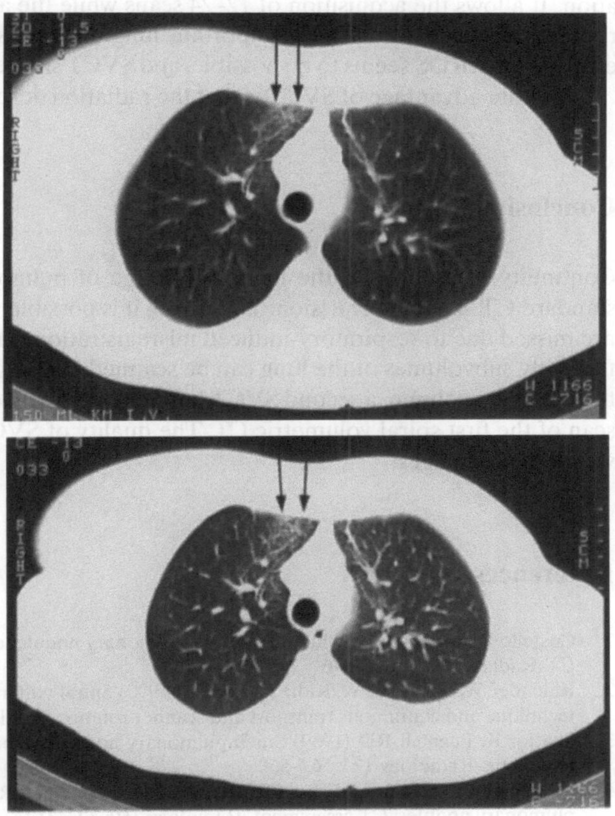

Fig. 3 a, b. Patient with radiation-induced fibrosis *(arrows)*. **a** Conventional CT; **b** Spiral volumetric CT: The fibrosis becomes blurred

Discussion

The main advantage of SVCT is the ability to survey a lung subvolume continuously. This avoids omission of nodules or other small pathologic changes. It allows retrospective reconstruction of any level within the volume, facilitating the demonstration of the center of a solitary pulmonary nodule for densitometry [2, 5]. Currently, up to 24 scans can be performed in a single breath hold and thus only the examination of a subvolume is possible. Several subsequent SVCT sequences may be used to screen the complete lung [1].

SVCT demonstrates the lesions in a continuous sequence and assists the morphologic analysis and differentiation of disease processes. It often improves the CT demonstration of small nodules. Nevertheless, the quality of SVCT scans is not equivalent to that obtained with conventional CT in the demonstration of normal anatomy. We noticed that a pleural membrane and hypostasis were missing, and radiation-induced fibrosis became blurred. But these disadvantages never aggravated the diagnosis. A new application for SVCT may be the examination of patients with artificial respiration. It allows the acquisition of 12–24 scans while the artificial respiration is interrupted. Diagnosis of the most important lung diseases such as pneumonia, pleural effusion, or ARDS seems to be possible, and SVCT shortens the examination time.

Another advantage of SVCT is that the radiation dose is significantly reduced [1].

Conclusion

Continuity of sections is the main advantage of pulmonary SVCT. In contrast to standard CT, it avoids omission. Therefore, it is possible to be certain that no lesions are missed due to respiratory-induced misregistration. The disadvantage of SVCT is that only subvolumes of the lung can be scanned in a single breath hold. To examine the complete volume, a second SVCT has to be performed in connection with the last scan of the first spiral volumetric CT. The quality of SVCT images is comparable to standard CT images.

References

1. Costello P, Anderson W, Blume D (1991) Pulmonary nodule: evaluation with spiral volumetric CT. Radiology 179: 875–876
2. Kalender WA, Seissler W, Klotz E, Vock P (1990) Spiral volumetric CT with single-breath-hold technique and continuous transport and scanner rotation. Radiology 176: 181–183
3. Shaffer K, Pugatch RD (1989) Small pulmonary nodules: dynamic CT with single-breath-hold technique. Radiology 173: 567–568
4. Siegelmann SS, Khouri NF, Lei FP, Fishman EK, Braverman RM, Zerhouni EA (1986) Solitary pulmonary nodules: CT assessment. Radiology 160: 307–312
5. Vock P, Soucek M, Daepp M, Kalender WA (1990) Lung: spiral volumetric CT with single-breath-hold technique. Radiology 176: 864–867
6. Zerhouni EA, Naidich DP, Stitik FP, Khouri NF, Siegelmann SS (1985) Computed tomography of the pulmonary parenchyma. II. Interstitial disease. J Thorac Imaging 1: 54–64

Quality Assessment of Continuous CT in the Thorax

M. Oudkerk, R. H. Kruyt, R. Bok, G. J. Kieft, and S. P. M. Mali

Introduction

Imaging techniques have improved dramatically over the past decade. Small structures, such as lymph nodes with a diameter of 10 mm or more, are routinely detected with scanners that offer a spatial resolution up to 0.30 mm or 14 line pairs per cm (volume resolution up to 0.12 mm^3) and a contrast resolution up to 2.2 mm discernable with 3 Hounsfield units (HU) and 20 mGy. Scan exposure times play an important role in the depiction of small structures in and around moving organs, such as in the thorax. Third generation CT scanners allow us scan exposure times of less than 3 s, but motion is still a major problem with a time resolution of 2 s, resulting in inconsistencies of the view data. The obvious way to reduce motion artifacts is to employ a shorter scan time. In many third generation scanners, the application of shorter scan times is possible, but at the cost of the acquisition of considerably fewer data, resulting in sharply diminished spatial and contrast resolution.

The Imatron – a nonrevolving ultrafast CT system – offers a very high time resolution of 50–100 ms also at the cost of a relatively low spatial resolution and contrast resolution [1]. At a time resolution of 0.6 s the Imatron produces a spatial resolution of 0.8 mm (6.2 lp/cm) and a volume resolution of 2 mm^3, and a contrast resolution of 5 mm discernable with 4 HU and 40 mGy. With the introduction of continuously rotating CT scanners, employing sliprings and rotating the tube and detector continuously, a scan time of 0.7 s became possible while retaining good values for spatial and contrast resolution. In order to determine if subsecond CT scanning improves the image quality, we performed a study of the thoracic hilum and mediastinum in 50 patients with lung cancer. Accurate evaluation of the hilum and mediastinum in patients with lung cancer is crucial for developing an appropriate treatment plan [2]. Multiple studies are now available that present various data and recommendations for using CT in the preoperative evaluation of lung cancer in which the presence or absence of nodal enlargement influences the staging of patients with these tumors [2–11].

Material and Methods

Fifty patients with lung cancer in different stages of their disease were evaluated by CCT (continuous computed tomography). All scans were obtained with a Somatom Plus (Siemens, Erlangen), a continuously rotating CT scanner wich offers scan times from 0.7 up to 4 s. After informed consent, all patients were studied twice with scan times of 0.7 and 2.0 s of the mediastinum and hilum with 5 mm slice thickness and

7 mm spacing. Scanning was started 45 s after the onset of injection of 100 ml Isopaque Cerebral 280 (Nycomed) in a 1:1 saline solution (140 mg I/ml) under a 150 PSI pressure limit at a flowrate of 0.65 ml/s continuously during a maximum of 145 s, programmed with a Liebel Flarsheim Angiomat CT injector system. No patients were excluded from the study. All images were evaluated separately by two observers from two different centers (Rotterdam Cancer Institute and Leyenburg Hospital in The Hague), and the interobserver variation was determined according to the blind scoring. The examinations were scored for (1) streak artifacts, (2) image distortion, and (3) detection of lymph nodes. A three-step scoring system was used for the presence of artifacts (free of artifacts, some artifacts, and many artifacts) and a two-step scoring system for the description of anatomical detail (good and bad). The number of lymph nodes and their location were scored in every case.

Results

Artifacts

Of the series obtained with the 0.7 s scanning time, 66% were free of artifacts and 34% showed some; no examination showed many artifacts. Of the series obtained with a 2.0 s scanning time, 8% showed no artifacts, 64% showed some, and 28% showed many (Table 1). The artifacts were mostly located near the aortic root and pulmonary hili. In total, artifacts were 58% more frequent and in 62% of the patients more severe with a 2.0 s scanning time compared with a 0.7 s scanning time. There was full interobserver agreement.

Image Distortion

With a 0.7 s scanning time, none of the images showed distortion, whereas 16 examinations (32%) with a 2.0 s scanning time showed a strongly impaired description of anatomical detail (Table 2), most frequently in the region of the heart. Also for this part of the evaluation there was full interobserver agreement.

Table 1. Artifacts in 2.0-s and in 0.7-s examinations of 50 patients

	2.0 s	0.7 s
Free of artifacts	4	33
Some artifacts	32	17
Many artifacts	14	None
Interobserver variation	None	None

Table 2. Image distortion in 2.0 s and in 0.7 s examinations of 50 patients

	2.0 s	0.7 s
No image distortion	16	50
Image distortion	34	None
Interobserver variation	None	None

Table 3. Lymph node (LN) detection in 2.0-s and 0.7-s examinations of 50 patients (PAT). The numbers between parentheses are the results of observer 2

	2.0 s		0.7 s	
	PAT	LN	PAT	LN
Negative for lymph nodes	25 (25)	x	17 (16)	x
Positive for lymph nodes	25 (25)	51 (51)	33 (34)	64 (65)
Equal results (pos + neg)	100%	100%	98%	98%
Interobserver variation	0%	0%	2%	2%

Lymph Node Detection

Observer 1 scored for the images obtained with a 0.7 s scanning time 33 examinations (66%) positive for lymph nodes. In these 33 examinations, 64 nodes were detected. With a 2.0 s scanning time, this observer scored 25 examinations (50%) positive for lymph nodes, and 51 nodes were detected. In 34 examinations (68%), the results (positive and negative) for the two scan times under considerations were equal. For positive detection this was the case in 24 examinations. Observer 2 disagreed on one patient of the 0.7 scan time series, whose scan was scored as having no lymph nodes by observer 1 and one lymph node by observer 2.

According to observer 1, eight examinations that were positive for lymph nodes on the 0.7-s scan were missed on the 2.0-s scans of these patients; observer 2 agreed on these eight but scored one examination more that was positive for lymph nodes on the 0.7-s and missed on the examination with the 2.0-s scan time (Table 3). To summarize, at least 13 lymph nodes (20%) of a total of 64 nodes which were diagnosed at the 0.7-s examinations were not detected with 2.0-s CT scanning. Upon 2.0-s CT scanning, at least eight patients (32%) out of 25 were regarded as negative for lymph nodes, in whom lymph nodes were detected at the 0.7-s CT scanning.

Discussion

It is obvious that our opinion about a normal CT examination of the mediastinum and hilum has changed during the past decade. The CT image quality has dramatically improved. The fastest scanning time of a second-generation scanner was 18 s; third generation scanners have scan times as short as 2 s. Spatial and contrast resolution were greatly improved, artifacts were reduced but unfortunately are still quite common with state-of-the-art scanners. Scan times of 1 s are considered rapid sequence scans in the recent literature [12]. We applied an even higher time resolution with a scan exposure of 0.7 s. In the present study, we found that anatomical detail in fast moving, pulsating structures like the heart, great vessels, and lung hilum is still difficult to depict with scan times of 2.0 s. Peripheral hilar structures are not reproducibly imaged, moving in and out of the slice during data sampling. One of the best and oldest ways to cope with motion in imaging is to reduce the exposure time.

In our series the combination of artifact-free examination with lack of image distortion has lead to a substantial improvement of the image quality if a 0.7-s scan time

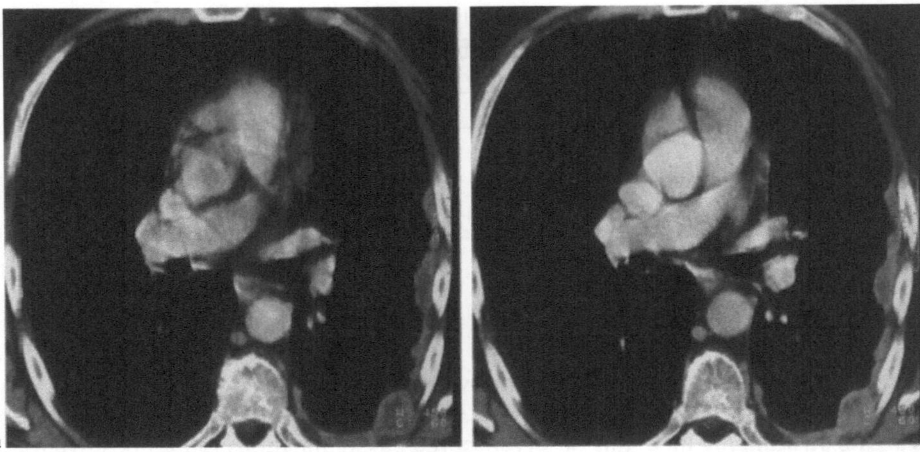

a b

Fig. 1. **a** A 2.0-s scan with streak artifacts in the area of the pericardium and pulmonary trunk, arteries, and aortic root. **b** A 0.7-s scan at the same level, in the same patient as in **a,** no artifacts are detected

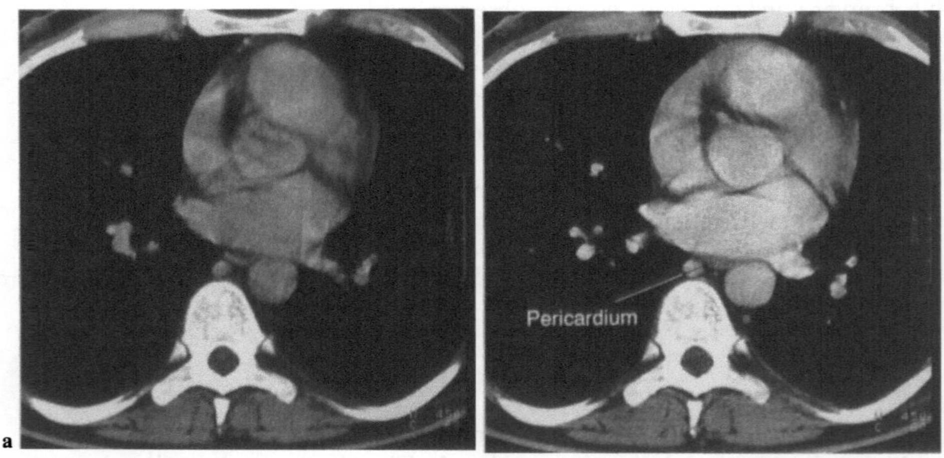

a b

Fig. 2. **a** A 2.0-s scan with streak artifacts in the area of the pericardium, aortic root, and left atrium. **b** A 0.7-s scan at the same level, in the same patient as in **a,** no artifacts are detected. Note pericardial fluid dorsal of left atrium, not detectable at 2.0 s

was used (Figs. 1, 2). With the 0.7-s scan time, more hilar lymph nodes were detected than with the 2.0-s scan time (Figs. 3–6). Interpretation problems which can lead to a false-positive description of lymph nodes were seen more often with the longer scanning time. Thus, with a shorter scanning time, the absence of lymphadenopathy can be predicted with more certainty and could eliminate an invasive surgical staging procedure in many patients. Furthermore, it should be noted that perception can mislead the interpreter. Smoothness is often regarded as synonymous with image quality, but images which look more granular can contain a lot more information,

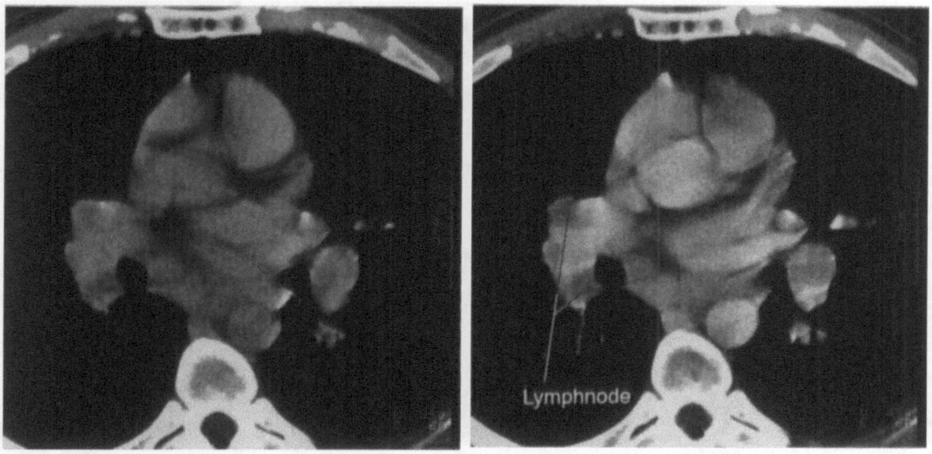

a b

Fig. 3. **a** A 2.0-s scan, no lymph nodes are detected in the enlarged hili either at this level or at the adjacent slice levels. **b** A 0.7-s scan, three lymph nodes are deteced in the right hilum at the same level and in the same patient as in **a**

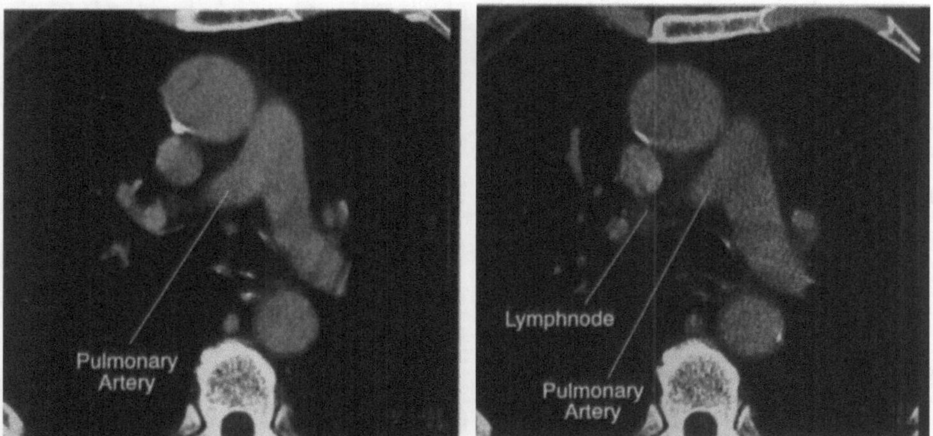

a b

Fig. 4. **a** A 2.0-s scan, no lymph nodes are detected. The adjacent slices were also negative for hilar lymph nodes. **b** A 0.7-s scan, one lymph node in the right hilum is detected at the same level and in the same patient as in **a.** The lymph node next to the pulmonary trunk is detected in the adjacent slice at 2.0 s

both in terms of border sharpness and tissue differentiation (compare a with of Figs. 1–6). With shorter scan times, we found better morphological differentiation, but the images showed a clearly increased graininess.

There is nearly universal agreement that enlarged lymph nodes would not exclude a patient from surgical consideration in the absence of histological proof [11–13], but the absence of detectable lymph nodes appears to make preoperative staging by mediastinoscopy superfluous [6–9]. Criteria for staging vary from 0.5 to 2.0 cm [5],

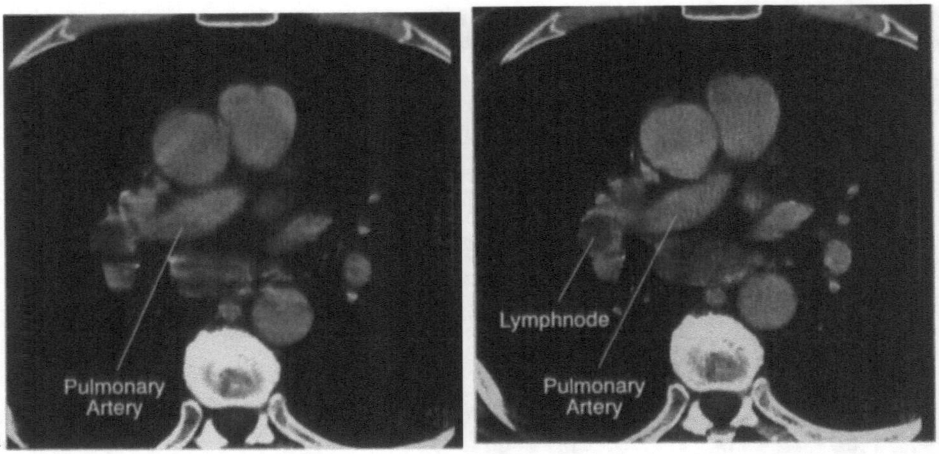

a b

Fig. 5. **a** A 2.0-s scan, no hilar lymph nodes are detected either at this level or at the adjacent slice levels due to prominent streak artifacts through both hili. **b** A 0.7-s scan, one lymph node in the right hilum is detected at the same level and in the same patient as in **a**

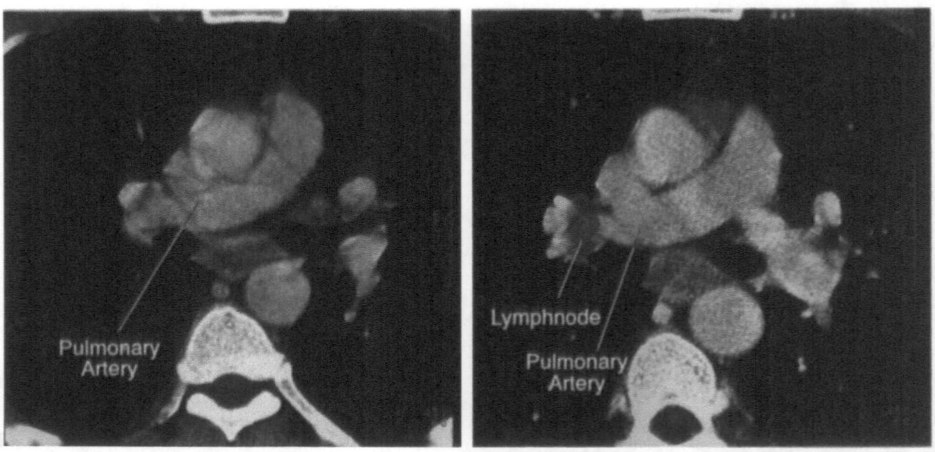

a b

Fig. 6. **a** A 2.0-s scan, no lymph nodes are detected either at this level or at the adjacent slice levels. There are some streak artifacts in the area of the pericardium. **b** A 0.7-s scan, one lymph node is detected at the same level and in the same patient as in **a**

and the difference in size between the ipsilateral and contralateral side may play a role [3].

In conclusion, shorter scan times improve spatial and contrast resolution and diminish the severity and frequency of motion artifacts. The diagnostic ability for hilar lymph node enlargement is significantly improved with 0.7–s scanning as compared with 2.0-s scanning. The combination of high temporal and high spatial resolution permits the delineation of hilar lymph nodes of less than 1 cm in diameter, and probably more importantly, lymphadenopathy may be excluded with more certainty.

References

1. Goldberg HI, Gould RG, Feuerstein IM et al. (1989) Evaluation of ultrafast CT scanning of the adult abdomen. Invest Radiol 24: 537
2. Platt JF, Glazer GM, Gross BH, Quint LE, Francis IR, Orringer MB (1987) CT evaluation of mediastinal lymph nodes in lung cancer: influence of the lobar site of the primary neoplasm. AJR 149: 683–686
3. Lewis WL, Pearlberg JL, Beute GH, Alpern M, Kvale PA, Gross BH, Magilligan DJ (1990) Can computed tomography of the chest stage lung cancer? – yes and no. Ann Thorac Surg 49: 591–596
4. Conte CC, Bucknam CA (1985) Role of computerised tomography in assessment of the mediastinum in patients with lung carcinoma. Am J Surg 149: 449–452
5. Libshitz HI (1990) Computed tomography in bronchogenic carcinoma. Semin Roentgenol XXV (1): 64–72
6. Vestring T, Achatzky R, Wahlers B, Macha HN, Peters PE (1990) Mediastinales Staging des nicht-kleinzelligen Bronchialkarzinoms. Stellenwert der Computertomographie und Mediastinoskopie. Radiologe 30: 178–184
7. Chiles C (1990) CT of the pulmonary hilum. Radiol Clin North Am 28: 3
8. Daly BDT, Faling J, Bite G, Gale ME, Bankoff MS, Jung-Legg Y, Cooper AG, Snider GL (1987) Mediastinal lymph node evaluation by computed tomography in lung cancer (an analysis of 345 patients grouped by TNM staging, tumor size, and tumor location). J Thorac Cardiovasc Surg 94: 664–672
9. Daly BDT, Faling LJ, Pugatch RD et al. (1984) Computed tomography; an effective technique for mediastinal staging in lung cancer. J Thorac Cardiovasc Surg 88: 486–494
10. Glazer HS, Kaiser LR, Anderson DJ, Molina PL, Emami B, Roper CL, Sagel SS (1989) Indeterminate mediastinal invasion in bronchogenic carcinoma: CT evaluation. Radiology 173: 37–42
11. Kiyono K. Sone S, Sakai F et al. (1988) The number and size of normal mediastinal lymph nodes: a postmortem study. AJR 150: 771–776
12. Onitsuka H, Tsukuda M, Araki A, Murakami J, Torii Y, Masuda K (1991) Differentiation of central lung tumor from postobstructive lobar collapse by rapid sequence computed tomography. J Thorac Imaging 6 (2): 28–31
13. Epstein DM, Stephensen LW, Gefter WB, Van der Voorde F, Archonik JM, Miller WT (1986) Value of CT in the preoperative assessment of lung cancer: a survey of thoracic surgeons. Radiology 161: 423–427

Spiral Volumetric CT in Follow-up Examinations of Children with Neuroblastoma

J.-P. Wakat, A. Rieber, T. Fleiter, H. J. Brambs, and C. D. Claussen

Introduction

Modern 1-s computed tomography (CT) scanners mostly avoid respiratory artifacts; however, especially in the case of reduced patient cooperation as in the examination of children, successive scans can cause an omission of anatomic levels. The purpose of this study was to avoid increased radiation doses in follow-up examinations in children with neuroblastoma without jeopardizing the success of staging, using spiral CT.

Material and Methods

For choosing the optimal reconstruction interval and scan mode, an Alderson Man phantom was used. Standard CT scans and spiral scans in different modes were carried out. Results were assessed by three experienced radiologists. In order to cover the largest possible scan volume, a table incrementation speed equal to the slice thickness was selected. For clinical studies the spiral mode "abdomen, 165 mA, slice

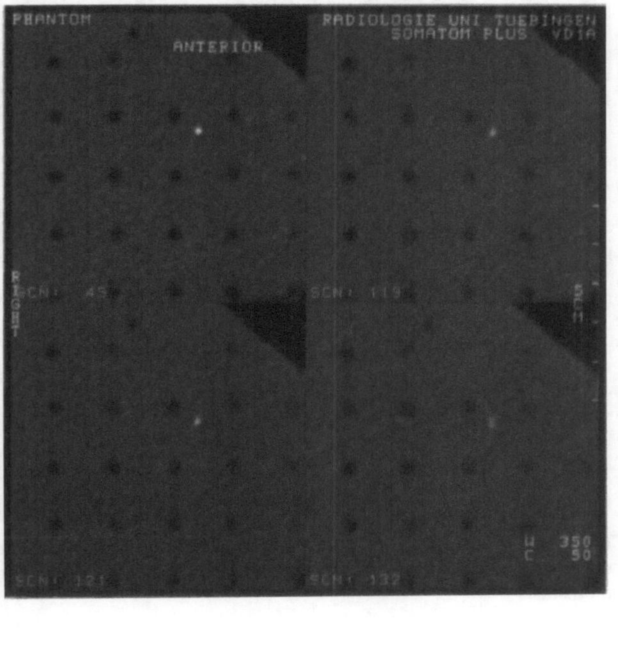

Fig. 1. Phantomstudy (selection). All scans were done at 120 kV. Reading clockwise: scan 45, standard CT, 210 mA, 10 mm slice thickness; scan 119, SVCT, 210 mA, 8 mm slice thickness; scan 132, SVCT, 85 mA, 10 mm slice thickness; scan 121, SVCT, 165 mA, 10 mm slice thickness. All spiral scans were reconstructed with intervals equal to the slice thickness and table incrementation

10 mm" was used, which permitted the examination of a section up to 10 cm long. The reconstructions are calculated in 10-mm intervals with a standard back-projection algorithm (Fig. 1). In the first three patients of our series, both standard CT and spiral volumetric (SV) CT were performed.

Nine children with neuroblastoma underwent follow-up examinations for restaging, with a total of 18 examinations during the course of their diagnostic evaluation and treatment. Diagnosis was confirmed by urine catechol levels, surgical resection, or biopsy. Patients were routinely sedated. In all children but one, the CT images were enhanced by intravenous contrast medium (Ultravist 300, 1 ml/kg), applied as a bolus (30%) with subsequent infusion. In 11 of 18 examinations, the stomach and bowel were opacified with meglumine diatrizoate. The initial examination was performed with standard CT (10 mm spacing and 10 mm slice thickness, 210 mA), and follow-up examinations with SVCT (10 mm/s, 165 mA); the interpolated data were reconstructed at 10 mm intervals. Magnetic resonance (MR) images were available for comparison. The volume scans were obtained with a commercially available, continuously rotating Somatom Plus scanner (Siemens Medical Systems, Erlangen, FRG).

Results

Neuroblastoma can occur anywhere along the sympathetic nervous system. The most common site of primary tumour is within the abdomen, either in an adrenal gland (40%) or in a paraspinal ganglion (25%); thoracic (15%) and pelvic (5%) primaries

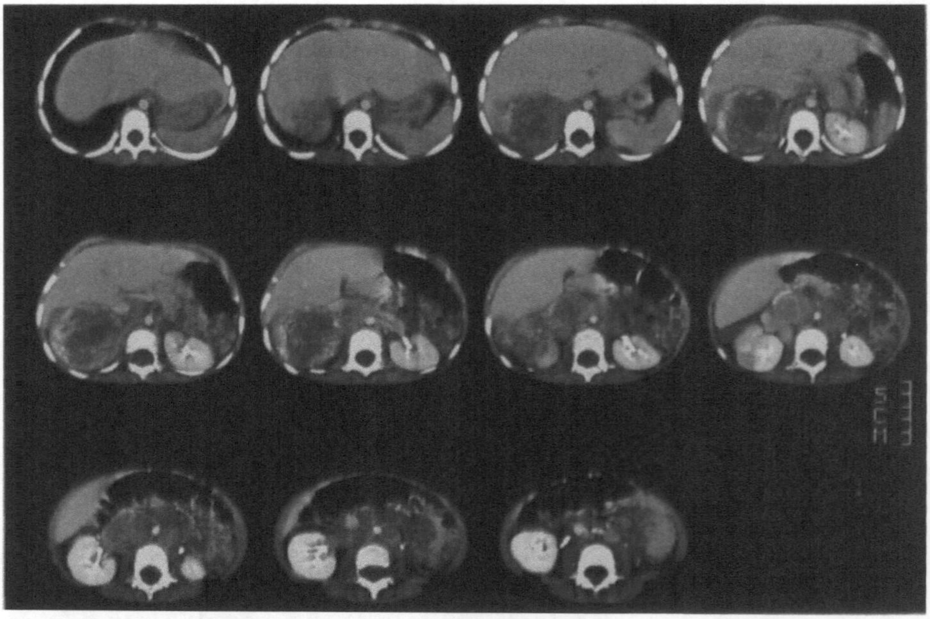

Fig. 2. Standard CT (120 kV, 210 mA, 10 mm slice thickness, 10-mm spacing). Adrenal gland tumor mass with calcifications infiltrating the right kidney, retroperitoneal lymphomas, solitary hepatic metastasis

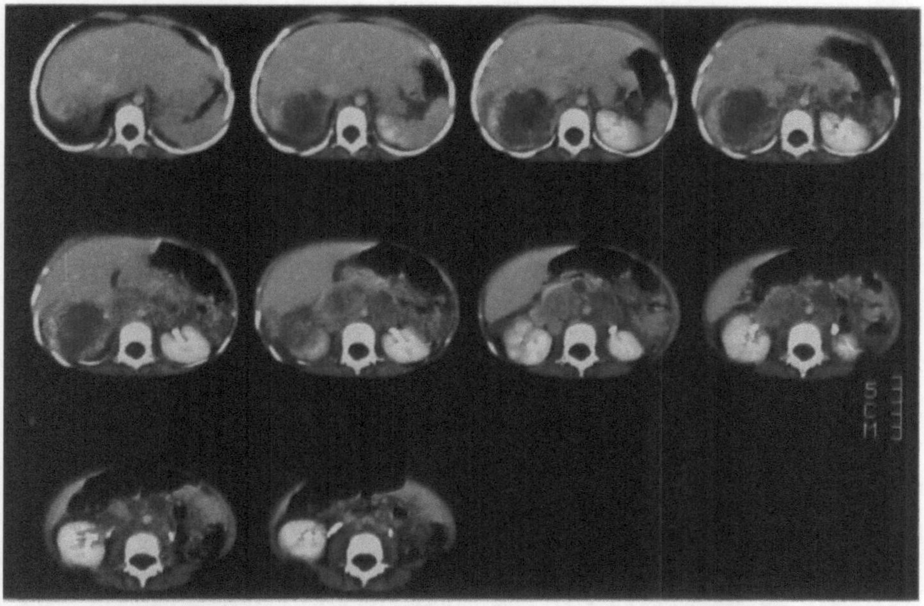

Fig. 3. Same patient as in Fig. 2: SVCT With 165 mA, 10 mm slice thickness, reconstruction interval, and table increment demonstrates the masses as well as standard CT

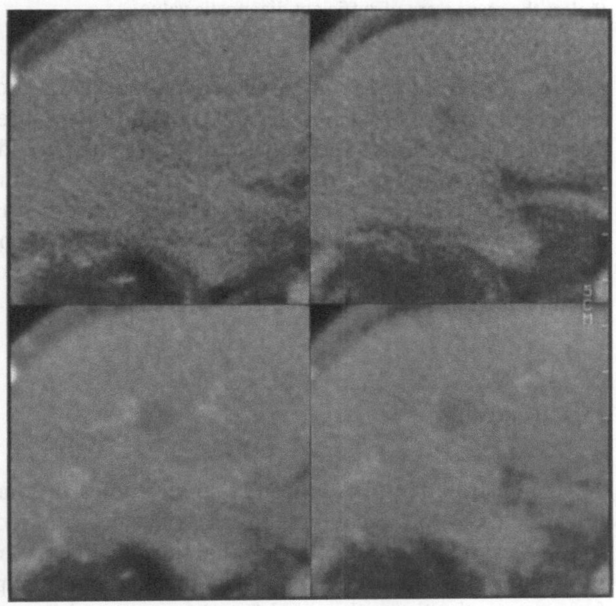

Fig. 4. Hepatic metastasis of a neuroblastoma. The lesion was demarcated as well as or even better on SVCT *(bottom)* as on standard CT *(top)*

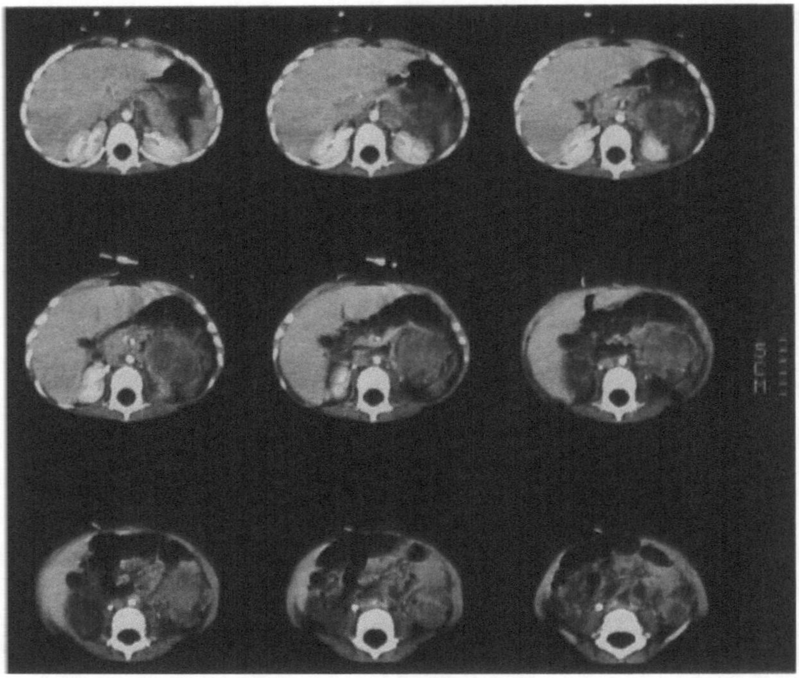

Fig. 5. Neuroblastoma, demonstrated by SVCT. The patient received insufficient sedation, but nevertheless the scans were of sufficient diagnostic value

account for the rest. In our series one patient had a thoracic manifestation, but the scans could not be presented because of technical failure. All lesions in the upper abdomen (nine patients) and pelvis (three patients) could be detected with SV CT as well as MRI. Abdominal masses could be detected within less than 30 s. Comparisons with standard CT (Fig. 2) reveals that masses are demonstrated as well as with SVCT (Figs. 3, 4). CT is, as is well known, superior to MRI in detecting calcifications and pulmonary nodules. Even in cases of insufficient sedation (Fig. 5), scans of sufficient diagnostic value could be obtained.

Discussion

As demonstrated by phantom and patient studies, the diagnostic value of the images is not affected by spiral scanning. In cases of insufficient sedation, SVCT can be superior to standard CT. Although the nominal slice thickness is increased by the interpolation procedure, this did not become a significant diagnostic problem. In comparison with former examinations, the need for repeat scans, increased procedure time, and subsequent higher radiation dose could be reduced, and likewise the time of patient sedation. In all patients, SVCT detected the size, location, calcification, composition, and contiguous spread of the lesions as well as standard CT did. SVCT appears to be a reliable technique for (re)staging and follow-up of children with neuroblastoma.

Clinical Application I

Chairmen: J. Lissner, U. Mödder, and K. J. Wolf

X-ray Computed Tomography Perfusion Imaging

M. P. Hayball, K. A. Miles, and A. K. Dixon

Introduction

Dynamic X-ray computed tomography (CT) is well established as a technique for enhancing information derived from CT investigations. In 1980, Axel produced a theoretical derivation of blood flow from dynamic CT, and a number of centres have investigated the derivation of functional data from time-density curves (TDCs) created from a region of interest (ROI) placed over an organ [2]. There has also been some interest in the production of parametric images from dynamic CT data [5].

In nuclear medicine it has long been possible to produce functional images from radioactive tracer dynamic studies, although the anatomical resolution has often been poor. Here we demonstrate that by applying techniques derived from nuclear medicine experience to CT it is possible to produce quantitative functional images from a single location dynamic CT sequence with the spatial resolution associated with CT.

Practice

A single location dynamic sequence of 1 s duration is performed immediately following the injection of 50 ml iopamidol (Niopam, Merck) 300 mg/ml into an antecubital vein. Images are acquired during quiet respiration – typically 10–12 images in 45–60 s with the exact timing chosen to suit the organ under study. The slice chosen should pass centrally through the organ under study to avoid partial volume effects and include a large artery passing perpendicularly through the slice.

Images are subsequently compressed into 256 × 256 pixel format and transferred onto a Acorn Archimides computer work station via a fast serial link for processing and colour display. Software has been developed to derive a TDC for those pixels which do not contain fat, bone or air. A perfusion map is produced representing perfusion on a colour scale in ml blood/min/ml tissue.

Theory

The theory used is derived from an extension of the use of radiolabelled microspheres in blood flow measurement [4, 6].

Following left-ventricular injection, the radiolabelled microspheres leave the circulation by lodging in capillaries. Organ perfusion can be measured by excision of the organ and measurement of the radioactive burden of the organ and hence the number of microspheres deposited. If a series of blood samples are taken following the injection, the cardiac output can be calculated. The proportion of total activity administered found in the organ gives the relative perfusion and hence the organ perfusion.

The arterial concentration in microspheres ($C_a(t)$) after injection will typically follow the shape shown in Fig. 1, which can be represented by a gamma-variant. The concentration within an organ can be derived by:

$$C_t(t) = \int_0^t C_a(t' - t_{lag})\, dt'$$

where t_{lag} is the time required for the tracer to travel from the site of measurement of $C_a(t)$ to the organ, and F is the tissue perfusion per unit volume of tissue (ml/min/ml) (Fig. 1). When all the microspheres have left the circulation, the organ activity per unit volume will be:

$$C_t = F I \quad \text{where} \quad I = \int_0^\infty C_a(t')\, dt'$$

Note: The area under the arterial TDC, I, is related to the cardiac output, CO, and the total mass of contrast medium, m, by:

$$CO = \frac{k\,m}{I}$$

where k is a conversion factor from mass of contrast to CT number.

Furthermore, since the shapes of $C_t(t)$ and the time integral of $C_a(t)$ are identical, differing only in magnitude, the maximum gradients of the two curves are also related by:

$$g_t = F g_a \quad \rightarrow \quad F = \frac{g_t}{g_a}$$

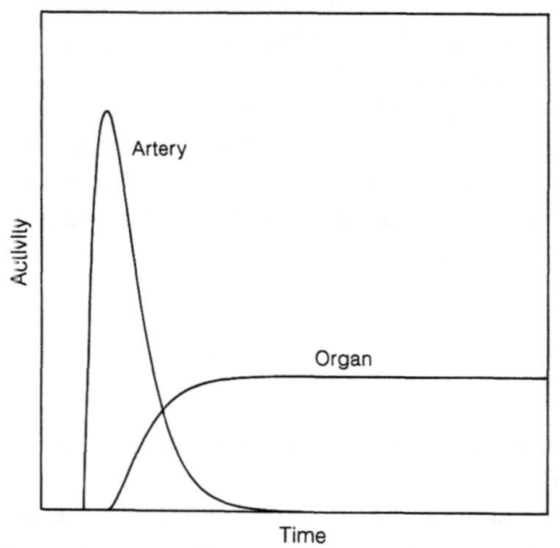

Fig. 1. Activity in the artery and an organ following injection of radiolabelled microspheres

where g_t and g_a are the maximum gradients of $Ct(t)$ and the time integral of $C_a(t)$, respectively. Thus, g_a can be simply calculated as the maximum value of $C_a(t)$.

In dynamic CT, C_a and C_t represent the contrast density in the artery and organ. Interpolation techniques are used to create a smoothly varying curve. $C_a(t)$ has the same initial shape as that for microspheres, but since the tracer is not trapped in the organs, it includes a recirculation component (Fig. 2). A tissue element not containing a blood vessel will have a tracer retention curve as shown in Fig. 3. The initial 'retention' phase represents the 'filling' of the capillaries in the tissue element. If this tissue element has as its input $C_t(t)$, the tissue TDC is as shown in Fig. 2.

Assuming that the retention phase is of sufficient duration for the maximum gradient to be visualised, then the perfusion can be calculated simply as:

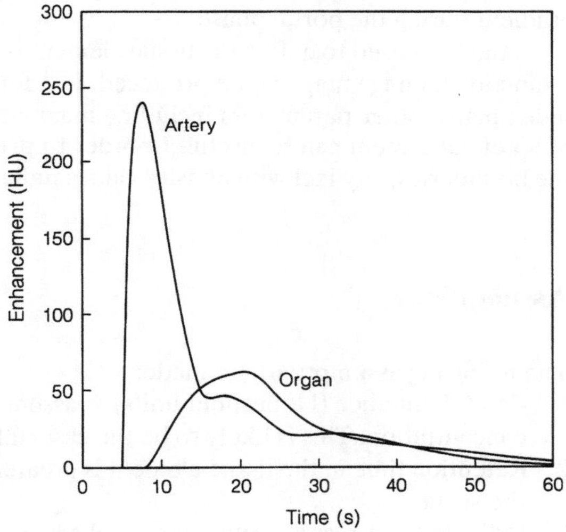

Fig. 2. Time-density curve for the artery and an organ following injection of iodinated contrast material

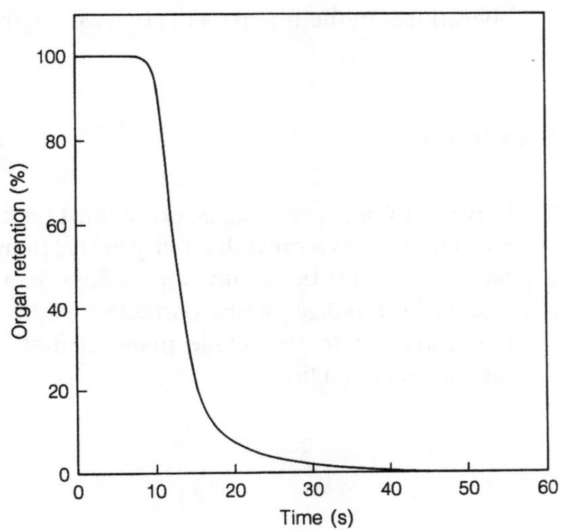

Fig. 3. A typical organ element retention curve

$$\text{Perfusion} = \frac{\text{Maximum slope of tissue TDC}}{\text{Peak of arterial TDC}}$$

This relationship can be used to provide further information. The liver has two distinct blood supplies: arterial and portal. The relationship between the maximum gradient and the perfusion can be used to create an index of relative perfusion. The spleen is used as a reference organ to identify the end of the arterial phase. The maximum gradient of the liver TDC is taken before and after the end of the arterial phase. The index can be created:

$$\text{hepatic perfusion index} = \frac{{}_{\mathrm{p}}g_t}{{}_{\mathrm{a}}g_t + {}_{\mathrm{p}}g_t}$$

where ${}_{\mathrm{a}}g_t$ is the maximum gradient during the arterial phase, and ${}_{\mathrm{p}}g_t$ is the maximum gradient during the portal phase.

If the ROI used to define the tissue element is reduced to the size of a single pixel, a functional image map can be produced. In addition to the perfusion and perfusion index maps, other parameters including maximum enhancement and time to maximum enhancement can be useful. In order to prevent artefacts due to movement at the boundaries, any ixel with density values indicating bone, fat or air is excluded.

Assumptions

The following assumptions are made:

1 The CT number (Hounsfield units) is assumed to be proportional to the iodine concentration. This is likely to be the case unless beam hardening is significant.

2 Retention time in the tissue element is greater than time to peak enhancement in the aorta.

3 Iodinated contrast is assumed to be pharmaceutically inert. It is unlikely that any of the theoretical effects of the contrast medium on organ flow would become operational in the first pass of contrast medium.

Conditions

1. In order to produce images, noise must be kept to a minimum. The Siemens Somatom Plus has a reproducibility better than ± 2 HU for a 256×256 matrix.
2. Movement must be ideally kept to less than pixel dimensions. Movement in the plane of the image can be corrected for by software techniques, but movement perpendicular to the image plane cannot be corrected for without full three-dimensional imaging.

Applications

Liver

There has long been keen interest in the perfusion characteristics of hepatic parenchyma and focal hepatic lesions. In the early days of CT, there were some rather extravagant claims about tissue specificity and various enhancement characteristics [1]. However, apart from a few near pathognomonic patterns (haemangioma, focal nodular hyperplasia, etc.), the overlap between benign and malignant tissues seems large. Nevertheless, machines providing high spatial and attenuation resolution, such as the Somatom Plus, have helped to further demonstrate these patterns.

Inherent in all studies of hepatic perfusion is the problem that the liver lies very close to the diaphragm. Because the patient may not maintain exactly similar phases of respiration, the ROI (e. g. a focal lesion) may not be captured in exactly the same anatomical slice on sequential images. Although some data can be obtained during the arterial phase during a single-breath-hold, dynamic, multi-sequence image, the interesting portal and late enhancement characteristics cannot be obtained in this way. We have been using a standard programme of data acquisition times (see above) following the short (ca. 10 s), hand-given, bolus, intravenous injection of 50 ml of standard contrast media into a large (cubital fossa) vein with a large bore cannula. This is done during gentle breathing, having first localised the area of maximal interest on a routine set of unenhanced images also obtained during gentle breathing. We have found attempts at getting the same phase of respiration on sequential images difficult.

We are currently evaluating the perfusion characteristics in supposedly normal livers. We have been able to separate arterial and portal perfusion and to assess their relative contribution in the left and right lobes using the hepatic perfusion index (Fig. 4). It would be interesting to evaluate this in patients before and after a meal to validate the findings from Doppler ultrasound studies, but the radiation and contrast medium risks would be hard to justify. The technique can also be used to study various forms of hepatic parenchymal disease. Again, ROIs can be drawn to suit the

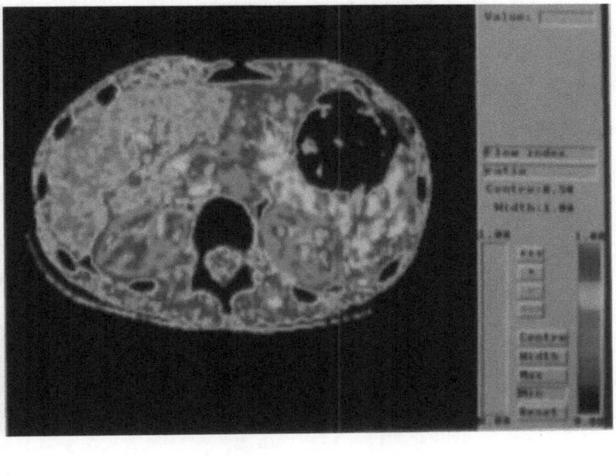

Fig. 4. Hepatic perfusion index image of a liver showing clearly different behaviour of the two lobes

pathological findings. Accordingly, perfusion characteristics of the caudate lobe could be differentiated from those elsewhere in the liver in conditions such the Budd–Chiari syndrome. The perfusion characteristics of various forms of cirrhosis are amenable to study. For example, the characteristic hypertrophy of the lateral segment of the left lobe of the liver in alcoholic cirrhosis [7] might appear as a result of vascular redistribution.

As regards hepatic tumours, the perfusion of various parts of the lesion can be assessed and peak enhancement shown in colour display. This information in itself is not particularly helpful, especially in tumours of known type. However, of considerable research interest is the behaviour of perfusion patterns following various forms of intervention. We are currently analysing the effect of chemotherapeutic regimens and hyperthermia in order to see the extent to which perfusion is altered.

Kidneys

By virtue of their relatively fixed retroperitoneal position, the kidneys are especially well suited for study by rapid CT. There is already some literature on the topic of regional blood flow [3]. However, the new perfusion technique offers exquisite anatomical mapping of peak perfusion and, in particular, accurate delineation of the boundary between cortex and medulla (Fig. 5). It is possible that alterations in this sharp demarcation might be early predictors of various forms of renal parenchymal abnormalities (e.g. diabetic renal disease).

Musculoskeletal System

The perfusion of muscles themselves is an area of great potential interest. Studies might provide useful data which could be extrapolated to the all-important myocardium. There is already considerable work on myocardial perfusion being undertaken in centres with access to Imatron CT systems which provide much faster data acquisi-

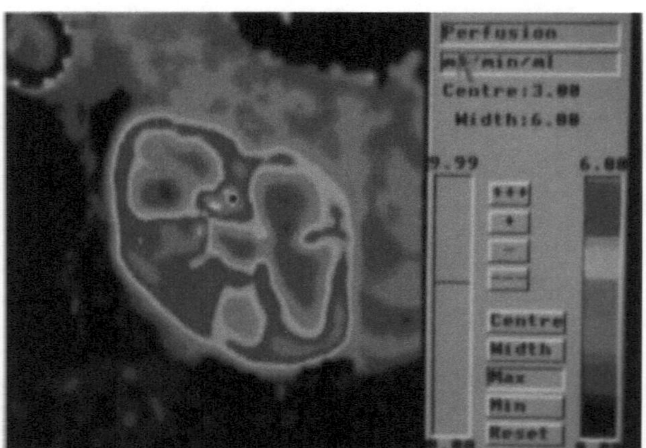

Fig. 5. Perfusion image of a kidney

tion than even the Somatom Plus. The normal muscle perfusion in the limbs can be measured using the Somatom Plus, although the perfusion is low at rest and therefore open to inaccuracies. Some centres have developed techniques to assess skeletal muscle perfusion following exercise, but we have not addressed this problem. We have assessed perfusion in tumours within skeletal muscle, again as a prelude to assessing the effect of chemotherapy or hyperthermia. Of course, such studies in the lower limb are fairly reproducible on account of the total absence of movement artefact.

Brain

There has been considerable work on brain perfusion using xenon CT techniques. However, these studies require careful supervision and special equipment. The perfusion technique described above is potentially much more widely applicable. Attenuation due to the skull and limitations on dose increase the noise, but movement artefacts are eliminated. Early experience suggests that the technique is of limited value in the normal brain, where the blood-brain barrier is intact. However, as in all cranial CT enhanced studies, it should be practical in lesions which have led to a defect in the blood-brain barrier. Again, perfusion characteristics before and after various interventions could be assessed.

Conclusion

The technique we have demonstrated is but one of the many functional imaging techniques available to a radiologist. Functional imaging has long been available from nuclear medicine where the wide choice of radiopharmaceuticals gives a corresponding wide range of functional images. In dynamic CT the iodinated contrast material labels blood and is then used in this first-pass study to demonstrate blood flow alone. Furthermore, it does not suffer from the limitations of nuclear medicine of poor resolution and often unquantified photon absorption. The tracer concentration can be calculated directly from the CT number. Doppler ultrasound provides blood velocity measurement, but it is difficult to relate this to tissue perfusion. Magnetic resonance imaging can now provide blood flow measurements by observing the movement of blood within tissues [8]. This should eventually provide the closest alternative to dynamic CT and is additionally valid within blood vessels, although it is a measurement of flow and will not necessarily indicate tissue perfusion as accurately as an uptake technique.

References

1. Araki T, Hai Y, Furui S, Tasaka A (1980) CT densitometry of hepatic tumours. AJR 135: 1037–1043
2. Axel L (1980) Cerebral blood flow determination by rapid-sequence computed tomography. Radiology 137: 679–686

3. Jaschke W, Sievers RS, Lipton MJ, Cogan MG (1989) Cine-computed tomographic assessment of regional renal blood flow. Acta Radiol 31: 77–81
4. Miles KA, Hayball MP, Dixon AK (1991) Colour perfusion imaging: a new application of computed tomography. Lancet 337: 643–645
5. Nagala K, Asono T (1990) Functional image of dynamic CT for evaluation of cerebral hemodynamics. Stroke 21 (6): 882–889
6. Peters AM, Brown J, Hartnell GG, et al (1987) Noninvasive measurement of renal blood flow with technetium-99 DTPA: a comparison with radiolabelled microspheres. Cardiovas Res 21: 830–834
7. Torres WE, Whitmore LF, Gedgaudes-McCleef K, Bernadino ME (1986) CT of hepatic morphological changes in cirrhosis of the liver. J Comput Assist Tomogr 10: 47–50
8. Young IR, Hall AS, Bryant DJ et al. (1988) Assessment of brain perfusion with MR imaging. J Comput Assist Tomogr 12: 721–727

Evaluation of Aortocoronary Graft Patency: A Comparative Study of CT Volume Scanning and Angiography

P. E. Huppert, H. Seboldt, J. Schulze, W. Vogl, S. H. Duda, and C. D. Claussen

Introduction

Computed tomography (CT) has been proven to be an useful method for the evaluation of patency in aortocoronary venous grafts (ACVG). Even though the quantification of graft perfusion is uncertain, and assessment of the supplied coronary arteries is impossible, the detection of graft occlusion in the early postoperative phase is of some interest. Enhancement of ACVG after the injection of contrast material is the criterion of graft patency. CT with a discontinuous rotating tube requires a step-by-step comparison of precontrast and postcontrast scans. Using this approach, the sensitivity and specificity in the evaluation of graft patency are limited due to variations of the volume inspired and exspired by the patient. The mode of continuous acquisition during table movement (spiral CT) provides complete scanning of a selected patient volume during one breath hold. Spiral CT was tested for the evaluation of patency in ACVG in this study.

Methods

In a prospective manner we evaluated 24 patients (20 men, 4 women) aged between 39 and 76 years (mean 62 years) who suffered from chronic ischemic heart disease and had undergone an implantation of ACVG ($n = 54$) or anastomoses between the internal mammarian artery (IMA) and left anterior descending coronary artery (LAD, $n = 9$). Two patients had one, nine patients had two, nine patients had three, and four patients had four ACVG and IMA-LAD anastomoses, respectively. Grafts to the following coronary arteries were present: LAD ($n = 15$), diagonal branches ($n = 10$), circumflex branch ($n = 1$), left marginal branches ($n = 16$), right coronary artery ($n = 8$), right posterior descending artery ($n = 3$), and right marginal branch ($n = 1$). The interval between operation and CT was 10–16 days (mean 14.3 days).

Spiral CT acquisition was performed before and after intravenous contrast medium injection. The scanning volume had a length of 12 cm and included the interesting parts of the heart and great vessels. Ten scans were obtained during 10 s after a delay of 3 s. The thickness of the reconstructed images was 10 mm. Via a cubital vein, 30 ml of contrast material (Ultravist 300, Schering AG, Berlin, FRG) was injected by means of a power injector (flow 1.5 ml/s). Acquisition was started after a delay of 15 s. In one patient, a second acquisition was necessary with a delay of 25 s.

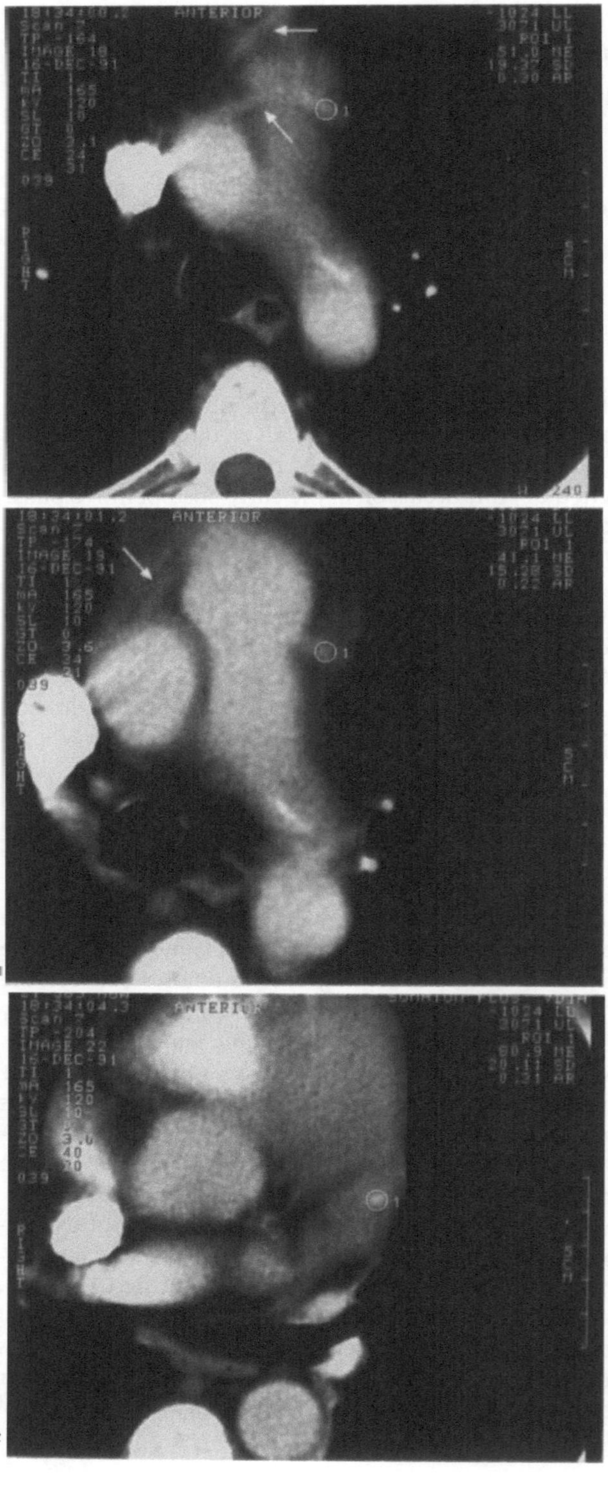

a b c

Fig. 1a–c. A 60-year old man had undergone implantation of ACVG to the left anterior descending artery and to the left marginal branch 17 days before angiography and CT. Spiral CT after contrast material injection: Demonstration of the proximal, middle and distal part of grafts. **a** Proximal both grafts (ventral LAD graft, dorsal marginal branch graft) are demonstrated in a longitudinal aspect *(arrows)*. **b** At 10 mm below, image demonstrates the marginal branch graft at the left side of the pulmonary trunk (density 41.1 HU) and the LAD graft ventral to the ascending aorta *(arrow)*. **c** Distal part of the marginal branch graft with a markedly increased density of 80.9 HU. This is probably due to a reduced run off (see Fig. 2)

CT images were reviewed by one experienced radiologist in two steps. In the first step he was unaware of the number and types of vessels implanted, and in a second step he had this information. Sensitivity was defined as the rate of correctly diagnosed patent vessels. Specificity was defined as the rate of correct diagnosed occluded vessels.

All patients underwent reference angiography on the day of CT examination ($n = 12$) or the day before ($n = 12$). High resolution digital subtraction angiography (Polytron, Siemens, Erlangen, FRG) was performed. Via 5 French pigtail-catheters a bolus of 35 ml of contrast material (Ultravist 300) was injected into the ascending aorta above the aortic valve. The flow rate was 25 ml/s (power injector, Siemens). Sagittal, left anterior oblique (45°), and right anterior oblique (45°) projections were used to obtain images at a frequency of 2 per second. For evaluation of the IMA-LAD anastomoses, 12 ml, of Ultravist 300 were injected (flow 5 ml/s) into the left subclavian artery. Selective angiography of ACVG was not performed.

Results

Angiography demonstrated 52 of 54 (96%) ACVG and all 9 IMA-LAD anastomoses to be patent. One diagonal branch graft and one marginal branch graft could not be detected angiographically, and occlusion was assumed. No complication was seen related to the angiography or CT examination.

Without knowledge of the number and types of ACVG and IMA-LAD anastomoses, sensitivity was 81% (42/52) for ACVG, 56% (5/9) for IMA-LAD anastomoses, and 77% (47/61) for both. With information about the vessels implanted, the sensitivity was 86% (45/52) for ACVG, 67% (6/9) for IMA-LAD anastomoses, and 84% (51/61) for both. One of the two angiographically occluded ACVG was judged occluded on CT, too; the other was judged as patent (specificity 50%). Of the 52 ACVG 23 (44%) were demonstrated on three or more consecutive scans and 47 (90%) ACVG on two scans. The typical aspect of the proximal and distal part of a left coronary ACVG in volume scanning images is shown in Fig. 1. The enhancement in the distal part of the marginal branch graft was increased due to an angiographically proven reduced run off (Fig. 2).

Without knowledge of the number and types of vessels implanted, five ACVG not present in reality were judged as patent. In eight patients true patent grafts were mistaken for each other (19%), but the identification of 34/42 (81%) true patent ACVB was correct.

Discussion

The spiral CT mode with continuous acquisition in a defined volume is useful to evaluate the patency of ACVB in the early postoperative phase. Despite several diagnostic difficulties, i.e., pericardial effusions and hematoma, a sensitivity of 86% was found compared with angiography. A sensitivity of 81 % was obtained even with-

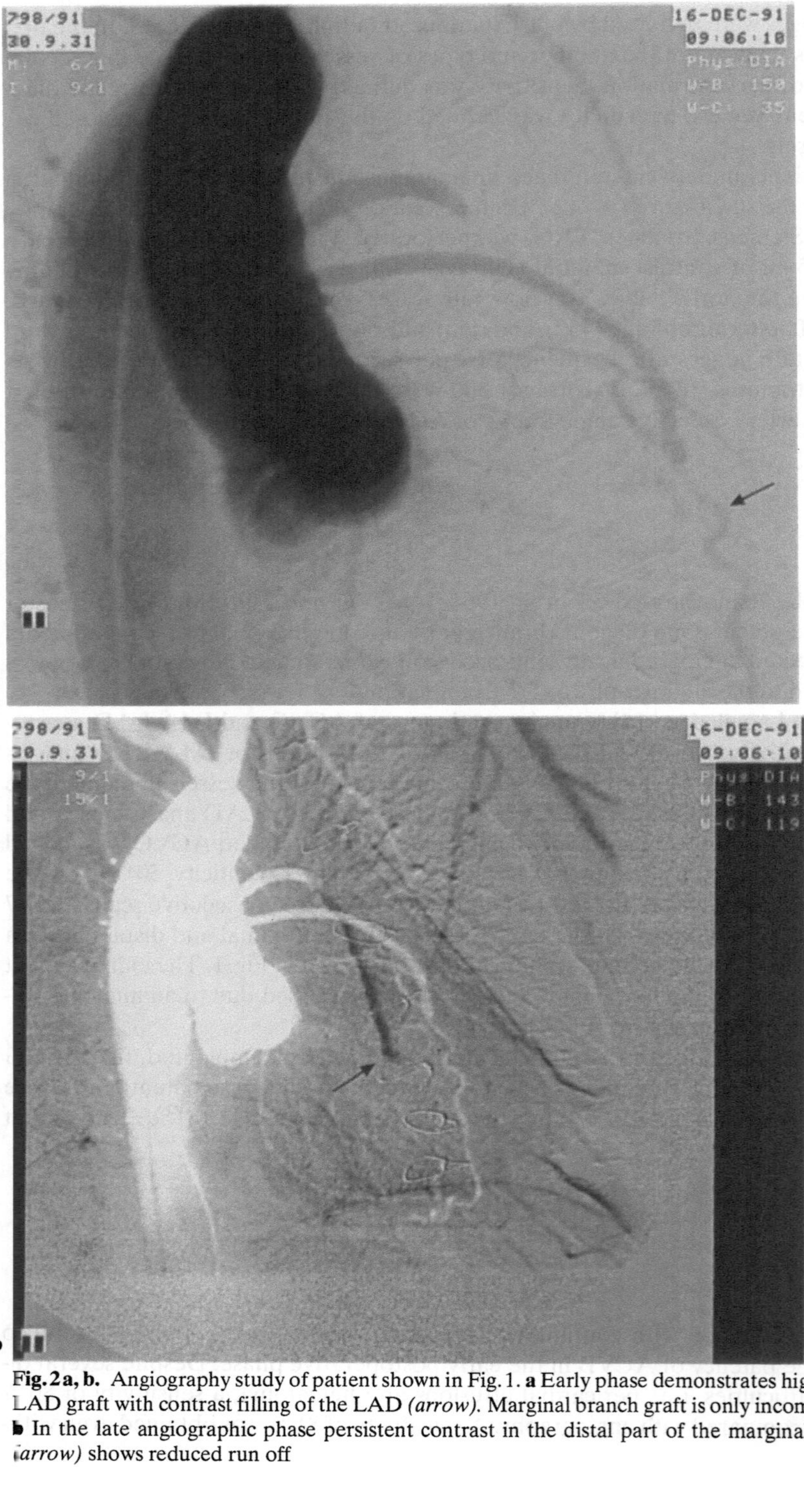

a

b

Fig. 2 a, b. Angiography study of patient shown in Fig. 1. **a** Early phase demonstrates high flow via the LAD graft with contrast filling of the LAD *(arrow)*. Marginal branch graft is only incompletely filled. **b** In the late angiographic phase persistent contrast in the distal part of the marginal branch graft *(arrow)* shows reduced run off out knowledge of the number and types of ACVG, and 81% of them were correctly identified according to their typical position and course. This shows the advantage of a volume scanning technique concerning the differentiation and identification of several types of ACVG and surrounding structures. The evaluation of IMA-LAD anastomoses in CT is uncertain compared with the results of ACVG. This is probably due to the smaller diameter of the arteries and their tortuous course.

Fast volume scanning resulted in a considerable reduction of the contrast material needed. CT examinations with discontinuous rotation of the tube require 100–150 ml of contrast material.

In this preliminary study, only two patients had occluded grafts. Therefore, the specificity has to be evaluated in a larger number of patients.

Preoperative CT Staging of Gastric and Colorectal Neoplasms with Water as Contrast Medium

J. Gaa, M. Georgi, and H. K. Deininger

Introduction

Conventional double-contrast barium studies and endoscopy continue to be the primary methods for examining tumors of the stomach and large bowel. In contrast to computed tomography (CT), however, these methods provide no information concerning tumor growth beyond the organ borders or the presence of regional lymph node and organ metastases. For more extensive diagnosis using CT, reliable opacification and adequate distension of the gastrointestinal tract are required. Aside from the commonly used iodine-containing contrast media and barium suspensions, some authors have recommended the use of water given orally or rectally as an alternative contrast medium [2, 3, 8].

The technical procedure and results of CT examinations of gastric and colorectal tumors with water as a gastrointestinal contrast agent are presented in the following report.

Material and Methods

In a pilot study, 38 patients between the ages of 31 and 84 years (mean 59) with histologically verified gastric or colorectal neoplasms were examined preoperatively by CT using water as a contrast medium. The focus of the ten gastric carcinomas was in the body of the stomach in six cases and in the antrum in four cases. Seven of the 28 tumors of the large bowel were found in the rectum and 21 in the colon (11 in the sigmoid, 5 in the ascending, 3 in the descending, and 1 in the transverse colon, and 1 in the cecum).

CT scans of the abdomen and the pelvis were performed following i.v. injection of 150 ml nonionic contrast medium (Solutrast 300, Byk Gulden, Constance, FRG) using a Somatom Plus (Siemens, Erlangen, FRG). Slice thicknesses and table feeds of 10 mm were used routinely. Additional scans with 8- or 5-mm slice thicknesses were performed in cases where the depth of tumor invasion was unclear.

Patients with gastric tumors fasted a minimum of 4 h before the examination. The stomach was generally emptied fully within this time period. Evacuation of the large bowel was achieved by administering three 10-mg doses of magnesium sulfate and 2.5 l of fluid orally. Patients with gastric tumors had to drink 600–800 ml of water immediately prior to scan begin. Gastrointestinal hypotension and a reduction in peristaltic artifacts were effected by i.v. injection of 40 mg Buscopan (Boehringer, Ingelheim, FRG) or 1 mg glucagon (Novo Industrie, Mainz, FRG). In order to display colorectal tumors, 1500 ml water (heated to 30–35 °C) was instilled rectally via a plastic tube. A balloon catheter was inserted in the event of an atonic anal sphincter. The rectally instilled water was withdrawn into the enema bag immediately following the examination in order to avoid intestinal water resorption or soiling of the examination table.

The 1987 TNM classification was used for staging of the tumors [9]. CT scans were analyzed for tumor size and depth of tumor invasion, lymph node involvement, and distant metastases. Lymph node enlargement greater than 1 cm in diameter or a cluster of three or more nodes each less than 1 cm was classified as pathologic. Lymph nodes larger than 8 mm in the gastrohepatic ligament and larger than 6 mm retrocrurally were also considered to be pathologic. The results of CT examinations were compared prospectively with surgical and histologic findings.

Results

Using water as a contrast agent, the normal wall thickness was found to be between 2 and 5 mm, with a mean of 3.6 mm for the stomach and 3.2 mm for the colon and rectum. All 38 tumors could be displayed in their full extension with CT, directly and unobscured by overlying structures. The maximum wall thicknesses of colorectal tumors varied from 1.1 cm to 2.5 cm (mean 1.7 cm) with the maximal tumor longitudinal extent being between 3.0 cm and 5.7 cm (mean 4.2 cm). For the gastric tumors, maximum wall thicknesses of 1.8–2.4 cm (mean 2.2 cm) and tumor longitudinal extents of 3.0–9.5 cm (mean 5.4 cm) were measured by means of CT.

Correct evaluation of the depth of tumor invasion was successfull using CT in 23 (82 %) of 28 colorectal tumors and in six (60 %) of ten gastric carcinomas (Figs. 1, 2). Since differentiation of submucosal infiltration (T1) or even infiltration of the muscularis (T2) itself was not possible with CT, these processes were classified as

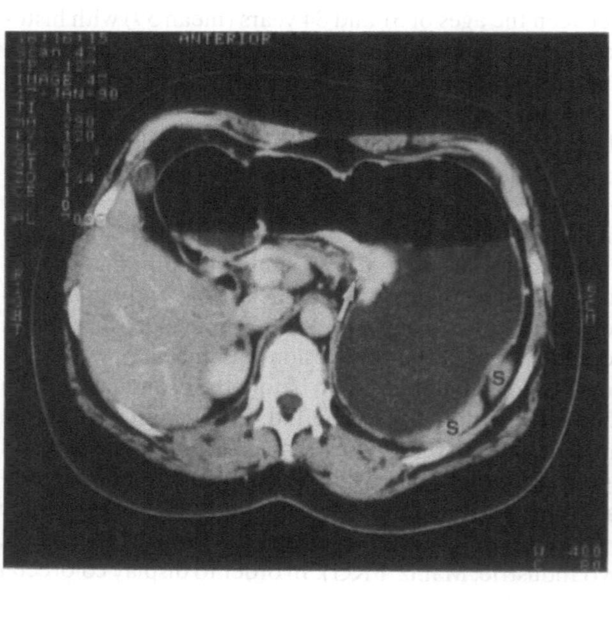

Fig. 1. Gastric adenocarcinoma. CT scan after oral administration of water shows localized thickening along the lesser curvature and infiltration of perigastric fat *(arrow)*. *S* spleen

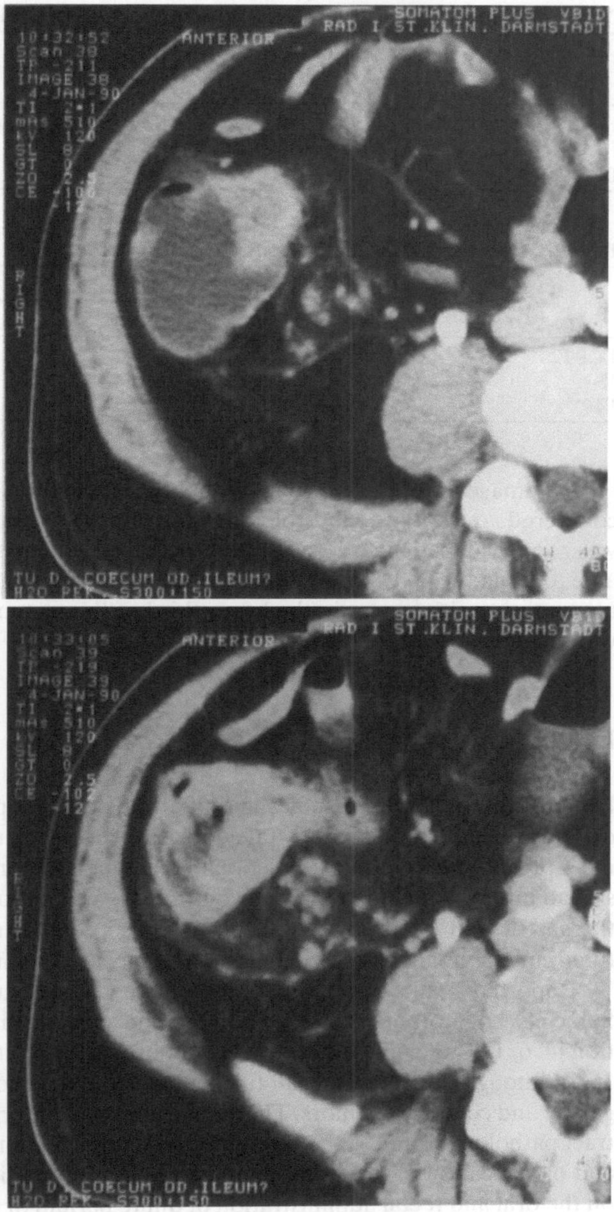

Fig. 2a, b. Carcinoma of ascending colon. CT scans after rectal administration of water reveal tumor invasion into pericolonic fat (**a**) and a considerably narrowed irregular lumen (**b**). A cluster of multiple lymph nodes each less than 1 cm in diameter is seen on both images. CT of the liver showed two hepatic metastases. CT staging (T3N2M1) was confirmed by pathologic studies

T1 + T2 tumors (Tables 1, 2). Regional lymph node metastases were demonstrated by CT in nine of the 11 colorectal tumors and evaluated correctly in seven (64%) patients. N staging with CT was correct in three (50%) of the six gastric tumors with lymph node involvement. Liver metastases were demonstrated by CT and subsequently confirmed surgically and histologically in seven patients with colorectal tumors and in one patient with gastric cancer.

Table 1. Accuracy of CT in the T classification of 28 colorectal carcinomas

	Histology	CT		
		correct	false >	false <
T1 + T2	7	5	2	–
T3	17	14	–	3
T4	4	4	–	–

Table 2. Accuracy of CT in the T classification of 10 gastric cancers

	Histology	CT		
		correct	false >	false <
T1 + T2	6	4	2	–
T3	3	1	1	1
T4	1	1	–	–

All images were of excellent quality. No motion-related artifacts were encountered. Acceptance and tolerance of water as a gastrointestinal contrast agent was good in all patients. No side effects occurred. Patients with gastric cancer were all able to drink the 600–800 ml water needed to obtain full gastric distension. However, two patients with cancer in the lower third of the rectum were unable to retain the water enema.

Discussion

Double-contrast barium studies and fiberoptic endoscopy are routinely used in the diagnosis of gastric and colorectal neoplasms. However, these modalities do not permit a precise preoperative prediction of whether a tumor is limited to the wall or has spread into surrounding tissue. In contrast, CT can not only be used to demonstrate the gastric and large bowel wall but can also demonstrate directly extension of a tumor into contiguous organs and the presence of distant metastases.

Reported results comparing preoperative CT with surgical findings are variable. Some investigators claim that CT can provide accurate preoperative staging information [4, 6, 12, 15], while others are less enthusiastic about the role of CT [5, 7, 10, 14, 16]. Although not specific, wall thickening is the only constant sign in patients with gastric and colorectal tumors. Therefore, successful interpretation of gastrointestinal tract pathology from CT scans requires meticulous care to ensure reliable distension and opacification of the stomach and large bowel. Traditional techniques are based on the oral and rectal administration of dilute barium or water-soluble contrast solutions [1]. The high densities of these positive contrast agents, however, restrict accurate evaluation of localized gastric and large bowel processes. Thus, the sensitivity of CT in detecting gastric and colorectal neoplasms varied between 61% and 97%. Negative contrast materials (e.g., air, oil emulsions) have proved superior not only in tumor detection, but also in providing a simple method for accurately assessing the thickness of the gastric and large bowel wall [11, 13]. However, air techniques require wide window settings and frequently cause partial volume and beam hardening artifacts (Fig. 3). Caution should be exercised in the use of fat-density oral contrast agents in patients with severe, symptomatic gallbladder disease or acute pancreatitis, because fat absorption may exacerbate symptoms [13].

Compared with these solutions, water is a much more physiologic and better accepted medium for opacifying and distending the stomach and large bowel wall. In conjunction with the high spatial resolution of the Somatom Plus, water provides a good depiction of the gastric and large bowel wall, and, above all, improves the depiction of the internal wall. It is therefore possible to recognize even a small degree of pathologic wall thickening (Fig. 4). Furthermore, the multiscan technique of the Somatom Plus makes it possible to obtain motion-free images of the gastrointestinal

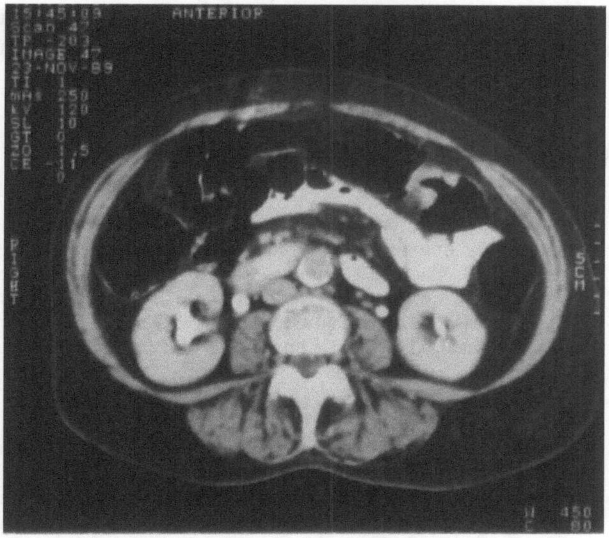

Fig. 3. Carcinoma of transverse colon (T3). CT examination was performed after oral administration of a dilute barium suspension and rectal air insufflation. The gut is well distended. However, compared with water, the large bowel wall stands out less clearly against the internal surface and pericolic fat. Note artifacts on the gas contrast image

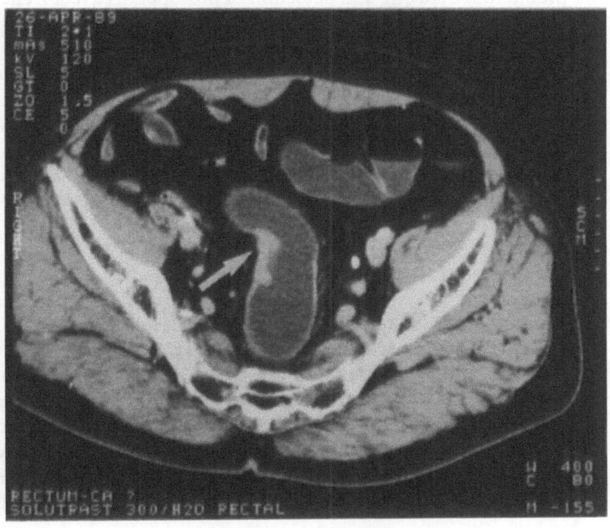

Fig. 4. Rectal carcinoma (T3N0M0). CT scan after rectal administration of water shows localized wall thickening with ulceration of the internal surface. The tumor extends into perirectal fat *(arrow)*

tract. Thus, using water as contrast agent, all 38 tumors could be detected without difficulties.

Despite its limitation in differentiating T1 from T2 tumors (which is important, because high-risk patients with intramucosal and intrasubmucosal colorectal tumors and no evidence of metastases can be treated with laser photocoagulation therapy) and the inability to detect metastases in normal-sized lymph nodes, CT is presently the only imaging technique for complete staging of gastrointestinal tract tumors according to the TNM classification. Using state-of-the-art equipment (like the Somatom Plus), the primary tumor's local expansion and the whole liver can be evaluated in the same investigation within a few minutes. On the basis of the simplicity of the method and the results obtained, water should be given routinely as a contrast agent for CT study of the stomach and large bowel wall if this method is used as a preoperative staging procedure in patients with known gastric and colorectal neoplasms.

References

1. Anderson DJ, Berland L (1989) CT techniques. In: Lee JKT, Sagel SS, Stanley RJ (eds) Computed body tomography, 2nd edn. Raven, New York, pp31–60
2. Angelelli G, Macarini L, Lupo L, Caputi-Jambrenghi O, Pannarale O, Memeo V (1990) Rectal carcinoma: CT staging with water as contrast medium. Radiology 177: 511–514
3. Baert AL, Roex L, Marchal G, Hermans P, Dewilde D, Wilms G (1989) Computed tomography of the stomach with water as an oral contrast agent: technique and preliminary results. J Comput Assist Tomogr 13: 633–636
4. Balthazar EJ, Megibow AJ, Hulnick DH, Naidich DP (1988) Carcinomas of the colon: detection and preoperative staging by CT. AJR 150: 301–306
5. Cook AO, Levine BA, Sirinek KR, Gaskill HV (1986) Evaluation of gastric adenocarcinoma: abdominal computed tomography does not replace celiotomy. Arch Surg 121: 603–606
6. Dehn TCB, Reznek RH, Nockler IB, White FE (1984) The preoperative assessment of advanced gastric cancer by computed tomography and surgery. Br J Surg 71: 413–417
7. Freeny PC, Marks WM, Ryan JA, Bolen JW (1986) Colorectal carcinoma evaluation with CT: preoperative staging and detection of postoperative recurrence. Radiology 158: 347–353
8. Gaa J, Deininger HK (1990) Methodische Optimierung der computertomographischen Dickdarmdiagnostik. Röntgenblätter 43: 80–82
9. Hermanek P, Sobin LH (1987) TNM classification of malignant tumours. Springer, Berlin Heidelberg New York
10. Komaki S, Toyoshima S (1983) CT's capibility in detecting advanced gastric cancer. Gastrointest Radiol 8: 307–308
11. Megibow AJ, Zerhouni EA, Hulnick DH, Beranbaum ER, Balthazar EJ (1984) Air insufflation of the colon as an adjunct to computed tomography of the pelvis. J Comput Assist Tomogr 8: 797–800
12. Moss AA, Schnyder P, Marks W, Margulis AR (1981) Gastric adenocarcinoma: a comparison of the accuracy and economics of staging by computed tomography and surgery. Gastroenterology 80: 45–50
13. Raptopoulos V, Davis MA, Davidoff A, Kazellas A, Hays D, D'Orsi CJ, Smith EH (1987) Fat density oral contrast agent for abdominal CT. Radiology 164: 653–656
14. Sussmann KS, Halvorsen RA, Illescas FF, Cohan RH, Saeed M, Silverman PM, Thompson WM, Meyers WC (1988) Gastric adenocarcinoma: CT versus surgical staging. Radiology 167: 335–340
15. Thoeni RF, Moss AA, Schnyder P, Margulis AR (1981) Detection and staging of primary rectal and rectosigmoid cancer by computed tomography. Radiology 141: 135–138
16. Thompson WM, Halvorsen RA, Foster WL, Roberts L, Gibbons R (1986) Preoperative and postoperative CT staging of rectosigmoid carcinoma. AJR 146: 703–710

Spiral CT – A Valuable Tool for Orthopedic Examinations?

H. Hirschfelder and P. Weber

Introduction

Classical computed tomography (CT) examinations are responsible for the clarification of such orthopedic problems as lumbar ischialgias and occupy as much as 40% of the scanner time. The position and arthrosis of the vertebral joints, osseous constrictions of the spinal column, as well as inflammatory or tumorous alterations can be differentiated without problems. Injuries of the myelon, on the other hand, are only possible with limitations using CT, being evaluated better with magnetic resonance imaging (MRI).

A display of peripheral joints is often required in the course of clinical orthopedic objectives. Here, the orthopedist is interested in structural disturbances in the joint and bone anatomy as well as in form and positional variations. Arthrotic changes with degenerative transformations (cysts, osteophytes, diminished joint space) are easily differentiated from arthritic destruction. Information concerning the quality of the affected joint partner with comparative thickness and density are available for deciding on therapeutic measures. Principally, this is also possible with conventional radiological methods, although a superimposition-free display of the anatomy, especially in combination with reformatted views, is an assistance provided by CT in the evaluation of joints. Instead of conventional tomography, we therefore make use of CT examinations in our clinic. The same information is available together with the advantages of soft tissue evaluation.

Finally, CT examinations of pure soft tissue alterations in the extremities are also required. Whereas bony structures can be evaluated without problems using CT, the differentiation of structural changes in muscle tissue is highly limited even with an optimization of the examination parameters. The application of MRI has today become an important possibility for the question of degenerative alterations, inflammatory disturbances, and tumorous infiltration of the soft tissues, so that the use of CT here has a greater role as a secondary, rather than as a primary, diagnostic method.

The CT diagnosis of orthopedic objectives on the extremities has today been reduced to the differentiation of bony structures. An optimal image can be provided with a minimum dose. This minimal dose for reduced patient exposure, in combination with the advantage of a more rapid examination, is possible with the spiral CT technique (Figs. 1, 2). The advantages of the spiral CT technique for orthopedic examinations are demonstrated herein based on 1 year's experience with 78 such examinations.

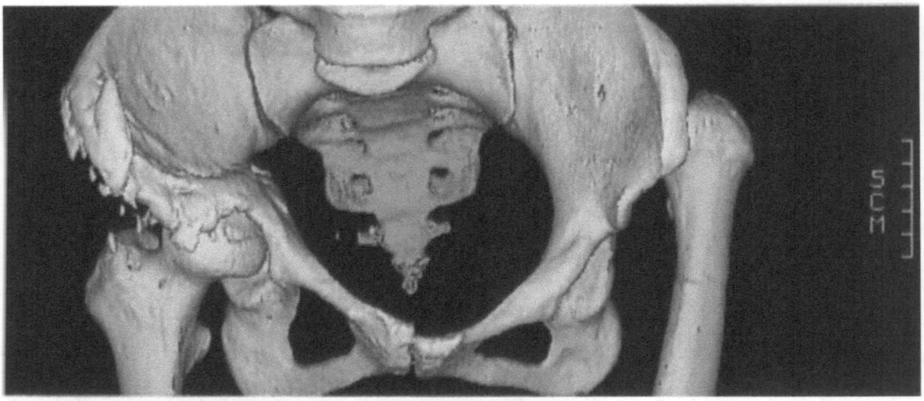

a

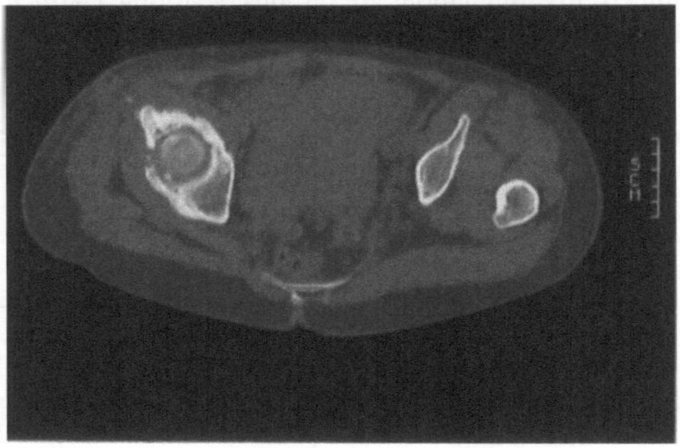

b

Fig. 1 a, b. 35-year-old woman. **a** Hip dysplasia *right* after Chiari osteotomy and hip dislocation *left:* three series of spiral CT, 2 mm slice thickness, 2 mm table feed. **b** Despite low dose, image quality allows good clinical interpretation (atrophy of muscles, asymmetry of joint space, osteochondrosis dissecans)

First Advantage: Large Examination Volumes

It is possible to evaluate large examination volumes with the spiral CT technique using freely selectable slice thicknesses. Aside from the short examination time for the patient, information of the region examined can be attained rapidly through a quick reconstruction of representative slices. Slice reconstructions can be performed not only contiguously but also additionally with overlapping slices for an evaluation of the entire examination region. An ideal data pool can thus be obtained for further processing of the data or three-dimensional surface reconstruction of joint structures in orthopedics, for example. This technique not only provides primary slices for the evaluation of structures, but at the same time makes possible the three-dimensional display of the anatomy for form and structural evaluation. These images can then be combined with the reformatting technique or multiplanar reformations as desired.

In the course of the intensive use of this method, a specific selection of examination parameters came to be developed for each important joint (Table 1). Today, nearly every examination of joints is done with the spiral technique and also with three-dimensional surface reconstruction.

The reconstruction of images was performed using a high-contrast resolution

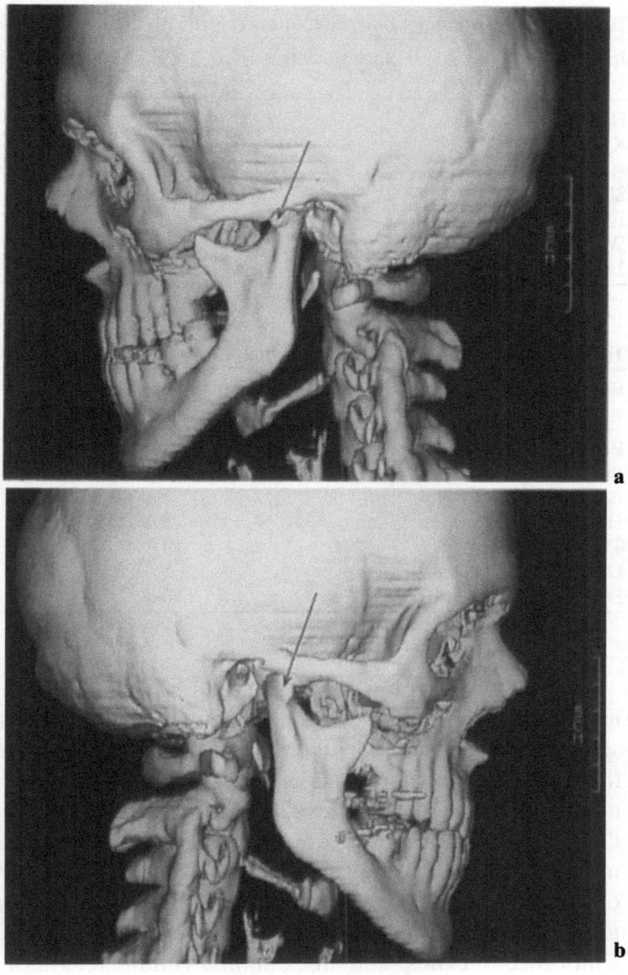

Fig. 2 a, b. A 26-year-old man with asymmetry of the facial skull caused by a different processus articularis of the temporal mandibular joint *(arrows)*: spiral technique with double table feed, 3 mm slice thickness, 6 mm table feed

algorithm if an evaluation of the bone structure was to be emphasized. The standard resolution algorithm was selected if the form and structure of the joint partners was important, since this permits three-dimensional surface reconstruction with a more harmonic image quality. A display of the soft tissue in the vicinity of the joint for differentiation of the capsule or of an effusion is possible even with a dose of 125 mA. Especially in the region of the shoulder, however, due to the low dose setting more artifacts may be expected, which nevertheless do not affect the clinical evaluation.

Should an evaluation of malpositioning and anatomical changes in form be more important than the detail-true evaluation of joint structures, the examination parameters will be selected in favor of a larger examination volume (Table 2).

It can also be seen here that the primary evaluation of the anatomical structures is sufficient so that no danger of a faulty interpretation of the images attained is present with these examination parameters.

Table 1. Typical examination parameters (each with the lowest possible milliamperes)

Joint	Slice thickness (mm)	Examination time (s)	Examination volume (mm)
Hip	2	32	60
Knee	1	32	30
Ankle	1	32	30
Shoulder	2	32	60
Elbow	2	32	60
Wrist	1	32	30
Jaw	1	22	40

Table 2. Examination parameters for malpositioning and anatomical changes

Region	Slice thickness (mm)	Examination volume (mm)
Pelvis	3	90 (possibly twice)
Patella	2	60
Foot	4	120
Hand	3	90
Thoracic deformities	10	300
Deformities adjacent to joint	5	150
Deformities distant from joint	10	300

The first impression was that the spiral technique could not be applied for examination of the vertebral column. Today, the indication for CT examination using the spiral technique is seen in over half of the cases. It does not appear to be suitable for the diagnosis of dislocations of a disk in the lumbar or cervical vertebrae, since the minute differentiation in the soft tissue structures also requires an evaluation of less densitometric differences, which causes problems due to increased artifacts from the minimal dose. If the clinical objective is the differentiation of an osseous constriction of the spinal column with a concomitant radicular syndrome and only one vertebra must be acquired, for instance, in degenerative spondylolithesis (with parameters of 2 mm slice thickness and an examined volume length of 60 mm), this technique can be applied without any problems. Should numerous vertebrae be examined, care must be taken that the morphometric measurements are made absolutely perpendicular to the spinal column. For the most part, this requirement is applicable for segments of the upper lumbar or middle and upper cervical spine (examination parameters: 3 mm slice thickness, examined volume length of 90 mm). On the other hand, should merely a positional control of the spinal column be necessary, the orthograde adjustment to the spine may be neglected. For atlantodental dislocations in rheumatic patients, spondylolisthesis, deformity following fracture, and scoliosis/kyphosis of the spinal column, for instance, one may again profit from the advantages of the spiral CT technique. The examination parameters are altered appropriately from 2 to 10 mm slice thickness, corresponding with an increase in the examined volume length of the vertebral deformity from 60 to 300 mm.

Numerous spiral examinations must occasionally be performed in order to evaluate structural disturbance and more extensive malpositioning concomitantly. The technique with double table feed which has only been performed on 11 patients so far promises to be more interesting here. With this technique, one sequence of examinations can be performed with constant slice thickness and the examined volume can be doubled. The calculation time required with the experimental version of this system is disproportionately long considering the time required for reconstruction of maximally 10 min in a simple examination using the spiral technique.

Second Advantage: Reduced Radiation Exposure

A minimal radiation dose can usually be taken advantage of for orthopedic examinations because of the reduced tube output required for the spiral CT technique. This is not only important for the examination of children, but also for examinations in the region of the lumbar spine and pelvis. Principally, this reduction in radiation exposure is also made possible by selecting the proper dose in "conventional" CT examinations, although experience has shown that a higher tube output is more likely to be required for examinations with single-slice scanning. Even overlapping slices – helpful for image reformatting – can be calculated from a spiral CT data set without the need of additional scans. With this in mind, the double table feed technique is especially interesting since it actually permits the scanning of twice the volume without increasing the dose (i.e., effectively reducing the radiation exposure by half). Because of this reduction in radiation exposure, the double spiral technique is appropriate for examinations of the acetabular, lumbar, or pelvic regions.

Third Advantage: Short Examination Times

The possibility of large-volume examinations with a reduced radiation exposure is principally possible even without using the spiral CT technique. The decisive advantage, however, is the extremely shortened examination time required for the patient: The total time necessary, including entering and leaving the examination room, need not exceed 5 min. This is important for infants and school children as we can now generally perform the CT examination without sedation. Even patients with claustrophobic problems (a disturbance seen less frequently with the larger gantry opening now possible) can benefit from the minimal examination time.

The short examination time, however, is more important for examinations in painful or unusual positions. Operative planning for hip-joint transposition is also supported by functional, three-dimensional CT examinations where the simulated, corrected position is occasionally only reached with difficulty. Every possibility of shortening the examination time is worthwhile, even for the examination of deliberately dislocated joints in the shoulder or patella. The multiscan method which, in principle, is technically similar can even be used to display the process of dislocation directly with temporal sequencing. Atlantoaxial dislocations in patients with rheumatism can be brought into neutral position, inclination, or reclination positions for quantifying the instability without any danger of myelogenic irritation, since the risk is reduced by the short examination times.

Artifacts which occur due to motion during the examination (swallowing, breathing) can also be avoided thanks to the short examination times. These artifact-free slices are especially suitable for the further processing of multiplanar or three-dimensional surface reconstructions.

The extremely short examination times must be emphasized for orthopedic examinations on traumatized patients. Medical treatment can even be continued without interruption during image documentation.

Conclusions

Interest in the spiral CT technique was initially limited. However, the advantages of this method have become so clear during the last year that we now use spiral CT in 90% of all joint examinations and 50% of all examinations on the spinal column with Somatom Plus-S. Other examinations of the spinal column will continue to be performed with different techniques, since contrast is low in examinations of the disks and because of the constant changes in gantry tilt required. A thin-slice spiral technique with an even larger examination volume would be desirable for the evaluation of structural disturbances as well as alterations in the form of entire anatomic regions, e.g., examinations of the facial skull or the entire pelvis. The spiral technique with a table feed of twice the slice thickness appears to offer a useful solution, although further developments are required to provide acceptable examination times.

CT Investigation of Traumatized Wrist Joints with Somatom Plus S

R. Frahm, H. Förstner, and B. Wimmer

Introduction

Despite subtle roentgen investigation combined with bone scintigraphy, conventional tomography and fluoroscopy in some patients, there are no correlative findings to clinical symptoms after trauma.

A computed tomography CT investigation of these patients started with Somatom 2 ans Somatom DRH shows the great advantage of CT. Scans with a slice thickness of 2 mm, high resolution and axial imaging without superimposition reveal more fractures and pathological changes than the roentgen-based methods mentioned above. Follow-up of this study with Somatom Plus S with its higher quality reveals improved results.

Material and Methods

CT is performed with high resolution (Somatom 2 and DRH) or ultrahigh resolution (Somatom Plus S). Slice thickness and feed are 2 mm or 1 mm with Somatom Plus S. The imaging planes were axial and longitudinal. The scaphoid was examined parallel to its length. To reveal subtle fractures or fissures, we used a "bone window" (4000/600). These images are not as "bright" as we are accustomed to seeing, but lesions in spongious and cortical bone are more clearly visible. We examined 49 patients by 51 CT investigations in two groups.

One group consisted of 19 patients, 14 of whom (11 Somatom 2 and DRH, three Somatom Plus S) had clinical symptoms of a scaphoid fracture following acute trauma while the remaining 5 (two Somatom 2 and DRH, three Somatom Plus S) had a long-standing scaphoid fracture, with persistent pain. Roentgenograms of all patients (wrist joint and carpal bones in two planes and special scaphoid projections) showed no pathology.

The second group of 30 patients with 32 CT investigations (17 with Somatom 2 or DRH, 15 with Somatom Plus S) had either clinical symptoms in the wrist joint or in the carpal region following acute trauma or symptoms remaining for a longer period (from 2 months up to 2 years), even after plaster immobilisation. Three patients had an existing trauma of the wrist joint or carpal bones with defined lesions and an acute trauma with sprain. Roentgenograms in projections relating to the symptoms showed no indication of acute bony lesions, nor did they reveal the fractures seen with CT. Sometimes scintigraphy showed a hot spot.

Two patients had an intraosseous ganglion of the scaphoid and the lunate with activity on bone scintigraphy study. Both patients underwent postoperative CT control scans.

Results

In the group with clinically suspected scaphoid fractures, CT revealed an acute lesion in 13 of 14 patients. Nine of these unexpectedly had additional fractures of the carpal bones. One patient was without any lesion. Four of five patients had a healed scaphoid fracture, three of them with badly dislocated fragments. One had a scaphoid pseudoarthrosis which was not delineated on roentgenograms.

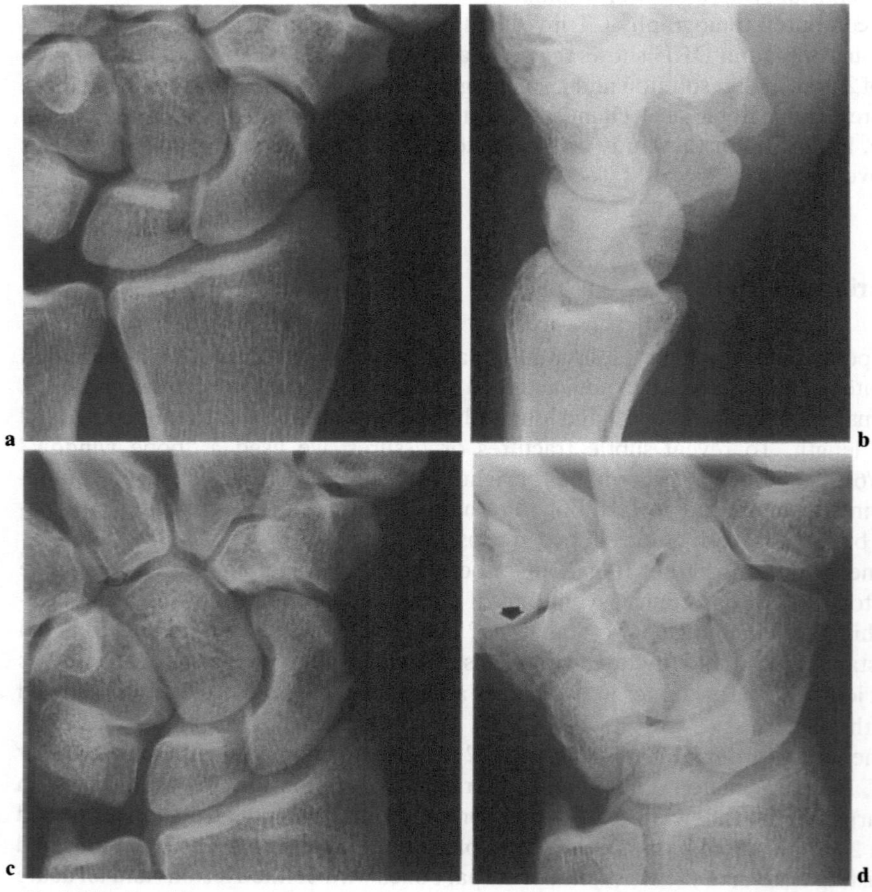

Fig. 1 a–d. Special roentgenogram projections of carpal bones (left hand) 2 weeks after trauma. **a, b** No fracture shown; **c** suspected cortical step of the capitate (correlation to clinical symptoms); **d** dorsal hamate fracture *(arrow)*

In the second group 23 patients had pathological findings on CT, including acute fractures of the carpal bones, ligament lesions or damaged ligament insertions, spurs or cortical steps after old, previously unrecognised fractures and degenerative arthrosis of carpal joint facets. CT in patients with intraosseous ganglions delineated the exact location for preoperative planning (dorsal or palmar approach). The widening of the ganglion connection to the synovial space can be evaluated exactly. Three dimensional reconstruction clarified the findings for operative intervention, and control scans documented the result after operation. Five patients with diffuse pain but normal roentgenography and scintigraphy results evidenced no CT pathological findings.

Discussion

Soon after beginning this investigation, we were surprised how many fractures of the wrist joint and carpal bones were not detected by current roentgenography methods including conventional tomography. CT with its excellent resolution and nonsuper-

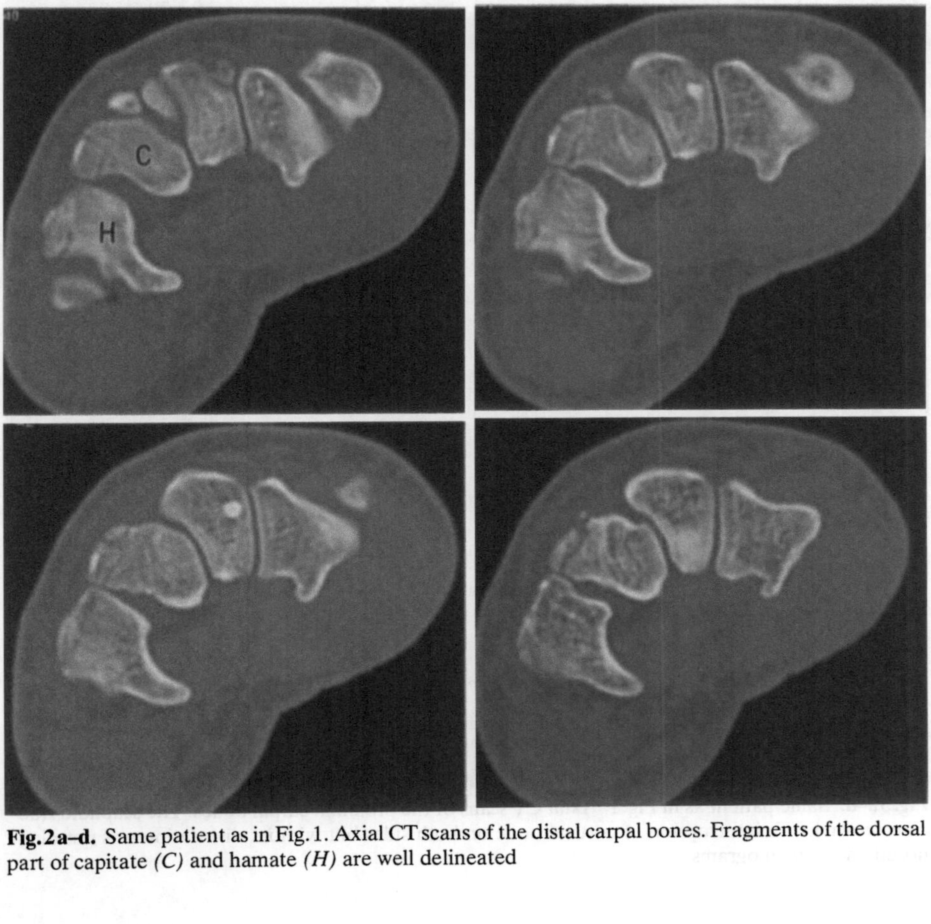

a b c d

Fig. 2 a–d. Same patient as in Fig. 1. Axial CT scans of the distal carpal bones. Fragments of the dorsal part of capitate *(C)* and hamate *(H)* are well delineated imposed images offers in these selected cases the chance to reveal fissures, fractures, bony fragments or ligament lesions. Upon knowing that there is not only "sprain" but actual damage of the wrist joint or carpal region, treatment can be modified to avoid further disability or degenerative arthrosis.

For example, a 35-year-old patient presented with a history of wrist and hand trauma, due to a heavy iron plate which had fallen on his flexed hand. There was swelling of the dorsal wrist and midcarpal region accompanied by pain. Immediate roentgenograms including scaphoid projections were without pathological findings. After 14 days of plaster immobilisation, the swelling was reduced, but pain over the whole dorsal wrist persisted. At that time, roentgenograms of the carpal bones (Fig. 1) suggested a dorsal hamate fracture (Fig. 1 d). There was a hint of a slight step in the distal capitate joint facet (Fig. 1 c).

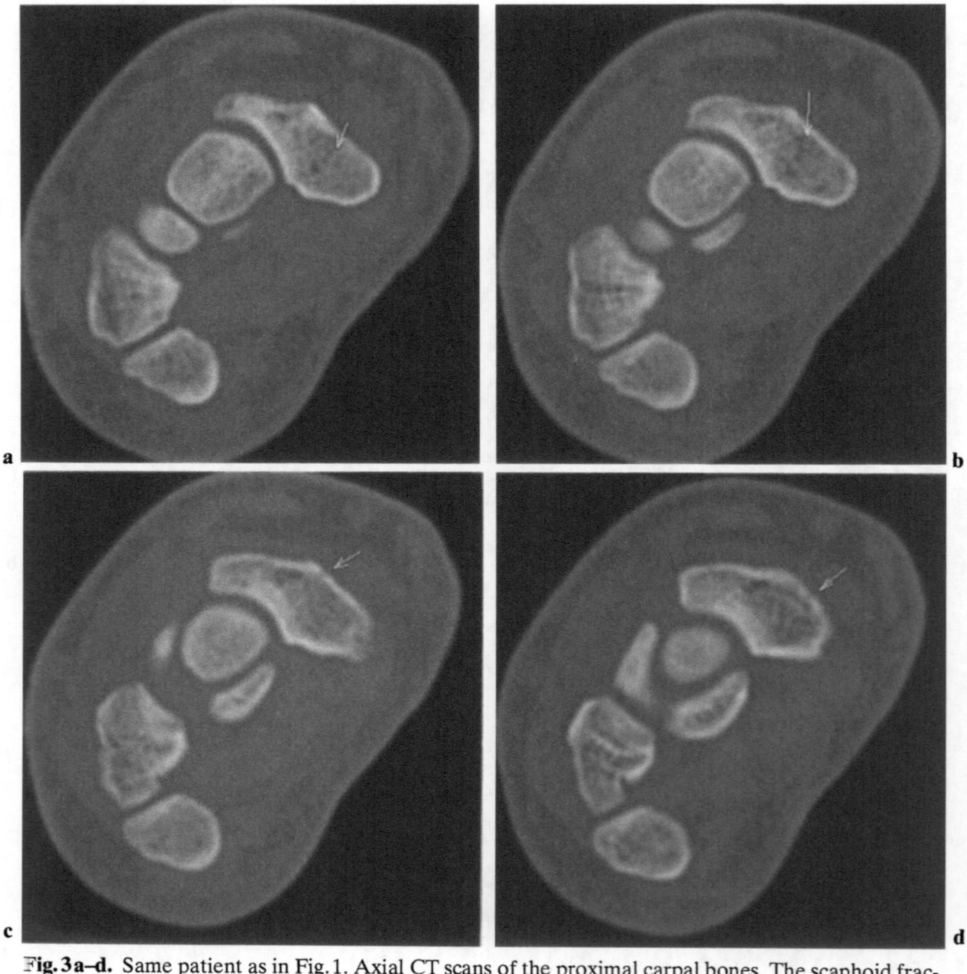

Fig. 3a–d. Same patient as in Fig. 1. Axial CT scans of the proximal carpal bones. The scaphoid fracture *(arrow)* with interruption of cortical bone on both sides but without dislocation was not diagnosed on roentgenograms

Axial CT images of the carpal bones revealed a dorsal hamate fracture with a slight fragment dislocation and a dorsal capitate fracture (Fig. 2). Surprisingly, scans of the proximal carpal bones showed a scaphoid fracture without dislocation in the palmar, distal part (Fig. 3).

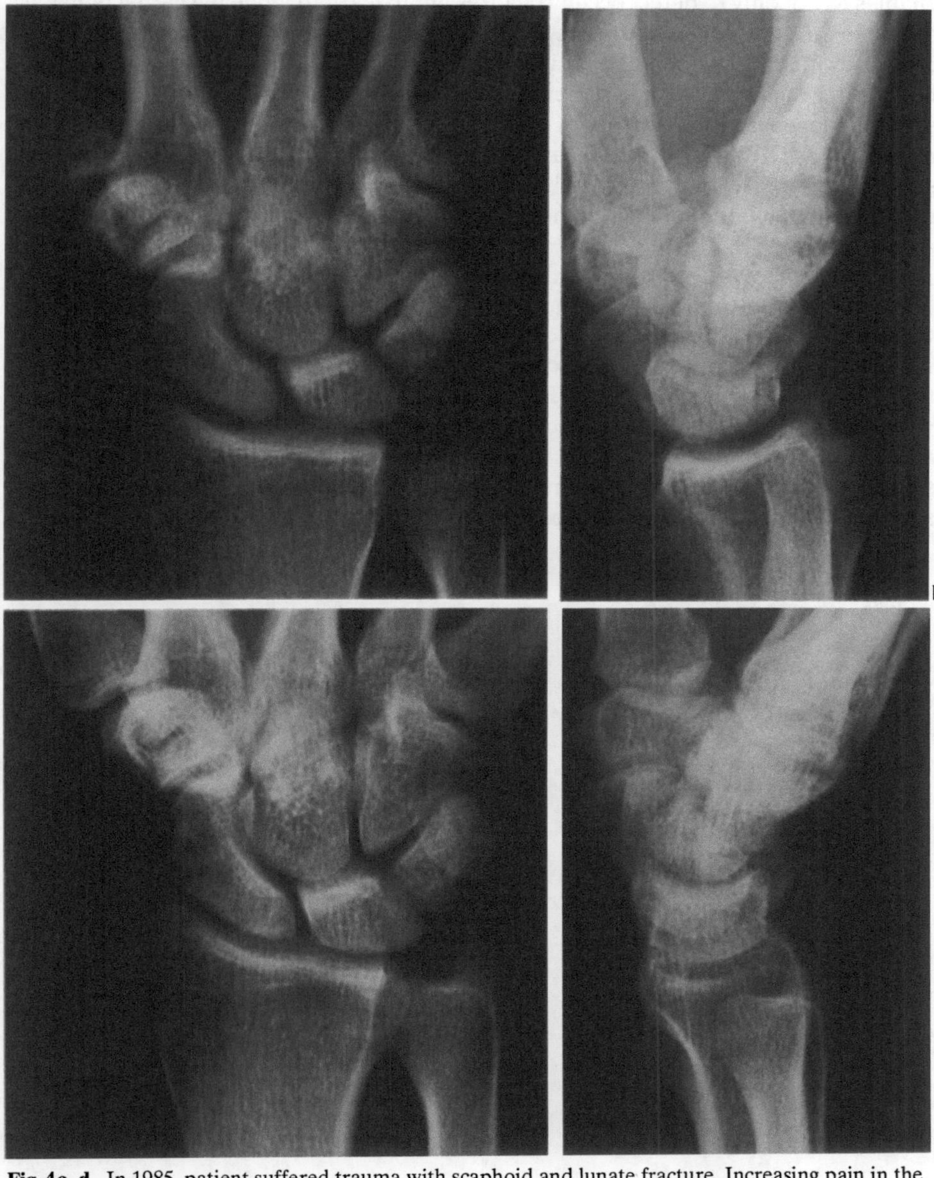

a b c d

Fig. 4a–d. In 1985, patient suffered trauma with scaphoid and lunate fracture. Increasing pain in the carpal region. **a, b** Carpal bones in two planes with almost healed fractures. Decreased bone mineral density after immobilization. A capitate fracture is not delineated. **c, d** Roentgenograms 6 years later. Increased subchondral mineralization of the lunate joint facet

This case demonstrates the importance of further investigation with CT when there is a difference between the clinical symptoms and roentgenography findings. Consequently, this patient requires a full-arm plaster cast including the thumb to prevent scaphoid pseudoarthrosis.

Images of high resolution and without superimposition, possible in three planes, enables us not only to detect occult fractures but to learn to judge the carpal bones as a functional unit. Any disturbance, e.g. lesions of ligaments or ligament insertions caused by trauma, is followed by incongruity of the joint facets among the carpal bones. More information and better and earlier delineation of resulting changes, for example degenerative arthrosis, is provided by CT. The primary diagnosis of such conditions as DISI (dorsal intercalated segment instability, PISI (palmar intercalated segment instability) or carpal instabilities relies on absolutely correct positioning for roentgenography. Video images under stress help to reveal instabilities not hitherto manifest.

As noted above, occult scaphoid fractures can clearly be detected by high resolution CT. Nine patients of 13 had unexpected additional fractures of the carpal bones. CT examination of the fractured scaphoid with persistent pain and with or without suggested pseudoarthrosis gives excellent information about the fragments, posttraumatic cysts and their dislocation. Partial healing can be demonstrated better than with roentgen-based techniques including tomography. Degenerative arthrosis after a healed dislocation is seen earlier than with roentgenograms. Residuals of bony lesions such as cortical steps or spurs not previously recognised can be seen without superimposition. Often, they can explain the patient's clinical symptoms.

a b c d

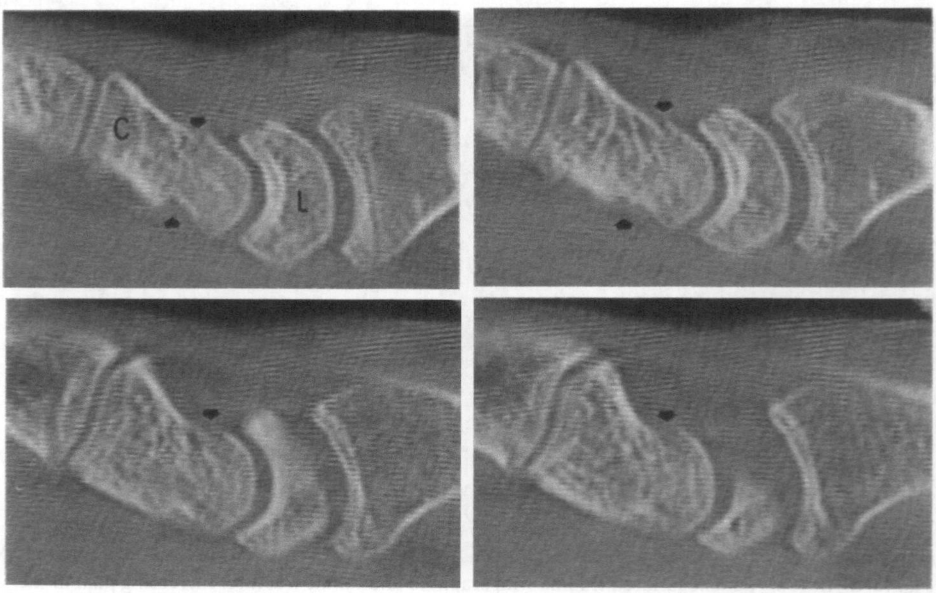

Fig. 5a–d. CT images of the same patient as in Fig. 4, plane parallel to hand/forearm axis. The lunate *(L)* shows a high density of the joint facet due to degenerative arthrosis. The capitate *(C)* has dorsal and palmar steps *(arrow)* after the healed fracture, which was not diagnosed by roentgenograms

The 35-year-old patient had suffered a proximal scaphoid and a lunate fracture in 1985, which had healed without complications (Fig. 4a, b). He had decreased pain in the carpal region for at least a further 6 months. After pain relief, the symptoms recurred 2 years ago, especially during heavy manual work. In 1991, roentgenograms showed an increased sclerosis of the lunate-capitate joint facet compared with 1985 (Fig. 4c, d). CT with Somatom Plus S revealed that the scaphoid and lunate fracture had healed in the correct position without pseudoarthrosis. However, a cortical step at the dorsal and palmar part of the capitate was obvious. There was a sclerotic change of the corresponding lunate joint facet (Fig. 5).

We must assume that there was an additional horizontal capitate fracture in 1985 which was not identified on roentgenograms. Now, visible degenerative arthrosis in the capitate-lunate joint facet and resultant disability were most probably caused by healing with a slight dislocation. Such findings are important for the patient's therapy, long-term damage assessment and insurance status.

A further indication for CT is the differentiation of accessory bones from bony lesions. The sclerotic rim of an accessory bone is easily defined with high resolution CT. CT has the same advantage in diagnosing congenital abnormalities, for example the "carpe boussue". This is an exostotic-like spur at the proximal end of the third metacarpal bone. Thin CT images reveal the intact cortical bone and visualise exactly the contact area of this "exostosis" to the dorsal capitate. Degenerative arthrosis in this

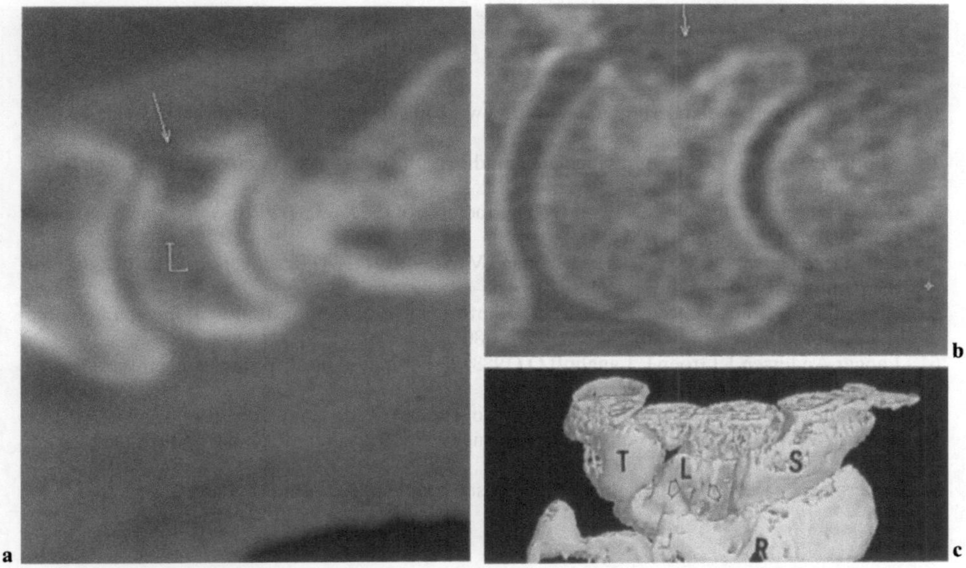

Fig. 6a–c. Patient with slight but persistent pain in the carpal region. Additional trauma with distorsion of the wrist. Clinical symptoms after trauma disappear, but preexisting pain remains. Roentgenograms show a cystic lesion of the lunate *(L)*. Scintigraphy reveals a hot spot. **a** High resolution CT with Somatom 2 parallel to hand/forearm axis. An intraosseous lunate ganglion is proven by dorsal connection to intraarticular space *(arrow)*. **b** Ultrahigh resolution CT with Somatom Plus S after operation. Ganglion is filled up with spongious bone. Slight irregularity of the lunate surface *(arrow)*. **c** Anatomic view by three-dimensional reconstruction. The surface irregularities are well shown *(arrows)*. *T*, triquetrum; *S*, scaphoid; *R*, radial bone

region due to pathological contact causes pain. Differential diagnosis from an acute traumatic lesion or older changes following an accident is easily obtainable by CT.

In addition to the above-mentioned CT indications following trauma of the carpal bones or wrist joint, CT images aid in diagnosing cysts or intraosseous ganglions and operative planning. Patients with ganglions can have constant pain; in these cases, scintigraphy shows increased activity in the ganglion region. Roentgenograms and conventional tomography reveal the lesion, but sometimes it is hard to find the cortical interruption and to decide whether a palmar or dorsal operation is better. CT clearly shows all the details (Fig. 6). The ganglion (lunate) has a dorsal connection to the intraarticular region (Fig. 6a). A control scan after the dorsal operation confirms total filling of the ganglion with spongious bone (Fig. 6b). A three-dimensional reconstruction demonstrates the anatomical situation after operation with slight irregularities of the dorsal lunate (Fig. 6c). This example reveals clearly the quality difference between images of Somatom 2, high resolution (Fig. 6a) and Somatom Plus S, ultrahigh resolution (Fig. 8b). To conclude, when looking for occult fractures or hidden bony lesions ultrahigh resolution is absolutely necessary when ever possible, if we want to detect more lesions than with conventional methods. Control images can be done with high resolution scans. Three-dimensional reconstructions assist in simplifying the discussion with nonradiologic colleagues, but they do not necessarily provide new information.

References

1. Brismar J (1988) Skeletal scintigraphy of the wrist in suggested scaphoid fracture. Acta Radiol 29: 101
2. Bourjat P, Foucher G (1990) Les incidences radiographicques en chirurgie de la main. Ann Radiol 33: 134–144
3. Gillespy T, Stork JJ, Dell PC (1988) Dorsal fractures of the hamate: distinctive radiographic appearance. Am J Radiol 15: 351–353
4. Gilula LA, Destouet JM, Weeks PM, Young LV, Wray RC (1984) Roentgenographic diagnosis of the painful wrist. Clin Orthop Rel Res 187: 53–64
5. Kindynis P, Resnick D, Kang HS, Haller J, Sartoris J (1990) Demonstration of the scapholunate space with radiography. Radiology 175: 278–280
6. Langer Andersen J, Groen P, Langhoff O (1988) The scaphoid fat stripe in the diagnosis of carpal trauma. Acta Radiol 29: 97–99
7. Lindequist S, Larsen CF (1986) Radiography of the carpal scaphoid. Acta Radiol 27: 97–99
8. Murray WT, Meuller PR, Rosenthal DI, Jauernek RR (1979) Fracture of the hook of the hamate. Am J Radiol 133: 899
9. Sollerman C (1988) Carpal trauma – a diagnostic problem. Acta Radiol 29: 95

The Use of CT in Traumatology of the Extremities

E. Tipold

Daily trauma therapy encompasses a range of extreme situations. The sudden appearance of a large number of persons with minor injuries as well as one or more severe or critically injured patients strains the functional capacity of the clinic. Organizational flexibility and the specific application of all diagnostic aids must always be the primary course of trauma clinics, so that a sensible therapy is provided for all patients. The mode of diagnosis, especially in emergency surgery, should therefore offer the highest level permitted by medical research, since one can never be exact enough, all the more because the injured person often arrives as an undocumented individual. Taking a patient history is often impossible, and even the details of the accident or the question as to whether it might have been an accident at all are often unanswerable.

The production and constant development of new surgical techniques (e.g. microsurgery of the blood vessels and nerves, replantation surgery, hand surgery, new osteosynthetic techniques, etc.) make an exact preoperative diagnosis mandatory, both as quickly as possible and at any time during the day.

Here, radiology provides the most important information. Without W.C. Roentgen's discovery of X-rays, the present state of emergency surgery could not be expected.

The XIIth District Traumatological Hospital of Vienna treats about 55000 injured patients each year. The patient population demonstrates injuries to all parts of the body, both polytrauma and trivial. The range of therapy includes not only those with recent injuries but also those undergoing reconstructive interventions. The worldwide problem of geriatric surgery also plays a role in emergency surgery. Elderly patients who are ill and have suffered an accident additionally confront the emergency surgeons with similar medical problems as do social patients.

Indeed, Houndsfield's discovery must necessarily have stimulated the interest of emergency surgeons. The hospital has had its own computed tomography (CT) system since January 1985. A Siemens Somatom Plus-S was purchased in July 1991. For our hospital, its rapid and extensive clarification of polytraumatized patients and the worthwhile, supplementary examinations, where conventional radiology cannot provide sufficient information, have quickly become indispensable.

The total number of CT examinations in 1991 was less than that in the previous years because of the change in systems. From the 2271 examinations, 784 (34.5%) were examinations of the cranium, 343 (15%) were spinal CTs, 98 (4.3%) were thoracic and 96 (4.2%) were abdominal CTs. In comparison with these "traditional" regions of CT examination, 950 (41.8%) of the CT scans were performed on the extremities. The greatest proportion of these were performed on the knee joints, with

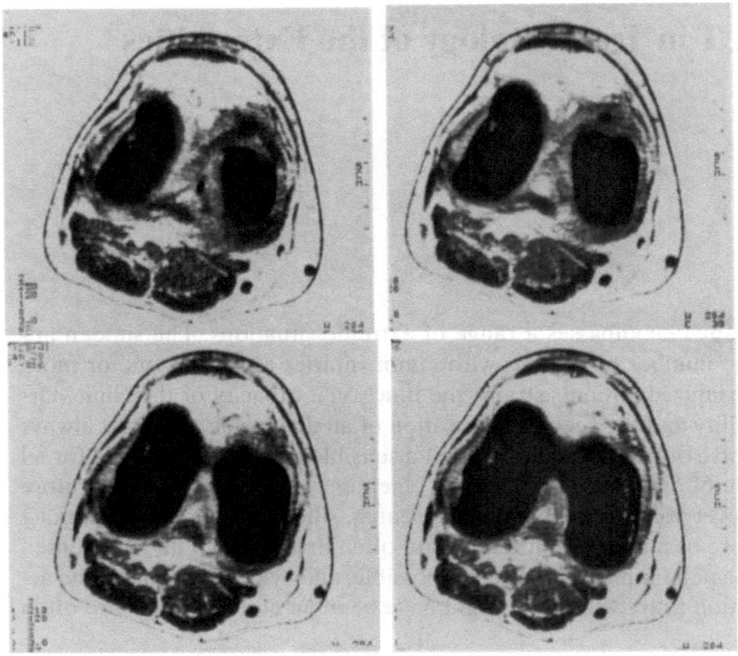

Fig. 1. A condition with an extensive longitudinal tear in the medial meniscus of the right knee. A large part of the meniscus is dislocated around an axis within the knee joint and located in the region of the anterior and posterior horns of the meniscus. It can also be seen how the dislocated meniscus within the knee joint displaces the posterior cruciate ligament

520 (22.9 %). CTs of the wrist, shoulder and other less common regions (ankle, elbow, tubular bones, etc.) account for about 5 % each (see Figs. 1–10 for four images of each of ten cases). The pelvis, with an examination rate of 3.3 %, was scanned least frequently.

A total of 17378 patients were examined from January 1985 to November 1991, whereby 2688 were of the knee joint. The majority came for a diagnosis of the extent of meniscus injury and that of the ligaments. The proportion of examinations of the extremities was only 17 % in 1989. The grounds for an increase in these examinations are numerous. Increased experience in evaluation with a concomitant elevation in diagnostic reliability and the inclusion of even marginal anatomical regions and diagnostic questions (inflammation, degenerative diseases, osteochondritis dissecans, etc.) are naturally substantial. A CT scan of the knee joint spares some of the patients an operation, although it can also be used to assist exact preoperative planning. Important for all CT examinations is the fact that a rapid feed-back is made possible concerning the site of operation and that every CT image is discussed thoroughly with the surgeon, both preoperatively and postoperatively.

CT examination of the knee joint is extremely complex since millimeter-thick slices are required in the region of the menisci. The region of the cruciate ligaments can be evaluated easily using 2- or 3-mm slices. Although the older CT units required a great deal of time for an examination of the knee joint, this examination can be

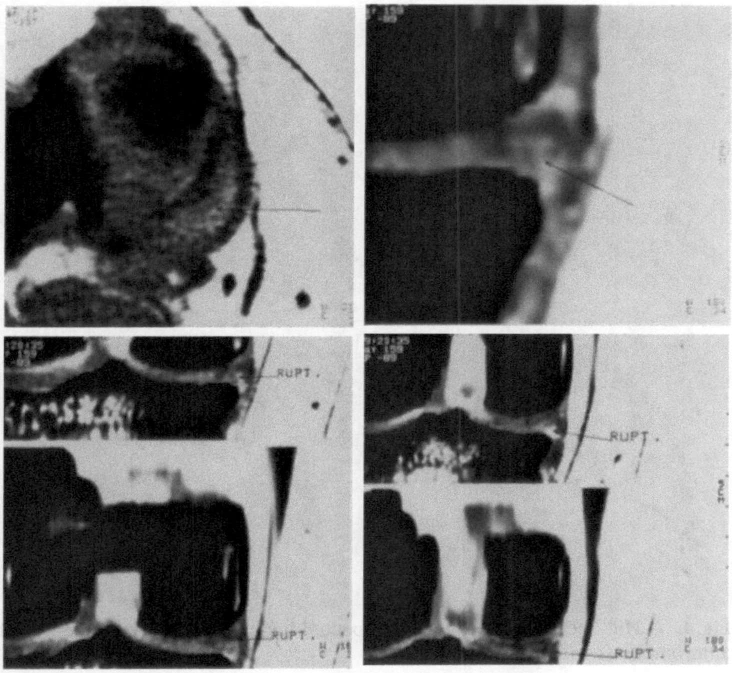

Fig. 2. An older rupture of the medial meniscus with secondary sequelae (pseudocysts, indentations)

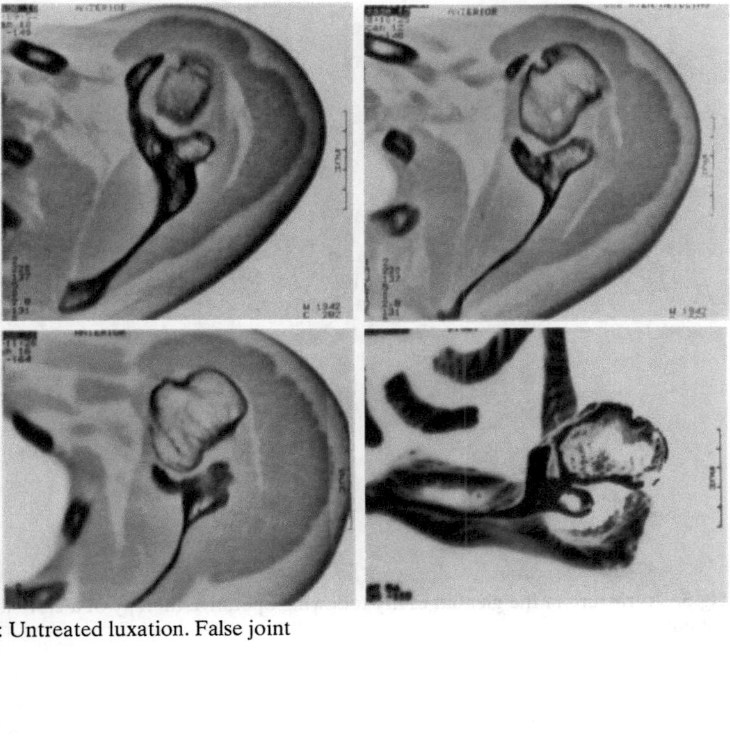

Fig. 3. Left shoulder: Untreated luxation. False joint

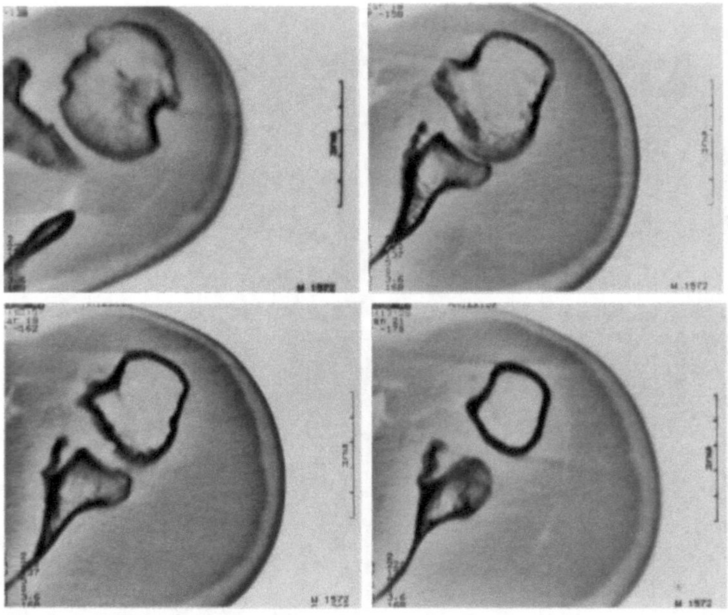

Fig. 4. A Hill-Sach's lesion following repeated luxations with involvement of the socket joint from anteromedial to anterocaudal

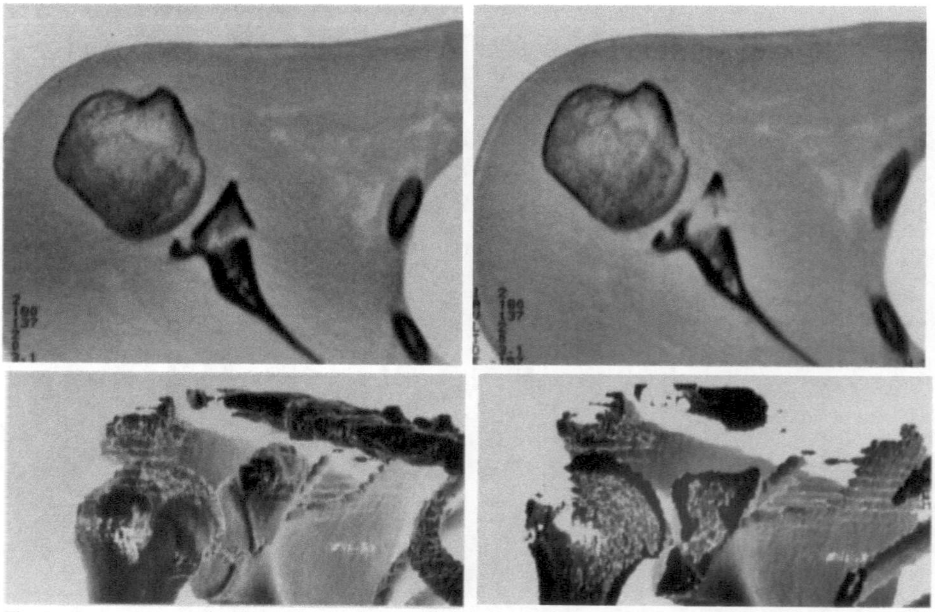

Fig. 5. A fracture in the glenoid cavity following operative therapy of a clavicle fracture in a young patient

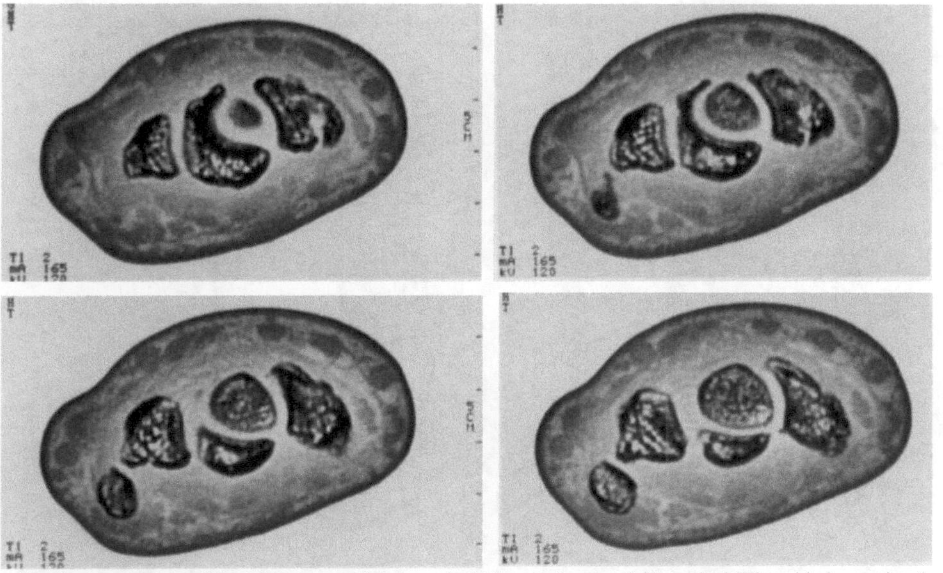

Fig. 6. A non-consolidated fracture of the scaphoid bone; the possibility of additional information is offered here when the conventional series cannot provide an adequate answer

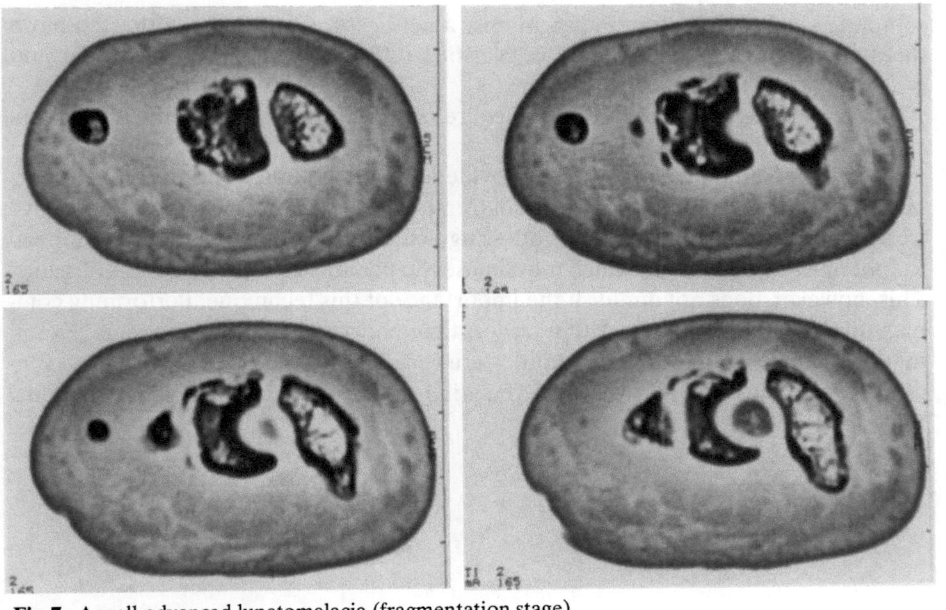

Fig. 7. A well-advanced lunatomalacia (fragmentation stage)

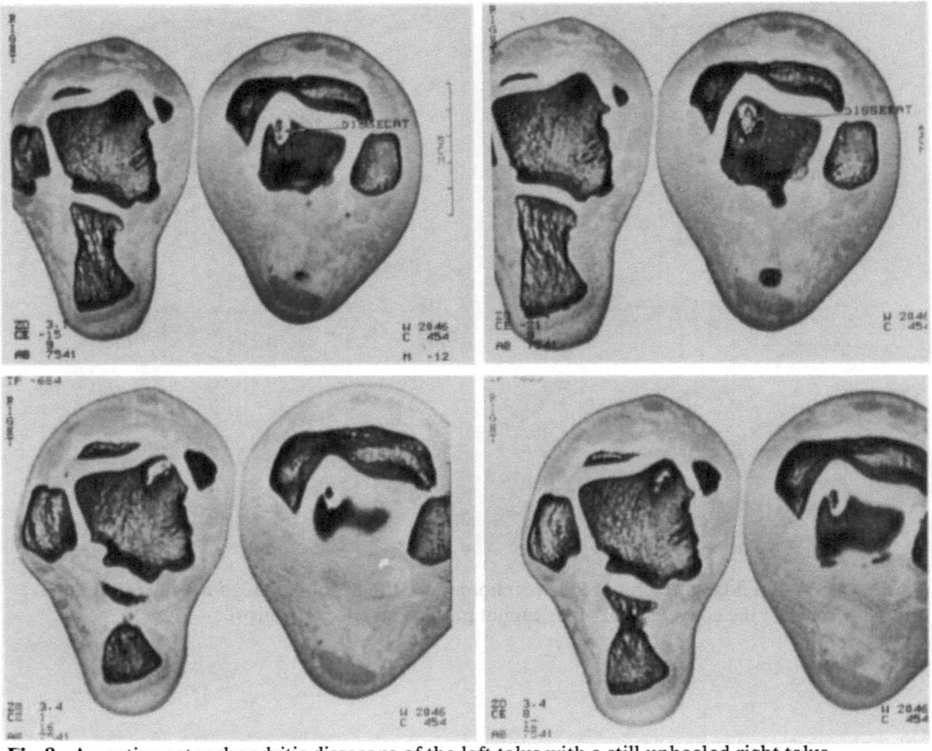

Fig. 8. An active osteochondritis dissecans of the left talus with a still unhealed right talus

completed with a Somatom Plus-S in only a matter of minutes and with even more slices than previously. Furthermore, various reformating provide additional and often important information.

Examinations of the sacroiliac joints are of special interest since they permit an exact differentiation of lesions.

I have only made an attempt to provide a highlighted description of the importance of CT in traumatology of the extremities. In patients undergoing intensive treatment as well as immediately following acute injuries, examinations from head to foot must be performed which must cause the patients as little distress as possible. This, however, does not diminish the importance of this technique. Performing complex thin-slice examinations within a short time period must also be possible. Examinations in the region of the extremities are certainly special cases in such emergencies. Nevertheless, they reveal the versatility of CT, especially in these marginal regions.

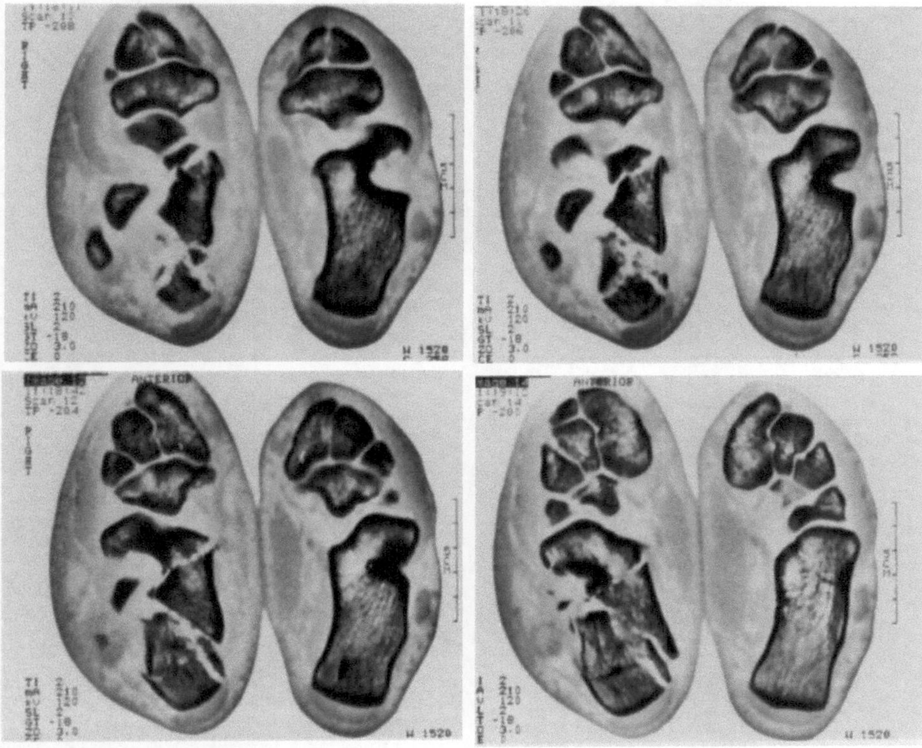

Fig. 9. A drastic comminuted fracture of the calcaneum which cannot be classified

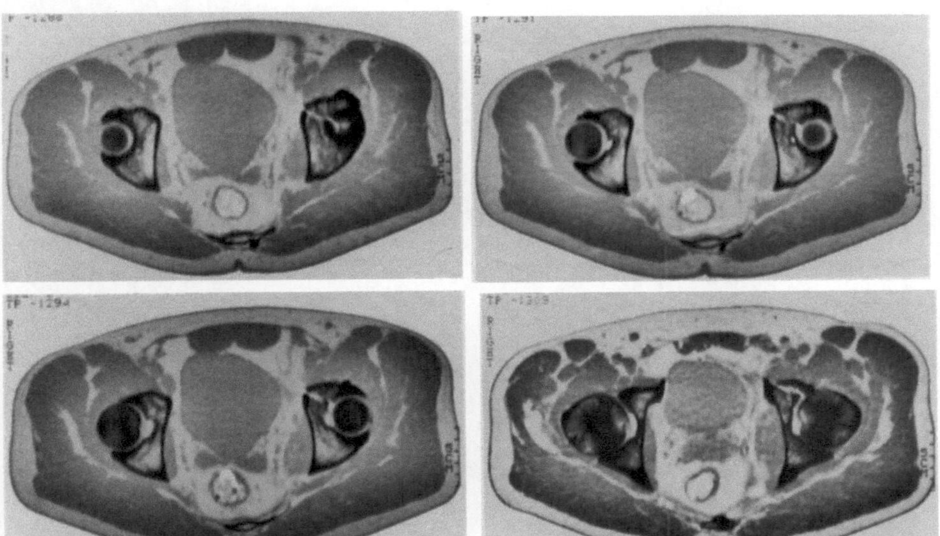

Fig. 10. A fracture of the acetabulum and of the anterior column. A hematoma of the internal obturator muscle is indicated on the margin

Spiral CT

Chairmen: E. Zeitler and M. Galanski

Current Status and New Perspectives in Spiral CT

W. Kalender, A. Polacin, G. Marchal, and A. L. Baert

Introduction

Spiral or continuous volume scanning is achieved when the patient is transported through the gantry while computed tomography (CT) data are being acquired simultaneously over a multitude of 360° rotations (Fig. 1). It was introduced into clinical practice in 1989 on Somatom Plus scanners [1–5] and gained acceptance immediately. Spiral CT has meanwhile been successfully applied and validated in a large number of clinical studies [6–19]. Such clinical applications are covered in other reports at this conference. Drawbacks were only reported with respect to X-ray power limitations and blurring of the slice sensitivity profiles [5, 20–25]. In this paper we will review the respective aspects of image quality, indicate possible improvements and discuss implications for clinical studies.

Spiral Scanning and Data Processing

All our measurements were taken on a Somatom Plus-S CT scanner (Siemens Medical Systems, Erlangen, FRG) which offers a spiral CT option with 32 s of continuous scanning. For these long exposure times, tube currents are limited. At present, a maximum of 165 mA can be selected at 120 kVp; it will be increased to 210 mA for a 32-s scan and 250 mA for up to 16 s in the near future. Slice widths can be chosen from 1 to 10 mm, and table feed values are available from 1 to 10 mm/s.

Spiral CT requires special data processing software since the direct reconstruction of images from data obtained over any 360° segment of a spiral scan would result in artefacts due to the patient transport. Data which would have been obtained in planar geometry have to be synthesized from the volume data set. This can be done in various ways. The most straightforward approach is given by linear interpolation (LI) between the two neighbouring data points obtained at the same angular position [5]. In Fig. 2 these are points z' and $z' + d$, with d denoting the table feed distance per 360° rotation. In this way, data from a range scanned during $2 \times 360°$ rotation are being used. We refer to this type of processing as 360° LI. Reduction of pixel noise and slice sensitivity profile (SSP) broadening have to be expected due to the interpolation.

By using data for interpolation from 180° opposite views the spiral scan range used for the reconstruction of one single image can be reduced significantly [22, 24, 25]. The procedure is equivalent to calculating a second spiral from the original

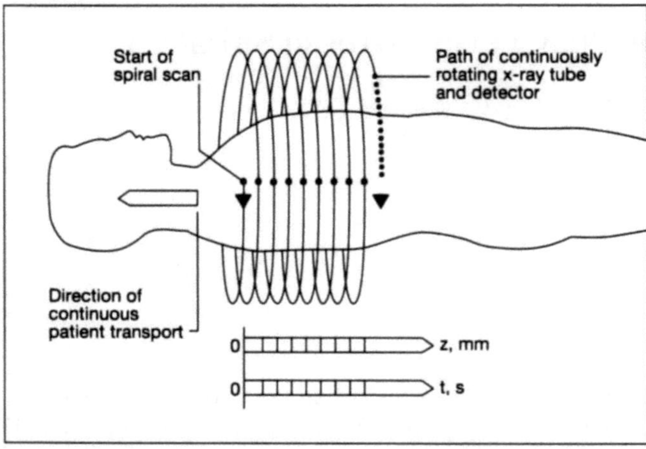

Fig. 1. Scanning geometry in spiral CT. Patient transport during continuous data acquisition results in a spiral path of the X-ray focus relative to the patient. (Figure reproduced with permission from [1, 5])

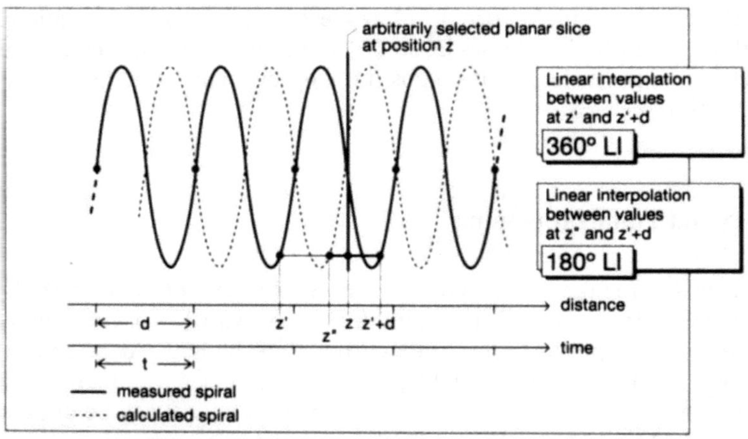

Fig. 2. Data processing algorithms in spiral CT. Linear interpolation between points z′ and z′ + *d* is most commonly used to synthesize data which would have been obtained in planar geometry; data from a range covered during two 360° scans are used (360° LI). Interpolation between data points z′ + *d* obtained at the desired angular position and data points z″ derived from 180° opposite views allows us to limit the scan range employed for image reconstruction (180° LI). The latter technique demands higher computational efforts but provides improved spiral slice profiles

which is offset by a distance *d*/2, as is depicted in Fig. 2. We use the term 180° LI when linear interpolation between points z″ and z′ + *d* is employed. The 180° algorithm was implemented as an experimental 'work-in-progress' software package which also allows selection of table feed values of up to 20 mm/s.

Image Quality with Spiral CT

The image quality with spiral CT is equivalent to that of standard CT with respect to most parameters. A primary example is spatial resolution, in which there is no difference between the two scanning modes. Differences only exist for image pixel noise and the shape of the SSP [5, 20–25].

Noise is measured as the standard deviation of pixel values in a homogeneous image. It depends on the X-ray dose, on slice collimation and on the algorithm chosen. These general considerations also apply to spiral CT without any restrictions. A relatively high noise level, which is sometimes noted, is predominantly due to the limited mA values available for long spiral scans. There is a small additional influence due to the interpolation process. In 360° LI, data from two 360° spiral segments are accessed for the interpolation procedure, which results in a reduction of

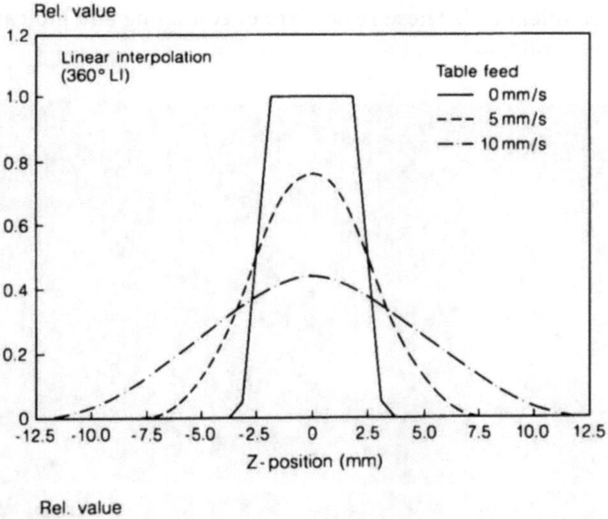

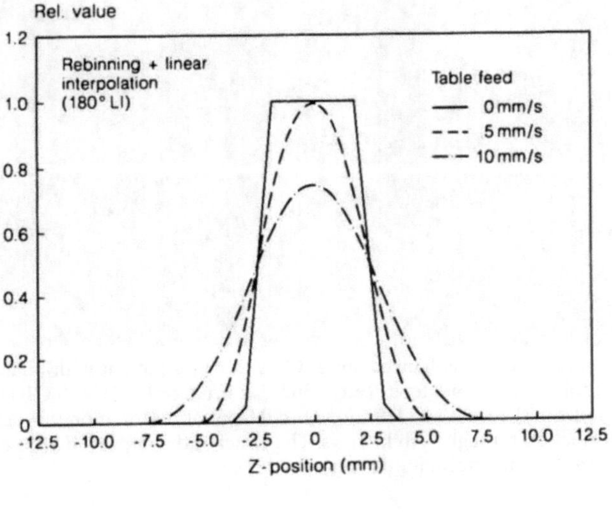

Fig. 3a, b. Slice sensitivity profiles (SSPs) in spiral CT. As compared with the original profile (table feed = 0 mm/s), spiral CT causes some SSP blurring. It becomes quite pronounced for 360° LI at higher table speeds (**a**). With 180° LI this effect is largely reduced; even table speeds greater than the nominal slice width appear practical (**b**)

noise by a factor of 0.82 when compared with a standard CT scan with otherwise identical parameter choices [5, 22, 23]. In 180° LI, which employs data from a reduced range, the noise is higher by a factor of about 1.12. Theoretical considerations are remarkably well confirmed by experimental results [23–25].

The same good agreement between predictions and results is given for the shape and width of the SSPs [23–25]. A full understanding of them is highly important in any volume scanning technique as they determine the spatial resolution in the longitudinal direction and thereby the quality of multiplanar reformations and three-dimensional displays.

Spiral CT will cause blurring of the original SSPs to a certain degree depending on the scan parameters and on the algorithm chosen. Simulation results are shown in Fig. 3 for both algorithms and for two different table feed values. SSP blurring is apparently much less severe for 180° LI than for 360° LI. It is of particular interest to note that, even at a table feed of twice the nominal slice thickness, the slice profile for 180° LI is as good as that for 360° LI with the standard choice of 'table feed equal to slice thickness'. These results are encouraging and indicate a potential for new scanning strategies.

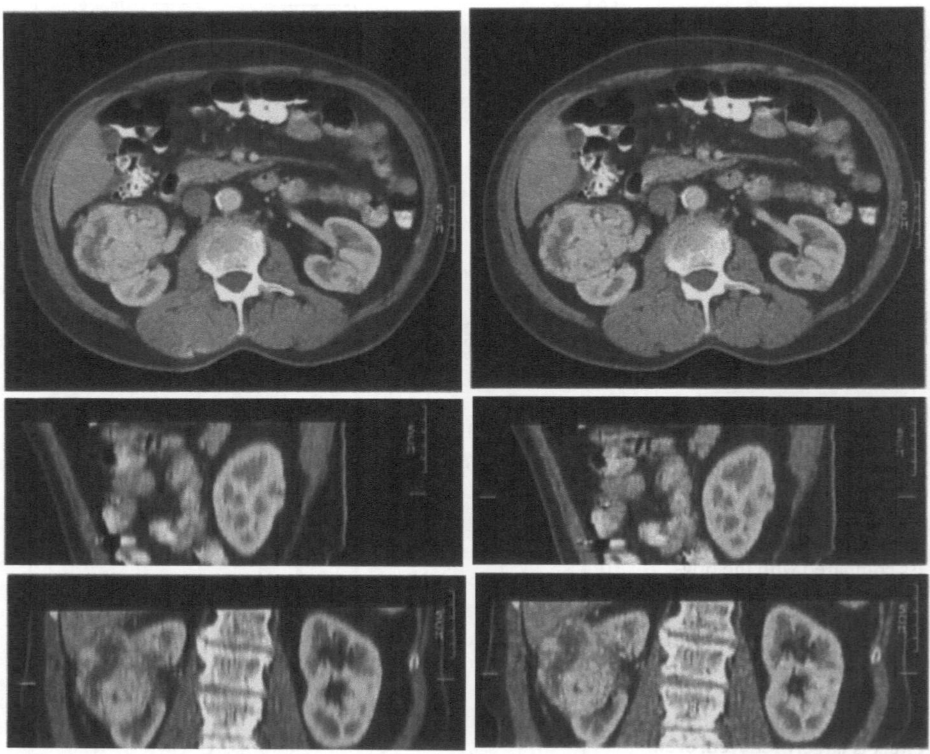

Fig. 4a–f. Bolus-enhanced spiral CT study in a patient with bilateral renal carcinoma (5 mm slice width, 5 mm/s table feed) (**a, c, e** 360° LI; **b, d, f** 180° LI). **a, b** CT images show the hypervascular tumours in the right and left kidney. **c, d** Sagittal reformation through the left kidney. **e, f** Coronal reformation through both kidneys. The effect of the improved SSPs of the 180° algorithm becomes apparent in the reformatted images

Implications for Clinical Studies

Spiral CT is now well established in radiological practice for a number of applications. Its universal use is above all precluded by the limitations in X-ray power. The selection of scan parameters in spiral CT will always constitute a trade-off between several goals: (1) low pixel noise which demands high mA values and thick slices; (2) large scan volumes which demand high table feed; (3) high spatial resolution in the longitudinal direction which demands thin slices and adequate table feed values. The selection of parameters depends on the clinical task.

For scan times the full 32 s will be chosen in most cases. With respect to mA values, the maximum value is also indicated in most applications. For slice thicknesses the choice is more complicated and constitutes a compromise between spatial

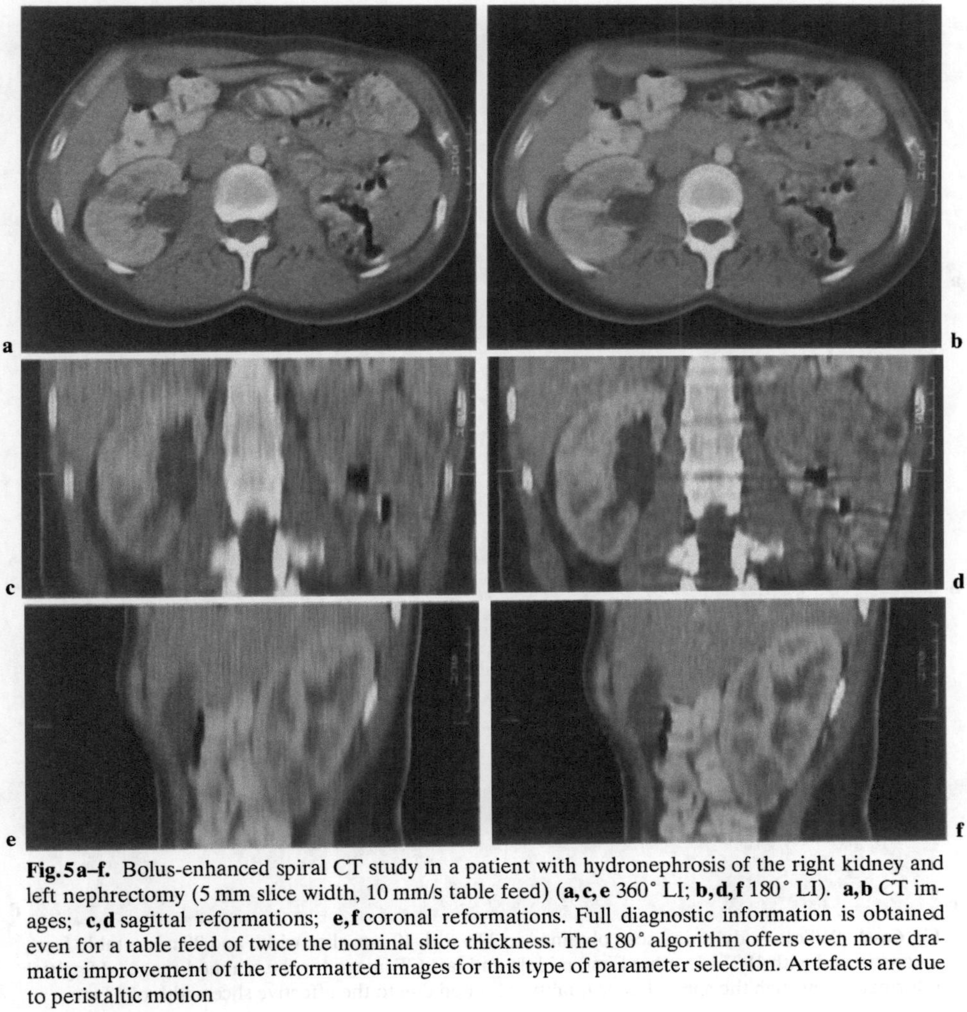

Fig. 5 a–f. Bolus-enhanced spiral CT study in a patient with hydronephrosis of the right kidney and left nephrectomy (5 mm slice width, 10 mm/s table feed) (**a, c, e** 360° LI; **b, d, f** 180° LI). **a, b** CT images; **c, d** sagittal reformations; **e, f** coronal reformations. Full diagnostic information is obtained even for a table feed of twice the nominal slice thickness. The 180° algorithm offers even more dramatic improvement of the reformatted images for this type of parameter selection. Artefacts are due to peristaltic motion resolution in the z-direction and pixel noise. For the abdomen, a 5 mm slice width appears to be the minimum to retain an adequate signal-to-noise ratio. Orthopaedic studies, in contrast, can be performed with 1-mm or 2-mm slices (see chapter by Hirschfelder). For table feed the standard choice is equal to the slice thickness. Greater table feed values appear possible now, with an influence on the SSP as described above.

The differences in image quality due to the SSPs are relatively difficult to assess in transverse CT reconstructions. SSP degradation often goes unnoticed when the table feed is less than or equal to the nominal slice thickness. Attention to detail such as small calcifications or bony structures will reveal this influence, however. The effect may become pronounced and intolerable when thick slices are chosen in combination with high table feed values.

Since SSPs determine the spatial resolution in the longitudinal direction, their effect can best be demonstrated in multiplanar reformations or cine loops. The 180° LI

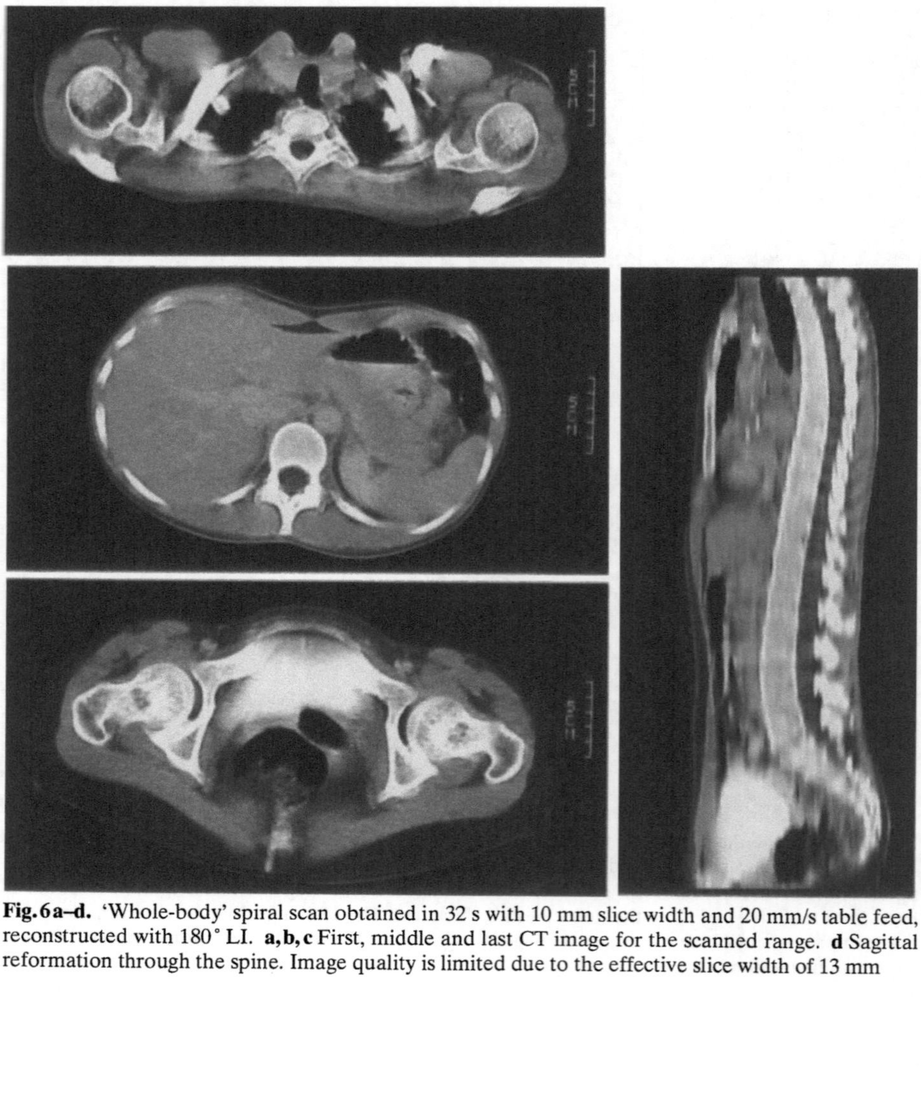

a b c d

Fig. 6 a–d. 'Whole-body' spiral scan obtained in 32 s with 10 mm slice width and 20 mm/s table feed, reconstructed with 180° LI. **a, b, c** First, middle and last CT image for the scanned range. **d** Sagittal reformation through the spine. Image quality is limited due to the effective slice width of 13 mm algorithm improves resolution significantly in these displays (Figs. 4–6). These findings were consistently obtained in a large number of clinical studies, confirming the superiority of spiral CT in scanning complete organs or anatomical regions without any gap (see chapter by Marchal et al.).

Results obtained at table feed values greater than the nominal slice thickness are slightly limited in image quality (Fig. 5). The effect may become intolerable for scans taken with large slice widths. To some degree, this is equivalent to stating that slice thicknesses beyond 10 mm are no longer considered acceptable nowadays. In the 32-s study taken with 10 mm slice width and 20 mm/s table feed, effective slice widths of 22.6 mm and 13.0 mm, respectively, result for the two algorithms (Fig. 6). The optimal choice of collimation and table feed for each clinical application have yet to be determined.

Conclusion

Spiral CT can in principle fulfill all the tasks of standard slice-by-slice CT scanning. The main drawback of the current equipment is given by the limitations in X-ray power. This is clearly outweighed by its ability to scan complete volumes in a minimal time without any gaps. Spatial resolution in the z-direction is effectively improved by 180° data interpolation, resulting in high quality of multiplanar reformations, three-dimensional and cine displays. It also offers the potential for scanning larger volumes by increasing the table feed to values greater than the nominal slice thickness, with a concomitant reduction in patient dose.

References

1. Kalender WA, Seißler W, Vock P (1989) Single-breathhold spiral volumetric CT by continuous patient translation and scanner rotation. Radiology 173 (P): 414
2. Vock P, Jung H, Kalender WA (1989) Single-breathhold volumetric CT of the hepatobiliary system. Radiology 173 (P): 377
3. Oudkerk M, Kalender WA (1989) CT of hilar adenopathy with 1-second and subsecond scan times. Radiology 173 (P): 452
4. Vock P, Soucek M, Daepp M, Kalender WA (1990) Lung: spiral volumetric CT with single-breathhold technique. Radiology 176: 864–867
5. Kalender WA, Seißler W, Klotz E, Vock P (1990) Spiral volumetric CT with single-breathhold technique, continuous transport, and continuous scanner rotation. Radiology 176: 181–183
6. Soucek M, Vock P, Daepp M, Kalender WA (1990) Spiral CT: Eine neue Technik für Volumenaufnahmen. II. Klinische Anwendungsmöglichkeiten. Rontgenpraxis 43: 365–375
7. Costello P, Anderson W, Blume D (1990) Spiral volumetric CT in the search for a pulmonary nodule. Radiology 177: 295
8. Bautz W, Skalej M, Kalender WA (1990) Diagnosis of pancreatic disease: clinical impact of spiral CT. Radiology 177 (P): 154
9. Bautz W, Skalej M, Thomas C, Kalender WA, Claussen CD (1990) New directions in CT of the pancreas. In: Fuchs W (ed) Advances in CT. Springer, Berlin Heidelberg New York, pp 37–47
10. Kalender WA, Vock P, Seißler W (1990) Spiral CT scanning for fast and continuous volume data acquisition. In: Fuchs W (ed) Advances in CT. Springer, Berlin Heidelberg New York, pp 55–64

11 Rigauts H, Marchal G, Baert AL, Hupke R (1990) Spiral scanning: phantom studies and patient material. In: Fuchs W (ed) Advances in CT. Springer, Berlin Heidelberg New York, pp 65–76
12. Vock P, Soucek M, Daepp M, Kalender WA (1990) Single-breathhold spiral volumetric computed tomography (SVCT) of the lung and the hepato-biliary system. In: Fuchs W (ed) Advances in CT. Springer, Berlin Heidelberg New York, pp 77–84
13. Dupuy DE, Costello P, Ecker CP (1991) Comparative study of spiral CT and conventional CT of the pancreas. Radiology 181 (P): 350
14. Bautz W, Strotzer M, Lenz M, Dittler HJ, Kalender WA (1991) Preoperative evaluation of the vessels of the upper abdomen with spiral CT: comparison with conventional CT and arterial DSA. Radiology 181 (P): 261
15. Remy-Jardin M, Deffontaines C, Remy J (1991) Chest evaluation with use of spiral volumetric CT with the single-breathhold technique. Radiology 181 (P): 273
16. Costello P, Dupuy DE, Ecker CP (1991) Spiral CT of the thorax with small volumes of contrast material: a comparative study. Radiology 181 (P): 274
17. Kuhlman JE, Ney DR, Fishman EK (1991) Two- and three-dimensional imaging of the in vivo lung: combining spiral CT with multiplanar and volumetric rendering techniques. Radiology 181 (P): 274
18. Schäfer CM, Prokop M, Döhring W, Schäfers F, Galanski M (1991) Spiral CT of the tracheobronchial system: optimized technique and clinical applications. Radiology 181 (P): 274
19. Anno H, Kondo T, Katada T, Ida Y, Tsujioka K, Koga S (1991) Three-dimensional coronary angio-imaging with helical scanning CT. Radiology 181 (P): 336
20. Kalender WA, Vock P, Polacin A, Soucek M (1990) Spiral CT: Eine neue Technik für Volumenaufnahmen. I. Grundlagen und Methodik. Rontgenpraxis 43: 323–330
21. Rigauts H, Marchal G, Baert AL, Hupke R (1990) Spiral scanning and the influence of the reconstruction algorithm on image quality. J Comput Assist Tomogr 14: 675–682
22. Crawford CR, King K (1990) Computed tomography scanning with simultaneous patient translation. Med Phys 17: 967–982
23. Kalender WA, Polacin A (1991) Physical performance characteristics of spiral CT scanning. Med Phys 18: 910–915
24. Polacin A, Kalender WA (1991) Simulation and measurement of image quality in spiral CT with different data processing algorithms. Radiology 181 (P): 111
25. Polacin A, Kalender WA, Marchal G (1992) Evaluation of slice sensitivity profiles and image noise in spiral CT with different data processing algorithms. Radiology (manuscript submitted)

Spiral CT and Conventional Incremental CT of the Lung

K. Rosenkranz, M. Langer, C. Zwicker, R. Langer, E. Schultz, and R. Felix

Introduction

The introduction of spiral volumetric computed tomography (CT) has opened up new perspectives in the examination of the lung [1–3, 6]. A major advantage is the ability to scan a large volume during a 12- (or 24-) s breath hold [3].

The purpose of this study was to compare the accuracy of spiral CT and conventional incremental CT in examination of the lung.

Patients and Methods

Fifteen patients, 13 men and two women (aged 52 ± 12 years) were examined by CT in order to exclude pulmonary metastatic disease due to colonic, pancreatic, and breast cancer. This study excluded patients with pathologic findings of the lung parenchyma.

The lungs were investigated by spiral CT (Somatom Plus, Siemens) in one breath hold (24 s, 137 kV, 75 mA) with a table feed of 10 mm/s and a slice thickness of 10 mm. Images were reconstructed in standard mode from the data set and compared with conventional incremental CT (137 kV, 145 mA) in standard mode with a slice thickness and a table feed of 10 mm and 10 mm/s, respectively.

The qualitative evaluation of image accuracy was performed by three radiologists. The quantitative analysis of CT scans at the level of the aortic arch, the carina, and the base of the heart included the assessment of ventrodorsal CT density gradients and a quantitative histogram analysis. The maximal density increase in the lung vessels and the integrals of three density peaks per patient (in mm^2) considered as representative were determined (Fig. 1).

Finally, we studied a Plexiglas phantom consisting of slices 0.5–2.5 mm thick (0.5, 0.6, 0.7, 0.8, 0.9, 1.0, 1.25, 2.0, 2.5 mm) by spiral CT (10-mm thickness, standard algo-

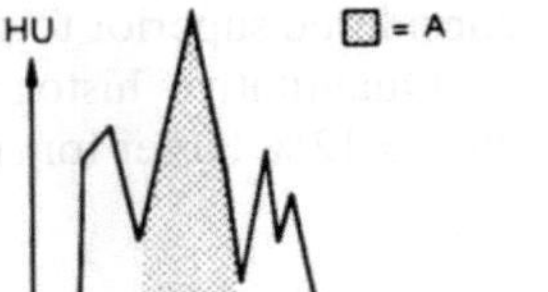

Fig. 1. Quantitative histogram analysis of CT density peaks in the lung vessels. The integrals of density peaks *(A)* were assessed (in mm^2) for spiral and conventional CT

Table 1. Image accuracy of spiral and conventional CT in the examination of the lung assessed qualitatively by three radiologists and quantitative histogram analysis of density peaks in the lung vessels (three per patient). The mean integrals of density peaks were assessed (in mm^2) for spiral CT (A_1) and conventional CT (A_2). In addition, the mean difference (δA) between A_2 and A_1 was calculated as percentage of A_2: $\delta A = A_1 - A_2/A_2 \times 100$ ($n = 15$)

	Qualitative analysis		
	Spiral CT	Conventional CT	
Accuracy superior	0	12	
Accuracy equal	3	3	
	Quantitative analysis		
	A_1/mm^2	A_2/mm^2	$\delta A/\% \pm SD$
	121	92	32 ± 12

rithm, 24 × 1 s, 137 kV, 75 mA) and conventional CT (10-mm thickness, standard algorithm, 137 kV, 145 mA). In addition to the assessment of spatial resolution, qualitative and quantitative evaluation of the image accuracy was performed, as mentioned above.

Results

Patient Study

Evaluation of conventional and spiral CT was possible in all cases. No patient failed to cooperate for the 24-s period of suspended respiration.

Concerning qualitative analysis, the image accuracy of conventional CT was considered as equal to spiral CT in three instances and superior in 12.

Table 1 summarizes the results of the quantitative histogram analysis. The mean CT density values of the lung parenchyma for spiral CT and conventional CT were -819 ± 49 HU and -828 ± 85 HU, respectively. The density increase in the lung vessels was 330 ± 77 HU for spiral CT and 355 ± 85 HU for conventional CT. The integrals of density peaks of the lung vessels were 32% larger for spiral CT than for conventional CT (Fig. 2).

Phantom Study

The spatial resolution of conventional CT was 0.6 mm and thus superior to the resolution of spiral CT with 0.8 mm (Fig. 3). The image accuracy of conventional CT was considered superior to that of spiral CT.

Quantitative histogram analysis showed the integrals of density peaks to be 39% ± 12% larger for spiral CT than for conventional CT.

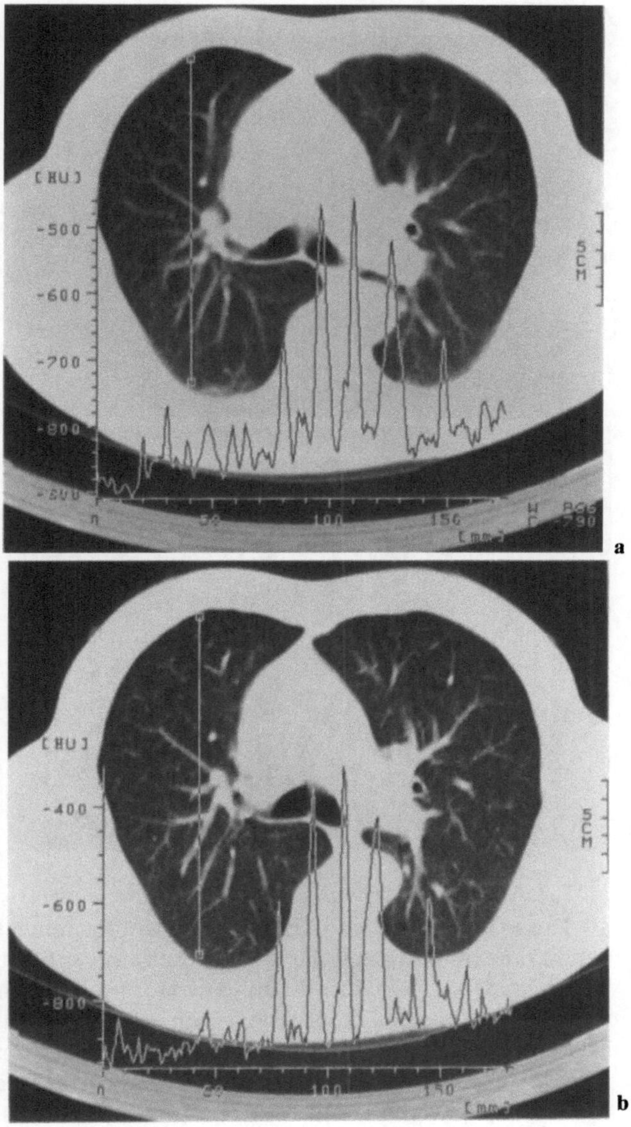

Fig. 2. **a** Spiral and **b** conventional CT scans at the level of the carina with assessment of ventrodorsal density gradients and quantitative histogram analysis. In comparison with spiral CT, the borders of the lung vessels and the respective density peaks are sharper on conventional CT

Discussion

Spiral volumetric CT is based on the new development of continuous measurement during several X-ray tube rotations in one breath hold and thus enables us to study an organ volume of up to 24 cm length. The artifacts resulting from the spiral scanning geometry are adequately removed by linear interpolation into the planar data [3, 4].

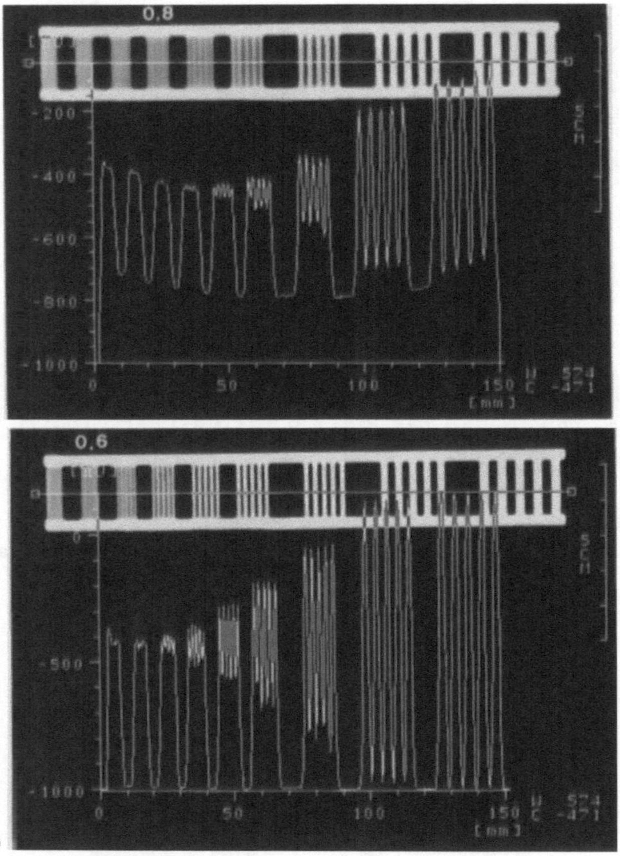

a b

Fig. 3. **a** Spiral CT (10-mm thickness, standard algorithm, 24 × 1 s, 137 kV, 75 mA) and **b** conventional CT (10-mm thickness, standard algorithm, 137 kV, 145 mA) of a Plexiglas phantom consisting of slices 0.5–2.5 mm thick. The spatial resolution of conventional CT was 0.6 mm and thus superior to the resolution of spiral CT with 0.8 mm. The quantitative histogram analysis of density gradients from the left to the right side of the phantom *(horizontal line)* shows the areas below the density peaks to be larger for spiral CT than for incremental CT

The *main advantages* in comparison with incremental CT are the short examination time of ≤ 24 s and the lack of respiratory artifacts due to examination in one breath hold [3, 6, 7, 8]. Inconstant respiratory volumes in incremental CT can lead to the omission of small focal lesions, for example, lung nodules < 1 cm [1, 3, 5, 7]. Therefore, it is often necessary to repeat scans or to examine with overlapping single slices [6]. Consequently, and due to the higher current than spiral CT, incremental CT involves a higher radiation dose. Respiratory artifacts must be considered as the main reason for the lower sensitivity of incremental CT in the detection of pulmonary nodules < 1 cm in comparison with spiral CT [1]. In addition, spiral CT offers a basis for secondary – for example, three-dimensional – reconstructions [2].

The *superior image accuracy of conventional CT* in the examination of the lung in comparison with spiral CT (as shown in this study) can be explained by the higher tube current (145 mA, spiral CT: 75 mA) with a consequently higher contrast resolution [9]. In addition, the increase of effective section thickness by a factor of 1.3 due to interpolation [4] in spiral CT (with a table movement of 10 mm/s) must be considered a reason for the superior image accuracy and also for the superior spatial resolution of incremental CT. According to our phantom study, the spatial resolution of spiral and incremental CT is 0.8 mm or 0.6 mm, respectively. Kalender et al. [3] showed a spatial resolution of 0.6 mm for spiral as well as incremental CT by a dot phantom, but with different examination parameters than those used in this study (120 kV instead of 137 kV used in this study).

The *most severe hardware limitation of spiral CT* is the heat capacity of the tube. Therefore, the number of rotations and thus the volume examined during one breath hold is currently limited [6].

According to our limited experience, suspended respiration for a 24-s period does not seem to be a severe problem, however, our study group did not include dyspneic or noncooperative patients.

Considering the advantages and current limitations of spiral CT mentioned above, we are convinced that this method has added a new dimension to the examination of the lungs and that its diagnostic significance will increase in the near future.

References

1. Costello P, Anderson W, Blume D (1991) Pulmonary nodule: evaluation with spiral volumetric CT. Radiology 179: 875–876
2. Gmeinwieser J, Wunderlich AP, Gerhardt P, Strotzer M (1991) Dreidimensionale Rekonstruktion von atemverschieblichen Organen und Gefäßstrukturen aus Spiral-CT-Datensätzen. Röntgenpraxis 44: 2–8
3. Kalender WA, Vock P, Polacin A, Soucek M (1990) Spiral-CT: Eine neue Technik für Volumenaufnahmen. I. Grundlagen und Methodik. Röntgenpraxis 43: 323–330
4. Kalender WA, Vock P, Seißler W (1990) Spiral volumetric CT with single-breathhold technique, continuous transport and continuous scanner rotation. Radiology 176: 181–183
5. Shaffer K, Pugatch RD (1989) Small pulmonary nodules: dynamic CT with a single breath technique. Radiology 173: 567–568
6. Soucek M, Vock P, Daepp M, Kalender WA (1990) Spiral-CT: Eine neue Technik für Volumenaufnahmen. II. Klinische Anwendungsmöglichkeiten. Röntgenpraxis 43: 365–375
7. Vock P, Soucek M, Daepp M, Kalender WA (1990) Lung: spiral volumetric CT with single-breath-hold technique. Radiology 176: 864–867
8. Zwicker C (1990) Spiral-CT. Habilitationsschrift, Berlin, pp 12–13
9. Zwicker C (1990) Prüfung der Abbildungseigenschaften des eingesetzten CT-Gerätes – eigene Untersuchungen. Habilitationsschrift, Berlin, p 14

Spiral Versus Dynamic Incremental CT

J. C. Hacking and A. K. Dixon

Introduction

The benefits of spiral volumetric computed tomography (SVCT) over dynamic incremental computed tomopraphy (DICT) have been well described [1–4]. They include the absolute contiguity of the reconstructed image. This overcomes the reliance on the patient reproducing an exactly identical respiratory excursion to produce sequential images. This should theoretically make it impossible to skip over small lesions. The lack of interslice delay means that all total data acquisition times are much shorter. This should lead to improved overall vascular and organ enhancement as more images will be obtained during peak levels of enhancement. This feature will be most noticeable when using a simple small bolus injection of contrast medium given by hand, as at our institution. These benefits are predicted to be available with little effect on image quality. Work on the CT investigation of pulmonary nodules is confirming the usefulness of slice contiguity [2, 3]. However, as regards image quality, there are certain inherent theoretical disadvantages attached to SVCT. In order to remain within present tube heating specifications, there are limitations on the available current, and these become more marked as the acquisition time increases. For example, when examining the liver in 1-cm thick slices on a standard algorithm using our version of the spiral Somatom Plus, the maximum allowable current for volumes up to 8 cm in length is 210 mA at 1 cm/s; for 8–12 cm this falls to 165 mA. For volumes between 12 and 24 cm in length a 'soft tissue' algorithm has to be used, with subsequent reconstruction using a standard algorithm. This allows 24-s of data acquisition but the permissible current is further reduced to 85 mA. This compares with the constant current of 210 mA which can be used for DICT. Increasing the table speed could help solve this problem, but a speed equal to the desired slice width per second has been shown to provide the optimal compromise between acquisition volume and level of artefact production [4].

Previous studies have shown no deterioration in spatial resolution, uniformity or pixel noise values, but these were performed using 210 or 170 mA [1–4]. Furthermore, good patient cooperation is required when examining large volumes, particularly for acquisitions in suspended expiration. To our knowledge no randomized trial comparing the possible benefits and disadvantages of SVCT has been performed. We have therefore performed a study to look particularly at the effects of spiral scanning on image quality and enhancement.

Material and Methods

Three regions of the body were selected for analysis: neck, thorax (comprising axillary and mediastinal problems) and abdomen (including liver, pancreas, kidney and adrenals). The abdominal group was subdivided into those where volumes less than or greater than 12 cm in length were examined; this identified the subgroup with the lowest current. One hundred consecutive patients in the above categories for whom enhanced images were required were randomly allocated to DICT or SVCT. For these sequences, it was important to maintain comparability between the techniques. A standard 10-mm slice thickness and incrementation was therefore adopted for all

Table 1. The technical parameters used in the 100 patients

Anatomical area	Numbers	Current ranges (mA)	Voltage ranges (kV)	Number of enhanced images obtained		Total time taken to obtain series of enhanced images (s)	
				Mean	range	Mean	range
Neck	DICT 7	165–250	120	9.6	4–13	60.4	38–125
	SVCT 6	120–145	120–137	6.7	5–13	6.8	5–12
Thorax	DICT 20	210	120	9.1	3–16	52.7	13–112
	SVCT 19	75–145	120–137	10.0	6–15	9.1	4–14
Liver	DICT 7	210	120	14.0	10–19	84.1	60–124
	SVCT 11	85–165	120	12.7	9–15	11.9	8–15
Pancreas	DICT 6	165–250	120	8.3	6–12	70.0	32–105
	SVCT 9	165	120	10.1	7–13	9.3	6–13
Kidney	DICT 3	210–250	120	10.5	8–14	72.5	52–88
	SVCT 5	85–165	120	12.8	9–15	11.8	10–14
Adrenal	DICT 4	210–250	120	11.0	7–15	65.5	41–91
	SVCT 3	165	120	11.0	9–13	10.0	8–12
Total	DICT 47	165–250	120	9.9	3–19	62.4	13–125
	SVCT 53	75–165	120–137	10.5	5–15	9.6	4–15

Table 2. Judged quality of images obtained with SVCT and DICT in terms of diagnostic image quality and enhancement (parentheses indicate a trend which did not reach statistical significance; where significance was reached the p value is shown)

	Better image quality	Better enhancement
Neck	(DICT)	(SVCT)
Thorax	(SVCT)	SVCT $p<0.01$
Abdomen	DICT $p<0.02$	(SVCT)
Liver	DICT $p<0.05$	(SVCT)
Pancreas	(DICT)	(DICT)
Kidney	(DICT)	(DICT)
Adrenal	(SVCT)	(SVCT)
Total	(DICT)	SVCT $p<0.01$

studies apart from the adrenal glands, where 5-mm contiguous slices were obtained. The numbers of patients in each group are shown in Table 1.

All subjects received 50 ml contrast medium by rapid hand injection (Iopamidol 300 mg iodine/ml, Niopam, Merck). Data acquisition commenced after approximately 35 ml for DICT and 45 ml for SVCT. The enhanced images were then subjectively reviewed by an observer (A.K.D.) and were scored for the overall image quality (0–10, 0 = nondiagnostic, 10 = excellent) and for the degree of contrast enhancement throughout the study (0–10, 0 = inadequate, 10 = excellent opacification). The number of slices obtained and the time of data acquisition were also recorded. Statistical analysis of the nonparametric data was effected by the Mann–Whitney U test.

Results and Discussion

The random number tables led to 53 of the 100 patients being examined by SVCT and 47 by DICT. The results of the various assessments form part of a larger study which is in preparation but summaries of the parameters and results are shown in Tables 1–3.

Neck

There were no statistically significant differences between SVCT and DICT here. The overall image quality was fractionally higher with DICT, but this was offset by slightly better enhancement using SVCT. Much depends, therefore, on the specific indication. If the whole neck (from the base of skull to sternal notch) is to be examined, it might be better to use DICT as the craniocaudal extent is likely to exceed 12 cm. However, if the examination is localized to a short segment of the neck where precise coverage without movement is essential (e.g. larynx), then SVCT might be the preferred option. For small lesions, higher resolution can be obtained using 5-mm slices. This, however, increases the graininess of the image still further. Should three-dimensional images be required, they should, theoretically, be better when using a spiral technique.

Table 3. The overall image quality in the abdomen

	Numbers		Mean score (0–10)	Standard deviation	Significance of difference
Total	48	DICT 20	8.0	1.1	$p < 0.02$
		SVCT 28	7.1	1.4	
< 12 cm	32	DICT 14	8.1	1.1	
		SVCT 18	7.4	1.2	N.S.
> 12 cm	16	DICT 6	7.8	1.2	
		SVCT 10	6.6	1.8	N.S.

Thorax

Axilla. Examinations of the axilla were all in patients with breast carcinoma with clinical problems in the axilla (pain, arm oedema or palpable mass). CT was being performed in order to distinguish between radiation effects and recurrent tumour. Obviously the mediastinum was assessed too. These patients were examined with their arms down by their sides.

Mediastinum. Examinations of mediastinum were usually to prove normality/abnormality of nodal status in cases of bronchial neoplasm or lymphoma. In these patients the arms were extended above their heads.

For these patients there was significantly ($p < 0.01$) better enhancement using the SVCT technique. There was no appreciable difference in image quality. Accordingly, for these clinical problems we now routinely use SVCT, as we do for nearly all localized (< 12 cm) problems in the thorax. The lower permissible current has very little effect here. Again, 5-mm-thick slices are used for higher resolution when examining small areas. The absolute contiguity of the images is yet another bonus. Of course, if the patient moves or breathes heavily during a SVCT study the effect is more deleterious than during a DICT run where only one or two images may be spoilt. However, most patients can be coerced into cooperating for a 12-s investigation.

Abdomen

Overall, there was a significant ($p < 0.02$) reduction in image quality with SVCT, largely due to current constraints leading to substantial graininess of the image. As can be seen from the mean scores (Table 3), this was most noticeable in those examinations of over 12 cm. However, due to the small numbers in this subgroup, statistical significance was not reached. It should be stressed that none of the studies was regarded as inadequate for diagnostic purposes and no patient required a second examination using the alternative technique.

Liver. The above comments regarding image quality were most applicable to the group undergoing liver examinations as it contained the largest number of studies over 12 cm in length (Fig. 1). The enhancement, as done in this study, was slightly better in the SVCT group. In practice, we now use DICT for nearly all enhanced hepatic studies, even though the patient may have difficulty taking very quick repeated respirations. However, a case could be made for using SVCT for a lesion abutting the diaphragm or in a patient who had already exhibited difficulty in obtaining consistent respiratory excursions. A major problem for hepatic SVCT, with our version of the product, is that the volume of interest is often longer than 12 cm.

Pancreas. In our technique, where there is almost always a set of unenhanced images of high quality for comparison, the slight (and insignificant) reduction in image quality using SVCT is of little importance. Respiration does not affect this retroperitoneal organ so much but, nevertheless, the assured contiguity of images is a helpful

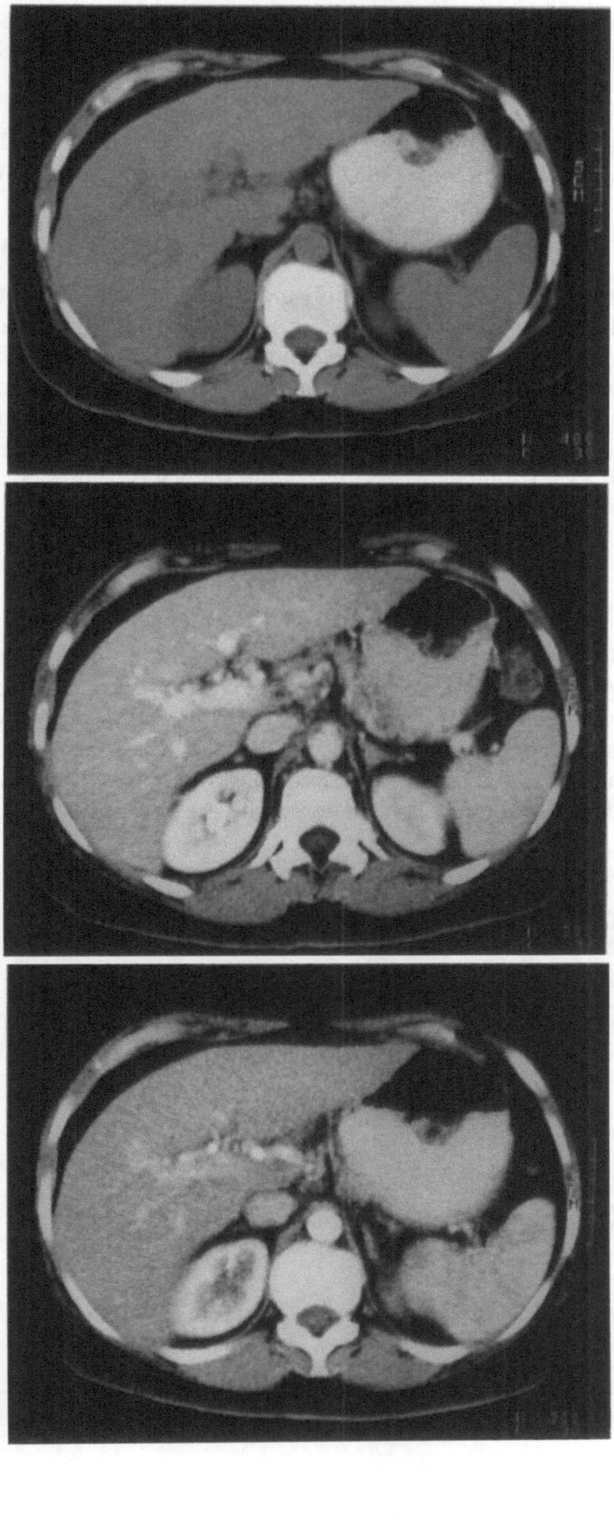

a

b

c

Fig. 1 a–c. Three images from the same patient suffering from hepatitis C-induced cirrhosis. **a** A precontrast initial image. Standard auto sequence: 210 mA, 120 kV, 2 × 1 s. **b** A dynamic (DICT) image: 210 mA, 120 kV, 1 s. Halving the data acquisition time has led to increased graininess of the image. The portal venous enhancement is very good although there has been some fading of the hepatic artery. **c** A spiral (SVCT) image: 85 mA, 120 kV, 1 s. There is excellent arterial and portal venous enhancement but the marked increase in graininess has given a blurred appearance to the margins of the vessels attribute of SVCT. Even if a 5-mm slice thickness is desired and a table movement of 5 mm/s is chosen, the volume of interest is unlikely to be large enough to cause a problem.

Kidneys. The small number of patients examined (3 DICT, 5 SVCT) precludes much comment here. For some clinical problems (e.g. renal vein involvement in renal carcinoma), absolute contiguity is again helpful. Only rarely will the volume of interest be over 12 cm in length.

Adrenals. There are probably more theories as to the optimal method of examining the adrenals than for any other organ [5, 6]. Suffice it to say that small adrenal lesions may be missed if the thickness of the cut is too large or if the respiration is uneven. Accordingly, the spiral technique should be ideal, in so far that it should be impossible to miss a small lesion between noncontiguous cuts. Unfortunately, the small number of patents in this group prevents much comment here, although further use of SVCT following cessation of the study has confirmed in our minds the usefulness of the technique in this application.

Overall

The overall image quality was fractionally, but not significantly, higher in the DICT group. However, the enhancement when using our rather unsophisticated technique was significantly ($p < 0.01$) better with SVCT. This, combined with the already proven benefit of contiguity, leads us to conclude that SVCT is a very useful technique (see Fig. 2). For dynamic studies we currently reserve DICT for imaging the entire liver and for those patients who are unable to maintain the long period of fixed

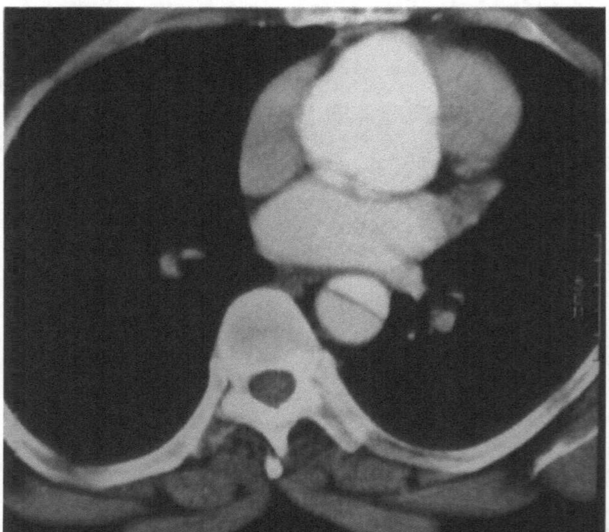

Fig. 2. A spiral (SVCT) image from a patient who previously had a surgical repair for a type A dissection of the aorta. A persistent flap is present in the descending aorta. Factors: 75 mA, 137 kV, 1 s. Although there is slight graininess, excellent image quality and opacification are seen

respiration. For hepatic studies of less than 12 cm and all other cases where enhancement is paramount, rather than image quality, we currently use SVCT.

References

1. Kalender WA, Seissler W, Klotz E, Vock P (1990) Spiral volumetric CT with single-breath-hold technique, continuous transport, and continuous scanner rotation. Radiology 176: 181–183
2. Vock P, Soucek M, Daepp M, Kalender WA (1990) Lung: spiral volumetric CT with single-breath-hold technique. Radiology 176: 864–867
3. Costello P, Anderson W, Blume D (1991) Pulmonary nodule: evaluation with spiral volumetric CT. Radiology 179: 875–876
4. Rigauts H, Marchal G, Baert AL, Hupke R (1990) Initial experience with volume CT scanning. J Comput Assist Tomogr 14: 675–682
5. Falke THM, van Seters AP (1989) Adrenal imaging. In: Husband JES (ed) CT review. Churchill Livingstone, Edinburgh
6. Siegelman SS, Fishman EK, Gatewood OMB, Goldman SM (1984) CT of the adrenal gland. In: Siegelman SS, Gatewood OMB, Goldman SM (eds) Computed tomography of the kidneys and adrenals. Churchill Livingstone, Edinburgh

Vascular Imaging with Spiral CT

C. Schaefer, M. Prokop, J. Nischelsky, P. Reimer, K. Bonk, and M. Galanski

Introduction

Angiography is still the method of choice for the evaluation of vascular structures. Due to a limited number of projections, complex vascular structures or vascular pathology may not always be sufficiently imaged with angiography. Spiral computed tomography (CT) allows for continuous volume acquisition within short scan times [1]. Thus, a high vascular contrast within the scan volume can be maintained, and subsequent three-dimensional (3D) reconstructions of vascular structures become feasible.

We present our experience with 3D vascular imaging using spiral CT scanning. The objective was to examine the influence of various technical parameters and to evaluate the clinical applicability of the technique.

Technical Specifications

Spiral CT was performed on a Somatom Plus scanner with a continuously rotating tube/detector unit. In the spiral CT mode, the scanner is able to acquire a maximum of 24 360° scans within 24 s. During data acquisition the patient is moved through the gantry at a speed of 1–10 mm/s. Therefore, the length of the volume that can be covered by one spiral scan is currently restricted to 24 cm. A linear interpolation algorithm compensates for the movement artifacts and calculates cross-sectional images of the planar geometry.

The variables of spiral CT imaging that determine the appearance of reconstructed 3D images are the slice profile, the dose per slice, the reconstruction interval, and the reconstruction algorithm [2]. The slice profile of a single spiral CT image is determined by the chosen slice thickness (collimation), table feed, and interpolation procedure. The slice profile determines the effective slice thickness. Three filter algorithms (standard, smooth, high) are available for image reconstruction from spiral CT raw data. Scans can be reconstructed with a minimum of 1-mm intervals. It has to be noted that the reconstruction interval does not influence the effective slice thickness.

The images obtained from a spiral CT study can be reformatted to multiplanar (two-dimensional, 2D) or 3D images. The 3D reconstructions are performed using a surface rendering algorithm with an interactively chosen threshold.

Phantom Study

A phantom study was carried out to evaluate qualitatively the impact of slice thickness and table feed on the appearance of 3D images. The objective was to define optimal parameters for vascular imaging. To simulate a vessel of known configuration, a contrast-filled infusion line with an inner diameter of 3 mm was scanned in a water basin of 20 cm diameter. The contrast filling in the line was adjusted to 200 HU. The infusion line was arranged in several loops. A knot and a simulated obstruction were added.

The slice thickness/table feed were increased from 2/2 to 3/3, 5/5, and 8/8 mm, and 3D reconstructions with various thresholds were performed.

The effects of increasing the slice thickness/table feed can be summarized as follows (Fig. 1 a–c):

1. Increasing distortion along the z-axis occurs.
2. Fine details (like the knot) become blurred.
3. All detrimental effects are strongest for structures parallel to the scan plane while those perpendicular to it are much less affected.
4. Due to increasing partial volume effects, the threshold for 3D reconstructions has to be lowered.

The influence of the threshold level was studied for a spiral CT scan with 5/5 mm slice thickness/table feed and a reconstruction interval of 2 mm (Fig. 2). We found:

1. The apparent diameter of the infusion line grows with decreasing threshold level.
2. Image distorsion along the z-axis grows with lower thresholds.

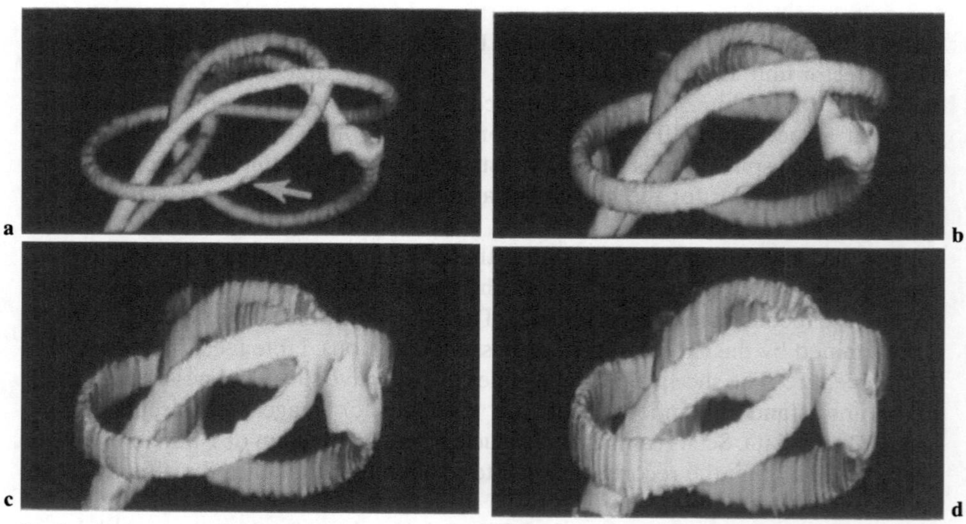

Fig. 1 a–d. A contrast-filled infusion line with a knot and an obstruction *(arrows)*. Increasing distorsion along the z-axis and progressive blurring of fine details occur with increasing slice thickness/table feed from 2/2 mm (**a**) to 3/3 mm (**b**), 5/5 mm (**c**), and 8/8 mm (**d**). All detrimental effects are strongest for structures parallel to the scan plane, while those perpendicular to it are much less affected

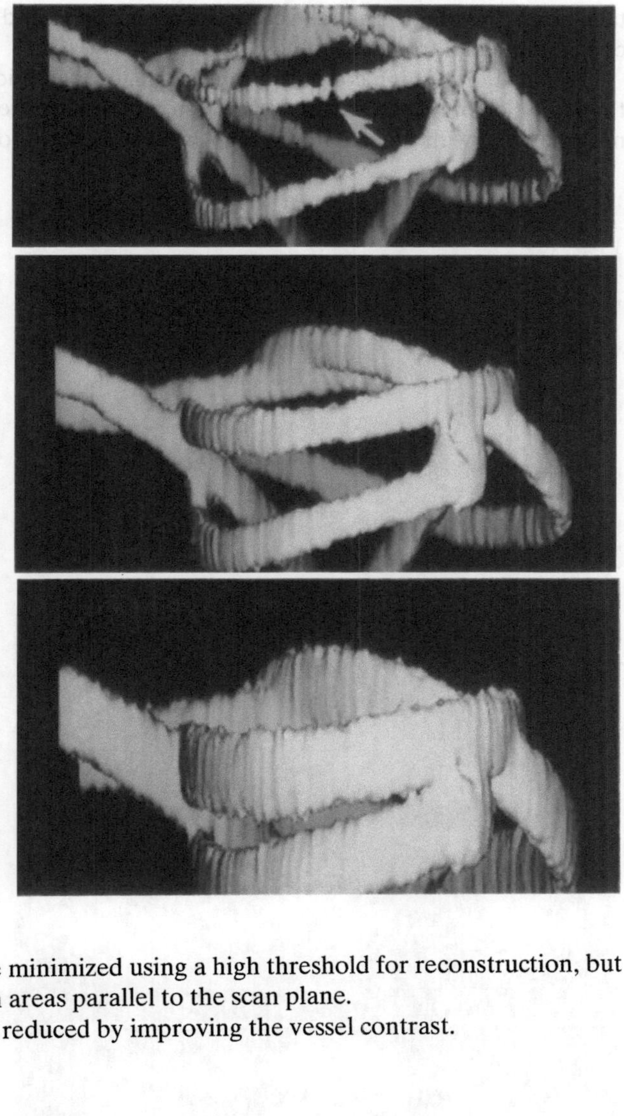

Fig. 2a–c. A spiral CT scan obtained with 5/5 mm slice thickness/table feed and a reconstruction interval of 2 mm that was reconstructed using three threshold levels of 100 HU (**a**), 75 HU (**b**), and 25 HU (**c**). Image distorsion along the z-axis and the apparent diameter of the infusion line grow with decreasing threshold level. Image distorsion can be minimized using a high threshold for reconstruction but pseudo-defects *(arrow)* occur in areas parallel to the scan plane

3. Image distorsion can be minimized using a high threshold for reconstruction, but pseudo-defects occur in areas parallel to the scan plane.
4. The latter effect can be reduced by improving the vessel contrast.

Application of Contrast Agents

A homogeneous and sufficiently high contrast enhancement of the vessels is the basic prerequisite to achieve diagnostic 3D images. Therefore, optimizing the way of contrast application is of utmost importance. We consider the following parameters to be optimal for the 'average' (middle-aged) patient and a broad range of applications: a total volume of 100–150 ml contrast medium, a flow rate of 3 ml/s, and a delay time of 30 s. In athletic young patients with a good cardiac function and a short circulation time, the flow rate should be increased and the delay time decreased. In uncertain cases, such as patients with low cardiac function, aortic valve regurgitation, or an ectatic aorta, the delay time between contrast injection and the start of the spiral scan can be estimated from a 10 ml test bolus.

Application of high concentrations (e.g., 300 mg/ml iodine) of i.v. contrast from the same side of the diaphragm as the lesion often leads to major streak artifacts that may interfere with the diagnosis (Fig. 4b). Instead, a venous approach from the con-

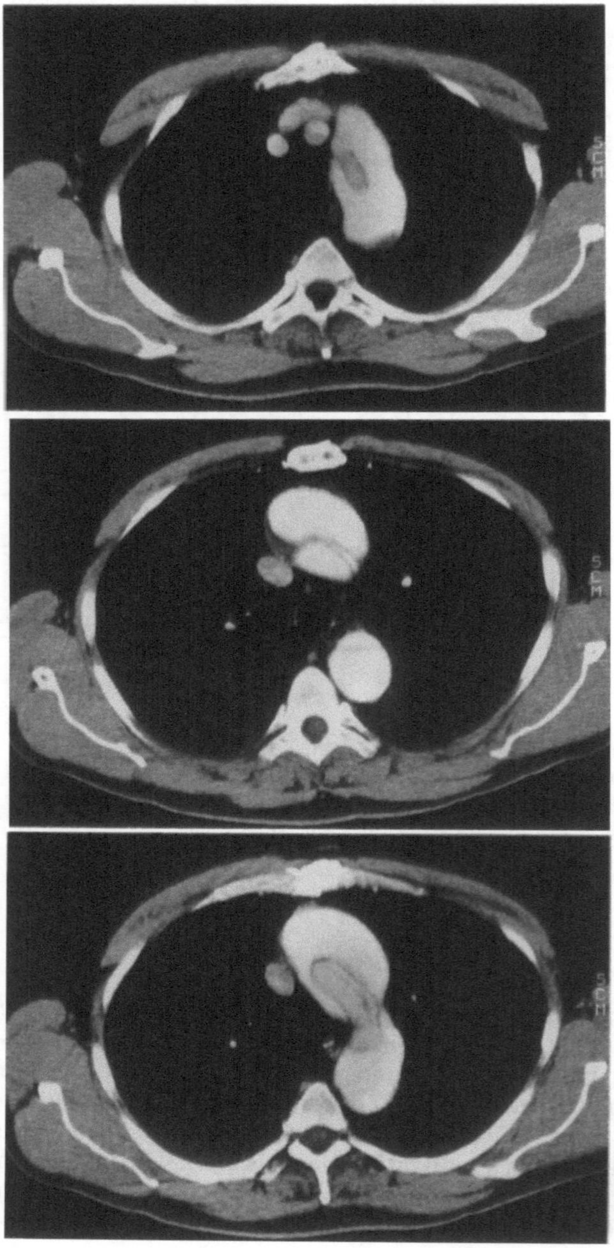

a

b

c

Fig. 3a–c. Images from a spiral CT scan of a patient with a composite graft of the ascending aorta following a type A dissection. The images demonstrate an elephant trunk that was placed in the true lumen at the level of the aortic arch. A persisting involvement of the brachiocephalic trunk was noted tralateral side of the diaphragm was found to be advantageous, such as a femoral injection for imaging of the aortic arch and the supraaortic branches, and a cubital injection for imaging of the abdominal vessels. In cases in which the contrast has to be injected from the same side as the region of interest, the contrast concentration should be markedly decreased, but the flow rate has to be increased.

Results and Clinical Applications

In general, all major vessels including the aorta and its supraaortic and visceral branches, the pulmonary arteries and veins, the superior and inferior vena cava, and the portal vein can be imaged by spiral CT. Clinical indications include stenoses as well as aneurysms, intravasal thrombi, and dissecting membranes, obstructions, and displacement of vessels caused by soft tissue masses.

Two major groups of applications can be differentiated.

Due to the short scan time, spiral CT can provide an optimal vascular contrast over the whole scan range. In addition to overlapping views, cross-sectional images can be reconstructed at any location within the scan range. Thus, complete information about the course of vessels and their relationship to adjacent soft tissues can be

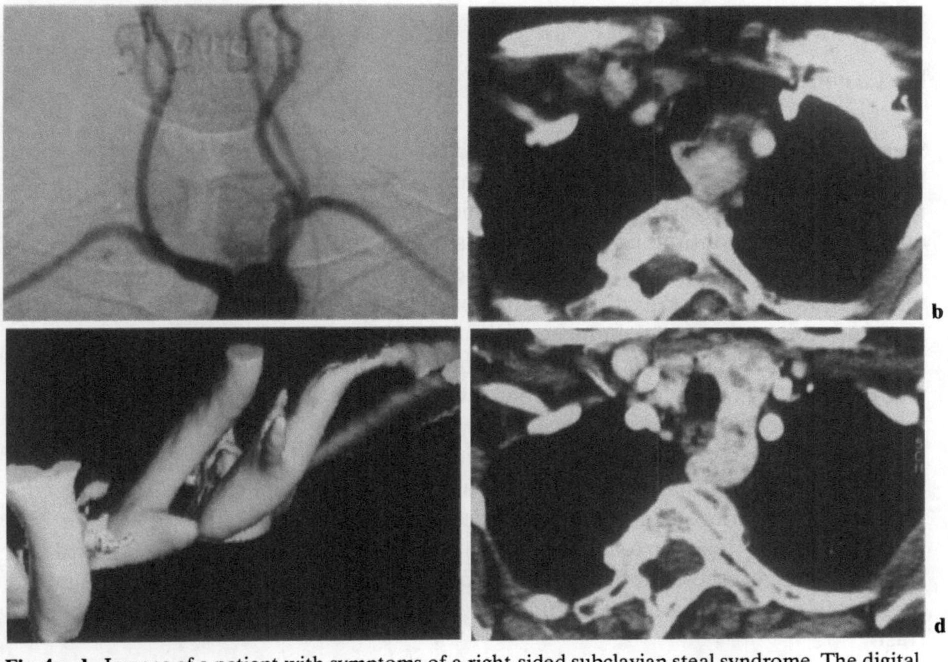

a b c d

Fig. 4a–d. Images of a patient with symptoms of a right-sided subclavian steal syndrome. The digital subtraction angiography (DSA) image suggests the diagnosis, although no unobscured view could be obtained. Injection of contrast media into the cubital vein led to marked streak artifacts (**b**). Images obtained after injection of contrast into the femoral vein (**c**) were used for 3D reconstructions (**d**) that easily demonstrate the circular stenosis of the subclavian artery with poststenotic dilatation provided by spiral CT. Intravasal pathology, like membranes or thrombi, as well as adjacent extravasal lesions can be clearly demonstrated. Because overlapping cross-sectional images basically contain all the diagnostic information, 2D and 3D images provide additional information only in selected cases. Review of the cross-sectional scans in a cine mode can simplify the evaluation of tortuous vascular structures. Clinical examples include aortic dissections or neoplastic disease.

In patients with aortic dissections, spiral CT not only demonstrates the presence of a membrane in the ascending aorta (thus distinguishing a type A from a type B dissection), but is also able to show the entry of the false lumen and to determine an involvement of the supraaortic or visceral branches (Fig. 3).

In neoplastic disease, the good contrast of vessels and adjacent soft tissues is able to improve staging and treatment planning. A displacement, obstruction, or encasement can easily be appreciated. For the diagnosis of infiltrations, however, the same limitations are true as for standard CT: An infiltration is suggested by irregular borders, intravasal material, and alterations in vessel diameter. The lack of these findings, however, does not exclude them.

The second group of clinical applications includes those cases that benefit from 3D reconstructions. Complex vascular situations may not always be sufficiently visualized by standard radiographic techniques. Using 3D imaging, optimal projections can be obtained with arbitrary angles, even if such views are not possible with conventional techniques (Fig. 4).

Discussion

Spiral CT proved to be superior to standard CT in the detection of lesions that rapidly change along the patient's longitudinal axis. Due to partial volume effects or a varying depth of inspiration, they may be missed on standard CT. Both effects can be overcome by the continuous volume acquisition of spiral CT.

For vascular imaging, spiral CT combines the advantages of angio-CT with that of incremental scanning. Potential advantages over the incremental dynamic CT technique are the continuous volume acquisition, a shorter scan time, and a continuously higher contrast. Clinical applications that benefit from these diagnostic potentials include aortic dissections and the preoperative staging of the anatomic relationship between the vasculature and neoplasms.

The need for continuous scanning drives the tube load to its limit. Especially for the long scan times that are most often used in clinical applications, the tube current has to be reduced to 75–165 mA (depending on slice thickness). Thus, a 24-s spiral CT usually leads to a decrease of patient dose as compared with standard CT. In most clinical cases, the increase in image noise (in comparison with standard examinations) can be compensated for by a signal increase due to higher vessel contrast.

The most striking advantage of spiral CT for vascular imaging is its potential for smooth multiplanar 2D and 3D reconstructions. The ability to interactively rotate 3D images in arbitrary, even unusual directions provides a clear visual concept of the anatomy. The 3D visualization may considerably simplify preoperative planning [3].

With spiral CT, there is a trade-off between 3D image distortion and length of the scan volume, both of which are closely dependent upon slice thickness and table feed. In most clinical settings, we found a table feed and slice thickness of 5 mm to be the best compromise. The table feed should be equal or only slightly larger than the selected slice thickness. A 8-mm slice profile leads to considerable image distorsion along the z-axis and appeared to be only suited for vessels (and pathology) perpendicular to the scan plane, e. g., a thrombus in the inferior vena cava. For small pathology in vessels running parallel to the scan plane, such as a stenosis in renal arteries or the subclavian artery, 2–3-mm scans should be used.

Next to the slice profile, image distortion depends on the size and contrast of the examined structure and on the threshold level used. In clinical cases, the threshold has to be chosen larger than the CT values of the surrounding soft tissues. As a result, the threshold is relatively high, and distorsion along the z-axis is not so much a problem as the pseudo-defects and lack of visualization of smaller vessels.

The ultimate role of spiral CT as a minimally invasive vascular imaging method in comparison with MR angiography still has to be evaluated.

References

1. Kalender WA, Seissler W, Klotz E, Vock P (1990) Spiral volumetric CT with single-breath-hold technique, continuous transport, and continuous scanner rotation. Radiology 176: 181–183
2. Kalender WA, Vock P, Polacin A, Soucek M (1990) Spiral CT: Eine Technik für Volumenaufnahmen. I. Grundlagen und Methodik. Rontgenpraxis 43: 323–330
3. Edwards FH, Wind G, Thompson I, Bellamy RF, Barry MJ, Schaefer PS (1990) Three-dimensional image reconstruction for planning of a complex cardiovascular procedure. Ann Thorac Surgery 49: 486–489

Spiral CT in the Preoperative Evaluation of Vessels of the Upper Abdomen

W. Bautz, H. Helmberger, M. Strotzer, M. Lenz, and P. Gerhardt

Introduction

Computed tomography (CT) plays an outstanding role in the diagnostic imaging of the upper abdomen. In many cases, therapeutic decisions are in part made on the findings of this examination. Diagnostic interest not only concentrates on the classification of pathological processes, but also on the evaluation of their operability.

Information concerning the localization and expansion of a process as well as possible complications (e.g., metastases) are important for solving clinical objectives. These findings can usually be displayed clearly with CT. A weakness of CT, however, has been the identification of such vascular complications as may result from tumor infiltration, for example. This kowledge may play an important role in therapeutic decisions. Preoperative planning would naturally be simplified if the vascular conditions and standard variations were known. Angiography of the vessels of the upper abdomen in the form of a celiacoportography and mesentericoportography are therefore often required additionally before surgery of the pancreas or liver. This may be supplemented by a survey aortography and cavography at the option of the therapist. Here, the most frequent clinical objectives (Table 1) are to clarify the anatomical relationships and to find the possibly infiltrative expansion of a process. With this in mind, the arterial supply of the liver and the anatomy of the gastroduodenal artery must be known, for instance, before initiating local chemotherapy. It is very important to know the relationship of malignant masses to the functional segments of the liver and the involvement of larger vascular structures in these masses before resection. The celiac artery, hepatic arteries, superior mesenteric artery, and the portal system may play a special role here.

The diagnosis of blood vessels with conventional CT is made more difficult because no contiguous coverage of the region of examination is guaranted. Contrast medium concentrations in the vessels are irregular and usually too low in the course of examinations with long procedural times. Spiral CT for the first time permits a contiguous evaluation of the organe of the upper abdomen during one apneic phase

Table 1. Preoperative diagnosis of vessels of the upper abdomen: frequent clinical objectives

- Tumor infiltration?
- Vascular supply of the tumor?
- Thrombosis of the portal vein?
- Standard vascular variations?
- Segmental anatomy of the liver?

[3]. High contrast medium concentrations allowing good imaging quality can also be attained in the blood vessels.

The present investigation is designed to determine whether and in which cases spiral CT might replace digital subtraction angiography (DSA; celiacography and mesentericography).

Material and Methods

In a prospective study, 45 patients underwent both a spiral CT and an arterial DSA examination preoperatively. The population included 16 pancreas tumors, 8 liver metastases, 7 carcinomas of the choledochus, 5 cases of pancreatic involvement, 5 hepatocellular carcinomas, 3 benign stenoses of the choledochus, and 1 duodenal carcinoma. Conventional CTs had been performed on 17 of these patients using various systems and for the most part at other institutions.

The most important imaging and evaluation parameters for spiral CT are summarized in Table 2. The patients drank 500–1000 ml of diluted iodine-containing contrast medium (3% meglumine diatrizoate) a minimum of $^1/_2$ an hour before the examination in order to visualize the stomach and small intestine. A further 250 ml of 3% meglumine diatrizoate was given directly before the examination in order to ensure adequate filling of the duodenum and thereby improve the differentiation from the head of the pancreas. After positioning the patient and locating the region of examination, intravenous injection of 200 ml iopamidol (300 mg I/ml, Solutrast-300, Byk-Gulden Co., Constance, FRG) was performed automatically 120 s before starting the spiral CT. We used a microprocessor-controlled infusion pump (CT Injektor XC 5500, Ulrich Co., Ulm, FRG) which permitted a programmed flow of contrast medium. The rate of infusion varied between 1 and 3 ml/s during the examination. The spiral CT was performed during an expiratory apneic phase of the patient in 24 s using a table feed of 10 mm/s. Reconstruction of the CT images proceeded immediately after collecting the data sample with a nominal slice thickness of 10 mm and a slice interval of 2 or 5 mm.

A celiacography and mesentericography was performed on all patients using the usual DSA technique (Polytron, Siemens AG). Selective probing of the celiac and the superior mesenteric artery was performed with a 5 F or 7 F sidewinder catheter. During each scan series 25–35 ml of contrast medium was injected automatically at a rate of 5–6 ml/s.

Two radiologist evaluated hardcopy documents of the spiral CT and DSA examinations. Displays of the most important vascular regions (celiac artery, common

Table 2. Spiral CT of the upper abdomen: technique

- CT unit: Somatom Plus-S
- 120 kV, 165 mA, 10 mm slice thickness
- Data acquisition: 24 s contiguous
- Table feed: 10 mm/s
- Contrast medium: 200 ml, 1–3 ml/s
- Image reconstruction with 2 or 5 mm slice intervals

hepatic artery, gastroduodenal artery, splenic artery, superior mesenteric artery, splenic vein, superior mesenteric vein, portal vein) were evaluated according to a diagnostically oriented evaluation schema. The individual responsible for the evaluation then had to establish whether the vessel was normal (= 1), likely to be normal (= 2), unkown (= 3), likely to be pathological (= 4), or definitely pathological (= 5). The type of change (e.g., displacement, infiltration, obstruction) was recorded.

Results

In four of the 45 patients, spiral CT revealed a lymphoma or a tumor surrounding the region of the celiac artery and a tumor surrounding the superior mesenteric artery in two cases. These findings were not recognized with DSA since the vascular lumen was unchanged. The spiral CT was seen to be superior to conventional CT in three cases.

Spiral CT revealed an infiltration of a liver metastasis into the portal vein in one case which could not be seen with DSA. The portal vein could not be diagnosed unequivocally in one case because of a large, highly vascularized gastrinoma in the head of the pancreas. Spiral CT revealed a portal vein with no pathological findings, a finding which was confirmed intraoperatively. In comparison with conventional CT, spiral CT additionally revealed an infiltration or compression of the portal vein in four cases.

A spasm of the superior mesenteric artery simulated an infiltration of the vessel by a tumor of the pancreas in one case. The spiral CT revealed normal findings with a distinct interval evident between the tumor and the vessel.

According to our experiences to date, standard variations in the vascular system can only be recognized with DSA. Three cases in which the right hepatic artery originated from the superior mesenteric artery were found in our patient population. Spiral CT revealed a suspicion of such a variation in two cases. The verification and interpretation of complex changes and small-caliber vessels in the sectional images were difficult or even impossible.

Imaging of the gastroduodenal artery with the described spiral CT technique was only sufficiently reliable in the region of the vessel's origin. Problems could be encountered in the differentiation of the common hepatic artery and the proper hepatic artery from the portal vein.

The vascular supply of a tumor can only be defined reliably with angiography, since spiral CT cannot resolve the fine vessels of the tumor. Only DSA displays the hemodynamics of a vessel or a mass adequately. Spiral CT is equal and in some cases even superior to angiography for verifying thromboses of the portal vein. Study of the collateral circulation revealed the same findings as standard variations of the vascular system.

The segmental anatomy of the liver can be displayed adequately with spiral CT (Fig. 2 a).

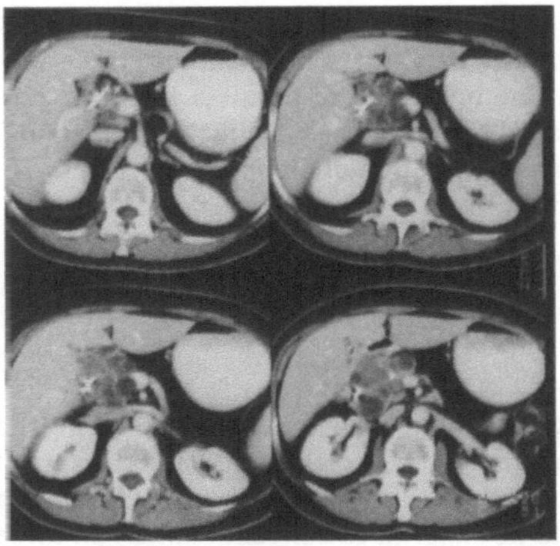

a

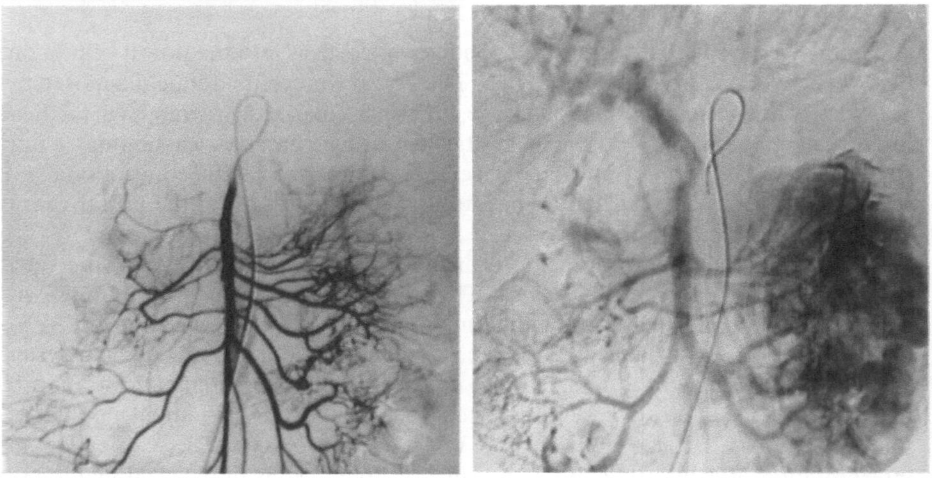

b

Fig. 1. a, b. Cystadenoma of the pancreas. Spiral CT (**a**) shows that the tumor surrounds the superior mesenteric vein and the confluence of the portal vein. Mesentericoportography (**b**) confirms these findings and provides no additional information

Discussion

An advantage of CT over DSA was seen in the fact that CT provides nonoverlapping anatomical slices. All vascular regions in the plane of section can be displayed simultaneously with their spatial relationship to the primary processes (Fig. 1). Results in our patient population reveal that more than 10% of the cases involved the incorporation of the celiac artery, the main trunk of the superior mesenteric artery, or the superior portal vein in a mass. This was not recognized with DSA since no constriction of the vascular lumen was present. Such findings are very important for therapeutic planning since surgical therapy will often prove to be superfluous. Because of the contiguous evaluation of the entire upper abdomen, with its nearly unchanging vascular and soft tissue contrast and its independence of reproducible respiratory position, spiral CT also demonstrates advantages over conventional CT here as well. With DSA, such highly vascular processes as hormonally active tumors, for instance,

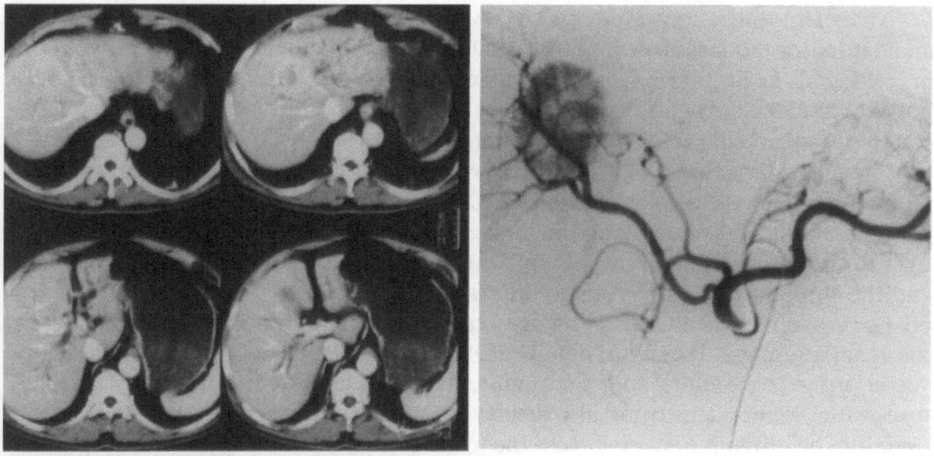

a b

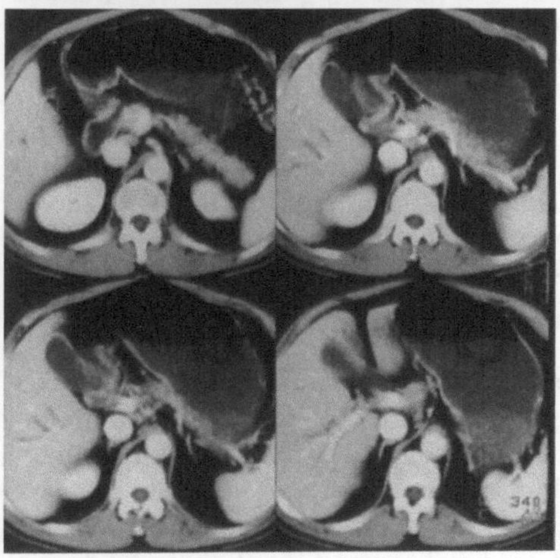

c

Fig. 2 a–c. Hepatocellular carcinoma. Spiral CT provides an exact display of the segmental anatomy of the liver. The course of the middle intersegmental vein reveals that the tumor is associated with both liver segment IV and VIII. The DSA study (**b**) confirms this finding. Additionally, the celiacography shows that the right hepatic artery originates from the celiac artery. This finding is especially important in the event of local chemotherapy. This standard variation is only realisable on the spiral CT (**c**) together with the knowledge of the DSA

can obscure a display of vessels or impair imaging of the vessels to such an extent that diagnostically valuable information is no longer available for evaluation. Even oblique projections may not always solve this problem. In such cases, spiral CT is clearly superior to DSA.

Sectional slice imaging of vessels also has its disadvantages, since it is difficult for the individual responsible for evaluation to follow the course of a vessel in the CT series, and small changes in the caliber of vascular lumina are therefore difficult to recognize.

Evaluation of the spiral CT is simplified by regarding the examination in the cine mode on the monitor of the console or at a workstation. Angiography generally displays the course of a vessel with its branches and changes in luminal diameter clearly in one single image. Standard variations in vascular anatomy can usually only be assumed with spiral CT when large-diameter vessels are involved. More complex variations can only be defined with angiography (Fig. 2b, c). This is practically only of special importance for liver surgery and for local chemotherapy, e.g., via a port.

An exact localization of the findings with a relationship to the liver segments is mandatory for modern liver surgery [2]. Definition of the liver segments is based on branching of the portal vein and the course of the hepatic veins. Using spiral CT, it is possible to make a diagnosis with practical significance, since both of these vascular systems can be recognized with this technique.

The great disadvantage of spiral CT over DSA is the reduced spatial resolution seen especially in the display of small vessels. Imaging a vessel with CT is not only dependent on the vessel diameter, the iodine concentration of the vessel, and the contrast to the surroundings, but also on the course of the vessel in the scanning plane and the subsequent partial-volume effects. These partial-volume effects do not appear or are minimal if the vessel progresses perpendicular or nearly perpendicular to the scanning plane. However, detail resolution can be reduced substantially if the vessel progresses parallel to the scanning plane and in certain cases in which structures with a higher density are also displayed in the direct vicinity of the vessel. It can therefore be difficult or even impossible to differentiate the common and proper hepatic arteries from the portal vein. For this reason, a celiacography will always be necessary when planning a port for local chemotherapy by way of the gastroduodenal artery.

The partial-volume effects can be reduced by using thinner slices. At the present time, this would mean a reduction in the measurement volume of the longitudinal axis of the body from 24 cm with a slice thickness of 10 mm, to 12 cm for 5-mm slices, for example. The image quality is also poorer because of increased image noise. Among other things, an improvement in slice profiles (a nominal slice thickness of 10 mm presently represents an effective thickness of 13 mm) is an advancement which can be expected in the future.

The intravenous administration of contrast medium is a technique which has gained importance for the diagnosis of vessels with spiral CT. However, the temporal course of contrast medium administration must be adapted to the circulatory characteristics of individual vascular regions and organs, and these are especially complex in the region of the liver. Since the portal circulation is responsible for about 75% for the circulation of the liver parenchyma [1], maximal contrast is not observed during the arterial phase, about 20 s after bolus contrast medium injection but instead after about 40 s, during the venoportal phase. The best display of hepatic foci is therefore 40–90 s after bolus administration. Since liver tumors over 1 cm in diameter are nearly all supplied arterially [4], the hypervascularization of these structures can only be perceived during the short arterial phase, 20–40 s after bolus administration. For the vessels of the liver, this implies that there are about 20 s between the maximal contrast of the hepatic arteries and that of the portal vein, for example. It can therefore be seen that any contrast medium administration represents a compromise, not only with respect to contrast of soft tissue structures, but also for the contrast of blood vessels. The type of i. v. contrast medium administration selected here provides a high tissue contrast and a relatively uniform contrast in all vessels. Further experiments will show whether the technique of contrast medium administration can be optimized. At any rate, automatic contrast medium administration is mandatory to ensure reproducible results. In the future, it is possible that certain cases will require two spiral CT examinations whith varying techniques of contrast medium administration. This is presently impossible because of the extensive time required.

References

1. Clark RA, Matsui O (1983) CT of liver tumors. Semin Roentgenol 18: 149–162
2. Claussen C, Lochner B (1983) Dynamische Computertomographie. Springer, Berlin Heidelberg New York
3. Kalender WA, Vock P, Seissler W (1990) Spiral CT scanning for fast and continuous volume data aquisition. In: Fuchs WA (ed.) Advances in CT. Springer, Berlin Heidelberg New York, pp 55–64
4. Lien WM, Ackerman NB (1970) The blood supply of experimental liver metastasis. Surgery 68: 334
5. Marchal GJ, Baert AL, Wilms GE (1980) CT of noncystic liver lesions: bolus enhancement. AJR 135: 57–65
6. Sugarbaker PH (1990) Surgical decision making for large bowel cancer metastatic to the liver. Radiology 174: 612–626

Spiral CT of the Liver: First Clinical Results

U. Keske, C. Zwicker, M. Langer, R. Langer, K. Rosenkranz, P. Neuhaus, and R. Felix

Introduction

In computed tomography (CT) systems with a continuately rotating tube and detector system, spiral CT has become available as a supportive method to fast dynamic CT [5, 6, 9]. Spiral CT enables us to scan a volume of 23 cm in length in a time of 24 s. Thus, the whole upper body may be scanned in a single breath hold. The method seems suitable to examine the early, mostly arterial perfusion phase of the entire liver in a single scan. In addition, the method might reduce breathing artifacts. The aim of this study was to examine which additional possibilities spiral CT offers compared with dynamic CT for the examination of the liver.

Patients and Methods

In all, 87 patients with a mean age of 42.5 years were examined (42 male, 25 female). CT was performed as part of a clinical check-up with a Somatom Plus (Siemens). Fourteen patients were examined as part of a routine follow-up after liver transplantation, 23 patients had liver cirrhosis and were being examined before liver transplantation, and 50 patients were examined in the search for a focal liver lesion.

Native CT was performed with a slice thickness of 10 mm and at a 10-mm scanning interval at 210 mA, 120 kV, and a scanning time of 1 s. Spiral CT was performed with 24 tube rotations and a slice thickness of 8 or 10 mm; the table increment varied between 7 and 10 mm. Due to the limited tube capacity, the 10-mm slices have to be performed at 85 mA and the 8-mm slices at 125 mA, resulting in a total of 2040 mA (10 mm) or 3000 mA (8 mm). Image reconstruction was performed with overlapping slices (interval 6 mm with 8-mm slices or 8 mm with 10-mm-slices). The movement artifacts caused by the continuous table movement are corrected by a special algorithm (linear interpolation [8, 9]. This leads to an enlarged slice thickness (for example, from nominally 10 mm to 13 mm). Starting 15 s before sanning, 100 ml contrast medium (cm) were injected at a flow rate of 3 ml/s into a cubital vein. A computer supported injection pump (XD 100, Ulrich) with nonionic contrast medium (Ultravist 370, Schering AG) was used. Angio-CT without the table increment were performed at the level of the intrahepatic portal vein or of focal liver lesions. An injection of 80 ml contrast medium at a rate of 4 ml/s was started. Ten seconds later, 15 scans with an interval of 2 s and afterwards single scans over 60 s with an interval of 10 s and further scans 120, 180 and 300 s p.i. were performed (scanning time always 1 s, compare [11]).

Dynamic CT scans with table increment were performed after an i.v. injection of 100 ml contrast medium with a flow of 1 ml/s and the scanning parameters described for native CT. Scanning was started 30 s after beginning the injection.

In a subgroup of 47 patients, all three contrast-enhanced methods were used. In order to remain below the limit of 200 ml contrast medium per day, the last contrast-enhanced CT was performed 24 or 48 h after the first two. Evaluation was performed independently by three examiners.

Results

Hepatic Artery

In spiral CT ($n = 87$), imaging of the intrahepatic segment of the hepatic artery was good in 48.3% and very good in 33.3% (Fig. 1). The extrahepatic segment was visualized well in 28.7% and very well in 71.3%. In angio-CT without table increment

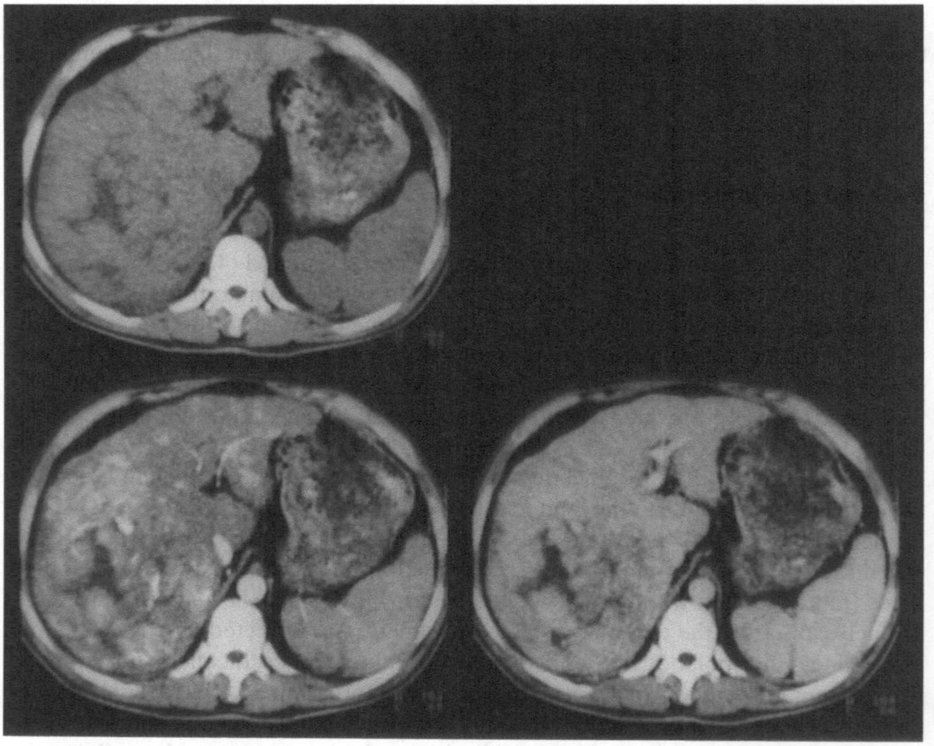

Fig. 1. A 50-year-old patient with liver cirrhosis and multifocal hepatocellular carcinoma. *Upper,* Native CT shows a hypodense lesion in the right liver lobe, which represents the tumor necosis. *Lower left,* Spiral CT reveals a large tumor in the right liver lobe and additional hyperperfused tumor manifestations in the left liver lobe. Note the good visualization of the intrahepatic segment of the hepatic artery. Lower right, Dynamic CT displays the tumor in the right liver lobe, but fails to show the involvement of the left liver lobe

Table 1. Documentation of the hepatic artery in spiral CT and angio-CT

	Poor	Good	Very good
Documentation in spiral CT ($n = 87$)			
Hepatic artery (extrahepatic)	0	25 (28.7%)	62 (71.3%)
Hepatic artery (intrahepatic)	16 (18.4%)	42 (48.3%)	29 (33.3%)
Peripheral segments	70 (80.5%)	17 (19.5%)	0
Documentation in angio-CT ($n = 29$)			
Hepatic artery (extrahepatic)	12 (41.4%)	7 (24.1%)	10 (34.5%)
Hepatic artery (intrahepatic)	6 (20.7%)	4 (13.8%)	19 (65.5%)
Peripheral segments	21 (72.4%)	8 (27.6%)	0
Documentation in spiral CT compared with angio-CT ($n = 18$)			
Hepatic artery (extrahepatic)	3 (10.0%)	8 (26.7%)	19 (63.3%)
Hepatic artery (intrahepatic)	16 (50.0%)	8 (26.7%)	7 (23.3%)
Peripheral segments	7 (23.3%)	20 (66.7%)	3 (10.0%)

($n = 29$), the intrahepatic segment of the hepatic artery was seen more reliably (65.5% very good, 13.8% good). The extrahepatic segment was seen less well (34.5% very good, 24.1% good), since it was mostly out of the imaging plane, which was chosen over the intrahepatic portal vein. Peripheral segments of the hepatic artery were seen better on angio-CT than on spiral CT (seen in 27.6% and 19.5%, respectively; Table 1).

The liver parenchyma showed almost no enhancement on the first spiral images (enhancement of an average of 4.7 HU after 2 s), whereas the later images showed a minute enhancement (8.6 HU after 12 s, 15 HU after 23 s; $n = 55$). Liver enhancement was much higher on dynamic CT (an average of 46.6 HU was found after 12 s, 71.5 HU after 120 s; $n = 35$). The portal vein and the liver veins were not contrasted during spiral CT.

Focal Liver Lesions

Focal liver lesions were seen in 29 patients. Thirteen had a hepatocellular carcinoma (four multifocal), 11 patients had liver metastases (four multifocal, etiology was colon carcinoma, $n = 7$; and mammary carcinoma, $n = 4$), and 5 patients had a cholangiocarcinoma.

In spiral CT, the hepatocellular carcinomas were visualized very well in 11/13 cases and well in 2/13 cases (15.4%). Thus, visualization was slightly worse than with angio-CT (very good in 8/8 cases). In dynamic CT, the tumors are visualized hypodense to the surrounding liver. Visualization was very good in 11/16 cases (84.6%), good in 4/16 (30.8%), and poor in 1/16 cases (7.7%). Hyperperfusion could only be demonstrated on spiral or angio-CT. Spiral CT provided advantages over angio-CT, since angio-CT could document hyperperfusion only in one slice, whereas spiral CT could document it over the whole organ. Furthermore, spiral CT showed more tumor lesions than angio-CT or dynamic CT in 10 patients (54 compared with 35 lesions; Fig. 1). Thus, spiral CT offers a higher sensitivity for the documentation of hepatocellular tumor lesions in the liver than the other CT methods.

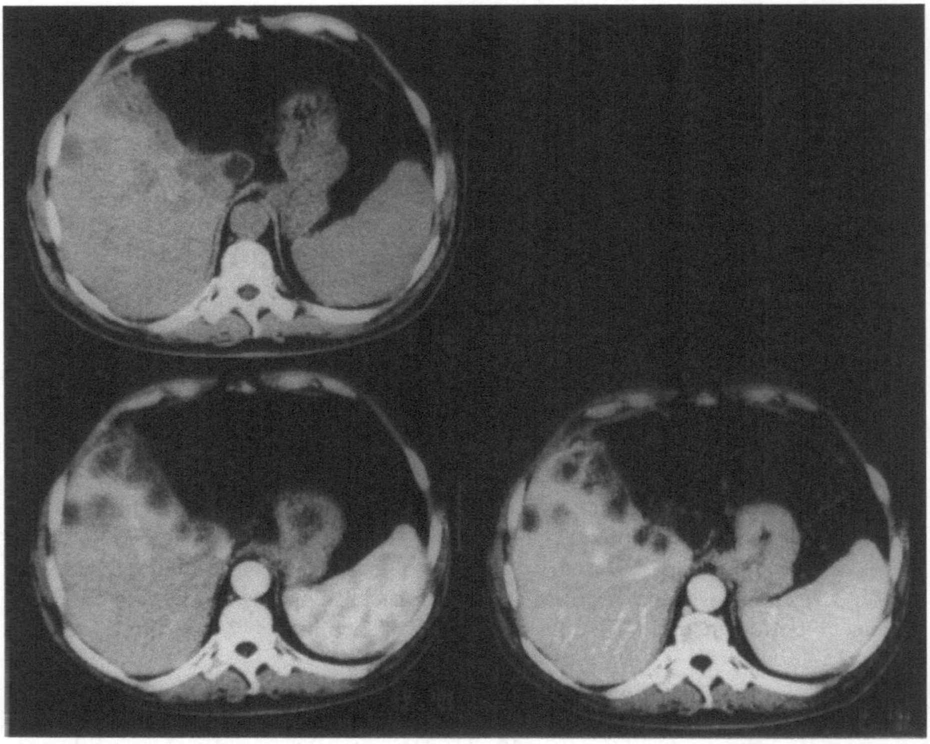

Fig. 2. A 64-year-old patient with colon carcinoma and multiple liver metastases. *Upper,* Native CT shows multiple liver lesions. *Lower left,* Improved imaging in spiral CT (10-mm slice thickness). *Lower right,* Excellent imaging of the metastases in dynamic CT with intermittent table movement, which shows best a hypervascular rim

For liver metastases and cholangiocarcinomas, spiral CT showed no advantages over the other contrast-enhanced CT methods. Both are hypovascularized liver tumors. For liver metastases, dynamic CT showed the best image quality (72.2% very good, 27.3% good; spiral CT: 27.3% very good, 63.6% good) and highest sensitivity (superior to spiral CT in 81.8%). In 8 cases, spiral CT showed a small hypervascular rim around the metastases; the rim was visible in 5 dynamic CTs (compare Fig. 2). In cholangiocarcinomas, dynamic CT with table increment was superior to all other methods, especially unenhanced CT (image quality very good in 5/5 cases; spiral CT: very good in 4/5 and good in 1/5 cases).

Spiral CTs show more scattered radiation and a decreased spatial resolution (compare Fig. 2). For the detection of small lesions, such as cysts or tumors that are relatively isodense to the liver, spiral CT has advantages over CT with intermittent table movement in uncooperative patients, who cannot or can only inconstantly follow the breathing commands. Here, the fast data acquisition in a single breath hold made in a few cases ($n = 3$) small lesions visible that were not seen on dynamic CT with intermittent table movement, since they were moved out of the plane as a consequence of inconstant breathing.

Discussion

Spiral CT is a supplementary method to angio-CT and dynamic CT for the investigation of liver perfusion. In 76.9%, spiral CT showed more tumor lesions than dynamic CT. This makes spiral CT a valuable method for the evaluation of patients before liver transplantation or partial liver resection, when the tumor extent or additional tumor manifestations need to be documented.

For the imaging of liver metastases, spiral CT has no advantages over dynamic CT. This is caused by the hypoperfusion of most metastases, which makes them best seen in the portal venous contrast phase. Only occasionally do they possess a hyperperfused rim [4, 7], which could be demonstrated more often on spiral CT than on dynamic CT. However, spiral CT may be helpful in hyperperfused metastases. This rare perfusion type is known for carcinoids, islet cell tumors, pheochromocytomas, and hypernephromas [1].

Angio-CT remains the method of choice for the detection of tumor etiology [3, 8, 11]. This technique enables the detection of hypervascularization, which characterizes lesions such as hepatocellular carcinomas or focal-nodular hyperplasia [4]. Spiral CT may give additional information since it may show hyperperfusion of liver lesions on more than a single CT slice.

The lower spatial resolution and a higher radiation scatter of spiral CT [9] are in most cases disadvantageous in the detection of very small liver lesions or lesions that are almost isodense to the liver. However, the fast data acquisition with spiral CT is helpful in patients who cannot or only inadequately hold their breath. In these patients, the detection of small lesions may be improved.

For the spiral CTs performed in this study, contrast injection was started 15 s before scanning. The portal venous system and the liver veins are not contrasted during the time of scanning. This was relevant in the patients examined since the documentation of the free perfusion of the portal vein is highly relevant in patients before and after liver transplantation [2, 10]. Thus, spiral CT cannot replace dynamic CT with intermittent table movement or angio-CT without table movement.

Conclusions

1. Spiral CT offers a reliable, noninvasive documentation of the central arterial system of the liver.
2. Spiral CT may show hypervascular tumors, such as hepatocellular carcinomas, with higher sensitivity than native CT, dynamic CT, or angio-CT.
3. Spiral CT is a supplementary method to native CT, dynamic CT, and angio-CT with additional information especially in hypervascularized liver lesions.
4. In most cases, dynamic CT or angio-CT remain necessary for the documentation of the portal vein and the portal venous phase of liver enhancement.

References

1. Bressler EL, Alpern MB, Glazer GM, Francis IR (1987) Hypervascular hepatic metastases: CT evaluation. Radiology 162: 49–51
2. Dalen K, Day DL, Ascher NL, Hunter DW, Thompson WM, Castaneda-Zuniga WRC, Letourneau JG (1988) Imaging of vascular complications after hepatic transplantation. AJR 150: 1285–1290
3. Freeny PC, Marks WM (1986) Patterns of contrast enhancement of benign and malignant hepatic neoplasms during bolus dynamic and delayed CT. Radiology 160: 613
4. Grabbe E, Bücheler E (1988) Diagnostik von Lebererkrankungen. In: Frommhold W (ed) Radiologische Diagnostik in Klinik und Praxis, Gastrointestinaltrakt II. Thieme, Stuttgart, pp 1-99
5. Hupke R (1990) The advantages of fast and continuously rotating CT systems. In: Fuchs WA (ed) Advances in CT. Springer, Berlin Heidelberg New York, pp 3–15
6. Kalender WA, Seißler W, Klotz E, Vock P (1990) Single breathholding spiral volumetric computed tomography (SVCT) by continuous patient translation and scanner rotation. Radiology 176: 181–183
7. Kober B, Gamroth A, Hermann HJ, zum Winkel K, Mende U, Kimming B (1983) Angio CT: Eine Erweiterung der Diagnostik maligner Leberprozesse. Fortschr Rontgenstr 139: 260–266
8. Kurtz B (1988) Leberdiagnostik I: Dynamische CT-Studien. In: Claussen CR, Felix R (ed) Quo Vadis CT? Springer, Berlin Heidelberg New York, pp 146–165
9. Rigauts H, Marchal G, Baert AL, Hupke R (1990) Spiral scanning: phantom studies and patient material. In: Fuchs WA (ed) Advances in CT. Springer, Berlin Heidelberg New York, pp 65–76
10. Zwicker C, Langer M, Felix R (1990) Computertomographie nach Lebertransplantation. Fortschr Rontgenstr 153 (4): 357–494
11. Zwicker C, Langer M, Astinet F, Langer R, Urich V, Felix R (1990) Differenzierung maligner Lebertumore mit schneller dynamischer CT. Fortschr Rontgenstr 152 (3): 293–302

Spiral CT of the Pelvic Organs

M. Oldendorf, P. Weber, R. Böhlke, and E. Zeitler

Introduction

Many tumors of the pelvis remain clinically quiescent for a long time. They can therefore first become manifest after having reached an advanced clinical stage. It is important for the operating surgeon to be given information concerning extension of the tumor and its relationship to the neighboring organs. The spiral computed tomography (CT) technique permits volumetric measurement in which overlapping image presentation enables secondary sagittal and coronary reformation. A report of experiences gained in the diagnosis of pelvic tumors using spiral CT in 30 patients follows.

Material and Methods

Thirty patients with tumorous processes of the minor pelvis were examined and subsequently evaluated with CT using the Somatom Plus-S and the spiral CT technique. Twenty-two patients were found to be in a substantially reduced general state of health, with severe symptoms of pain as well as fecal and urinary incontinence.

Two standard spiral measurements were performed per patient. The purely volumetric times were 32 s for one spiral procedure. The maximal tube loading was taken advantage of for each spiral measurement. The first spiral examination began on the upper border of the liver and was performed with the maximal scanning time of 32 s and resulted in a total scanning path of 32 cm, using a slice thickness of 10 mm. In order to achieve this measured scan path, the tube current must be limited to 165 mA.

A second spiral CT measurement followed directly and was compared with this first spiral examination. Here, a smaller slice thickness of 5 mm was selected in order to improve the detail resolution. With the same low current of 165 mA, an additional scan path of 16 cm could thus be attained. In order to reduce the examination time as much as possible for the patients, the data attained were stored individually as raw data sets and only reformatted to image data after the examination had been completed.

Each patient received an intravenous drip of contrast medium (70 ml of a nonionic contrast medium over a period of approximately 10 min) to ensure an optimal filling of the urinary bladder. An additional bolus administration of 25 ml contrast medium was performed on the examination table before each spiral examination in order to optimize contrast of the abdominal arteries. The full examination time, during which the patient must lie still upon the CT table, is thereby reduced to about 4.5 min: positioning of the patient (30 s), performance of the tomogram (60 s), loading of the spiral mode (30 s), first spiral measurement (32 s), data collection for the first spiral examination (approximately 90 s), performance of the second spiral examination (32 s). The subsequent image reconstruction was performed between the individual patients (time required: 10–15 min).

In oder to improve the detail resolution, overlapping image sequences were reformatted from the individual raw data sets: We selected an overlap of 5 mm for slice thicknesses of 10 mm in the first spiral examination and an overlap of 2 mm for slice thicknesses of 5 mm in the second spiral examination. A total of between 98 and 112 individual images was produced for each patient with the possibility of good sagittal and coronary image reconstructions. Image documentation was performed with an Agfa laser camera.

Results

Thirty patients were examined with the spiral CT technique. Twelve patients had tumors in the region of the urinary bladder, six had tumors of the prostate (exclusively prostate carcinomas), six had a tumor of the female genitals (ovary), four patients had tumors originating in the rectum or anus, and two had soft tissue sarcomas.

The criterion aimed for was the determination of tumor expansion, classified according to the TNM system (UICC). A direct comparision could be performed between the operative findings and the CT diagnosis in patients who underwent surgery.

Ten of the 12 patients with tumors of the urinary bladder underwent surgery, and nine of them revealed an agreement of the diagnosed stage and the operative findings, whereby an exact differentiation between stage T1 (invasion of the lamina propria) and stage T2 (superficial invasion of the muscle) or stage T3a (deep invasion of the muscle) was not possible. One patient had a substantially trabeculated bladder as well as a carcinoma in situ (T1s). Here, suspicion of a T2 tumor was expressed after examination with CT. Evaluation of the posterior wall of the urinary bladder, the perivascular fatty tissue and the form and size of the seminal vesicles, as important in-

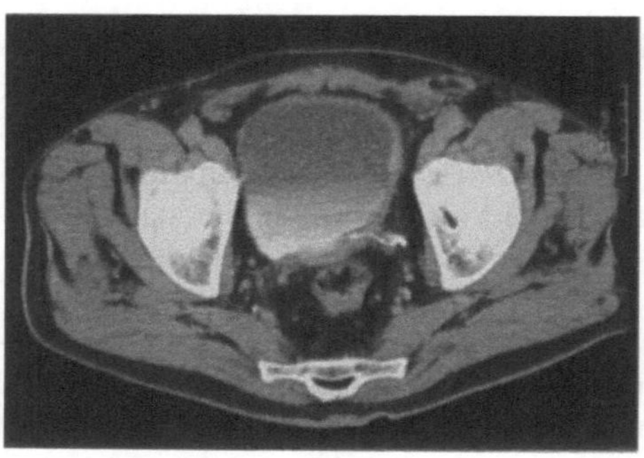

Fig. 1. A 71-year-old man with carcinoma of the urinary bladder, pT1N0M0, histologically no infiltration of the muscular structures, clearly visible left ostium of the ureter

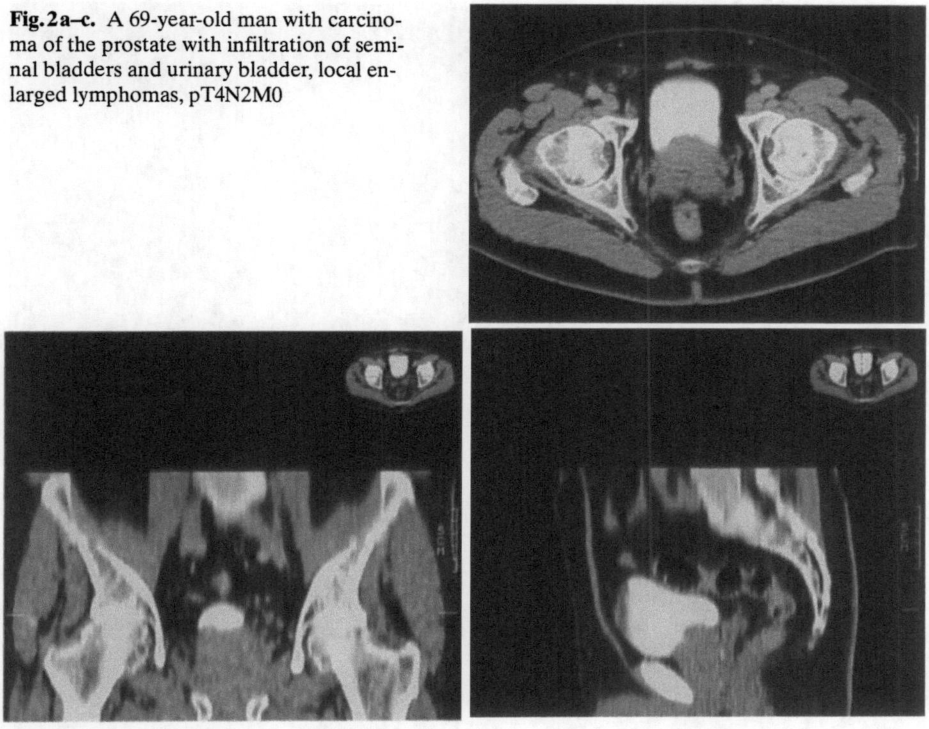

Fig. 2 a–c. A 69-year-old man with carcinoma of the prostate with infiltration of seminal bladders and urinary bladder, local enlarged lymphomas, pT4N2M0

dications for the resectability of the tumor, could be performed well to very well in all patients (Fig. 1).

The six patients with tumors of the prostate all had histologically verified carcinomas; paraaortal lymph node metastases were found in only one patient (pT3N4MO). If the tumor growth does not extend beyond the capsule (stage T1 = small node maximally 1.5 cm in size, stage T2 = tumor larger than 1.5 cm without capsule involvement), a differentiation between T1 and T2 is not possible. An evaluation of the tumor extension with respect to the seminal vesicles as well as to the periprostatic fatty tissue was nevertheless clearly possible (stage T3 or T4. Fig. 2).

Six female patients were examined for the suspicion of tumors in the region iof the ovaries. Five had an ovarial carcinoma (four cystadenocarcinomas and one chorionepithelioma), one had a stenosis of the ureter at the level of the ovary brought about by the regional inflammatory reaction to a pathological vascular finding. A differentiation of stage T1 (tumor limited to one ovary) from stage T2 tumors (both ovaries involved and tumor growth extends beyond the ovary and into the minor pelvis) is possible with spiral CT. Using spiral CT and with the help of an arterial bolus injection of contrast medium, changes in the iliac lymph nodes can be recognized and distinguished clearly from vascular structures. The ascites which is already seen in stage pT1c of ovarial carcinomas can be recognized at early stages with CT and is additional information to the other findings. Preoperative staging in patients with rectal or anal tumor formations is unproblematic (pT2 to pT4), as is the information con-

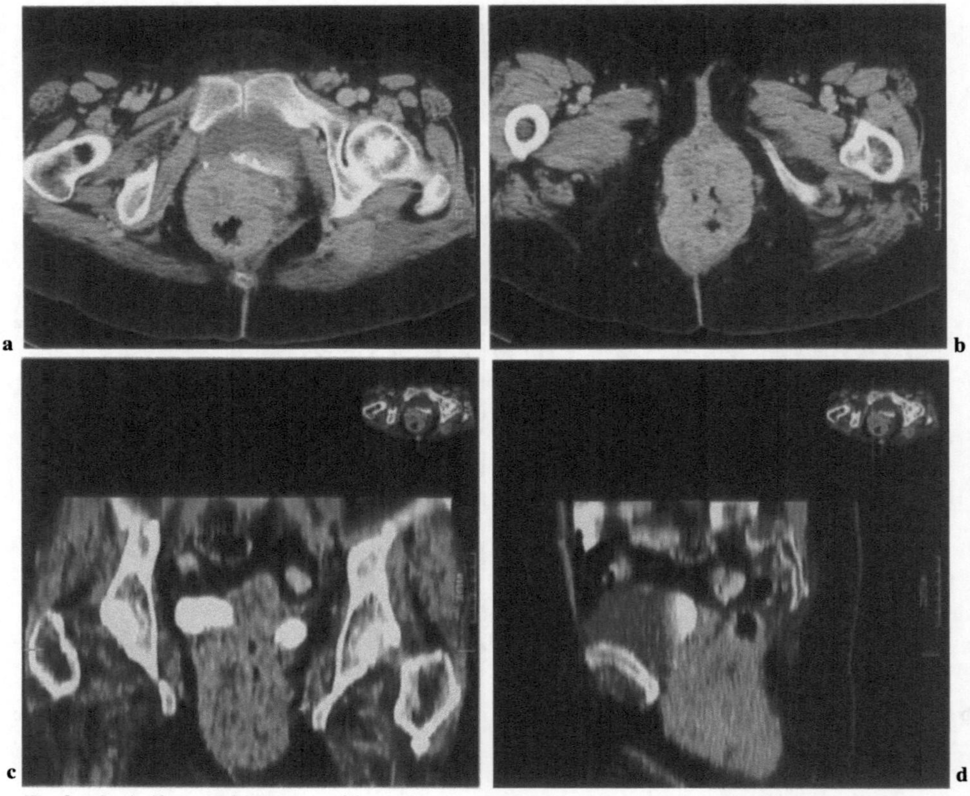

Fig. 3a–d. A 49-year-old woman with carcinoma of the anal region, pT4 N3M0, infiltration of all surrounding structures; in addition an abscess in M. gluteus caused by intramuscular injection is evident

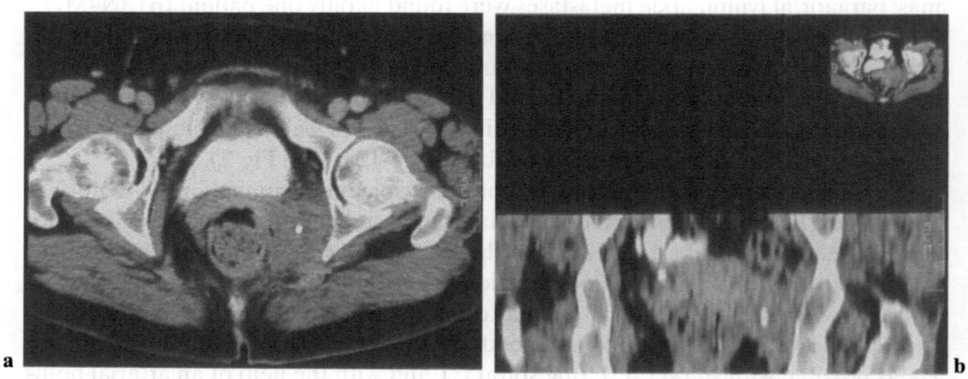

Fig. 4a, b. A 52-year-old woman with malignant sarcoma with infiltration of the muscular structures, rectum and uterus, pT3N1

cerning lymph node changes which are expected to be pathological and the presence of distant metastases. With the clinical question of recurrent tumors, changes occurring postoperatively cannot be differentiated clearly from scarred structures (Fig. 3).

Both patients examined with soft tissue sarcomas (rhabdomyosarcoma and malignant fibrous histiocytoma) could be classified with the proper staging because of the growth behavior of the tumors (T1 = tumor smaller than 5 cm, T2 = tumor larger than 5 cm, T3 = tumor infiltration into bone, blood vessels, etc.) (Fig. 4).

Discussion

Tumorous masses in the pelvic region can be evaluated noninvasively with the spiral CT technique. The danger of respiratory artifacts in the region of the pelvis is minimal. An advantage over the single scan technique is the distinctly shorter examination time (3.5–4 min as compared with 20 min), which represents substantially less distress for the patient. Because reformatting was performed subsequently, the total number of patients examined could only be increased slightly.

The volumetric measurement technique permits reformatting of the existent raw data sets to overlapping slices in critical organ regions. This procedure serves to alleviate the poorer spatial resolution resulting from the lower power required for the individual segment in comparison with that required for the single scan technique.

Good to very good image documentation is possible, especially for tumors of the prostate and urinary bladder. The posterior wall and floor of the urinary bladder as well as the ostia of the ureters, in combination with the question of infiltration into the seminal vesicles, can be evaluated especially well. Even minute iliacal and paravascular changes in the region of the ovaries can be documented clearly and differentiated from iliacal vascular changes and smaller changes in the lymph nodes. Tumor staging according to the TNM classification, with determination of the T stage starting with T2 and information concerning pathological changes in the lymph nodes as well as distant metastasis, is always possible.

Based upon our results, the following advantages to spiral CT examinations in the region of the pelvis are seen: short examination times, large image capacity, good vascular contrast with a short contrast medium bolus, good to very good sagittal and coronary image reconstruction, and low radiation exposure.

The following indications for spiral CT examination can be derived from this:

- Poor general condition of the patient with fecal and urinary incontinence.
- For tumor staging (TNM classification) of tumorous processes of the urinary bladder, prostate, ovary, rectum, and anus
- Clarification of abdominal lymph node metastasis

Due to its better spatial resolution, an additional examination using the single scan technique may eventually be decisive for the critical evaluation of recurrences on the pelvic wall of any origin.

3D-CT and Clinical Application II

Chairmen: H. E. Riemann and D. zur Nedden

Differentiation of Benign and Malignant Liver Lesions with Fast Angio-CT

J. Gaa, H. K. Deininger, and M. Georgi

Introduction

A definite computed tomography (CT) diagnosis of benign and malignant liver lesions can be made by obtaining dynamic, serial images at a single level (angio-CT) after intravenous bolus injection of iodinated contrast agents. In the past, differentiation between benign and malignant liver tumors by angio-CT was based on the analysis of dynamic and delayed patterns of lesion contrast enhancement [1, 4, 5, 9, 10]. However, owing to the short intravascular lifetime of iodinated contrast agents fast imaging techniques are necessary to provide temporal resolution of the tumor's enhancing characteristics. This study was performed to examine the early perfusion characteristics of various hepatic tumors using a fast angio-CT technique.

Material and Methods

Fifty-six patients with benign and malignant liver lesions were included in our prospective study. These included 33 patients with 35 hepatic hemangiomas, 16 patients with 43 liver metastases, and seven patients with four focal nodular hyperplasias and three liver abscesses. In the 16 patients with metastatic disease the primary tumor occured in the colon ($n = 9$), breast ($n = 4$), lung ($n = 2$), or ovary ($n = 1$). Lesion sizes ranged from 0.7 to 12 cm in benign tumors and from 0.8 to 10 cm in metastases. There was a total of seven subcentimeter lesions (four metastases, three hemangiomas).

CT studies were performed using a Somatom Plus (Siemens, Erlangen, FRG). After contiguous precontrast scans of the whole liver with 10-mm slice thickness, the slice level was selected at the largest tumor diameter. Fast angio-CT was initiated 10 s after bolus injection of 50 ml nonionic contrast agent (Solutrast 300, Byk Gulden, Constance, FRG) with a flow rate of 6 ml/s. A total of 15 scans were obtained in the first 30 s. In patients with suspected hemangiomas additional delayed scans were obtained at a rate of 2 scans/s up to a maximum of 30 min, unless the lesion became hypodense, at which time the delayed scan sequence was discontinued.

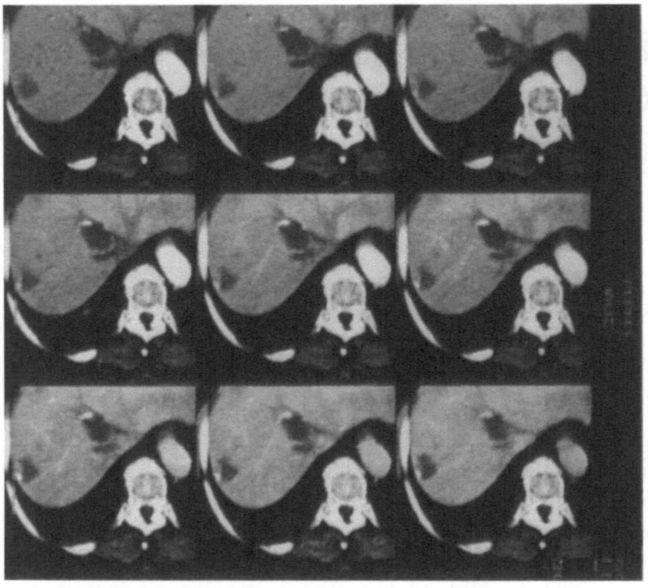

Fig. 1. Fast angio-CT (scan every 2 s with first image at 10 s) shows two hepatic hemangiomas with intense, sharply circumscribed, nodular enhancement along the mural edge during arterial and early portal phases

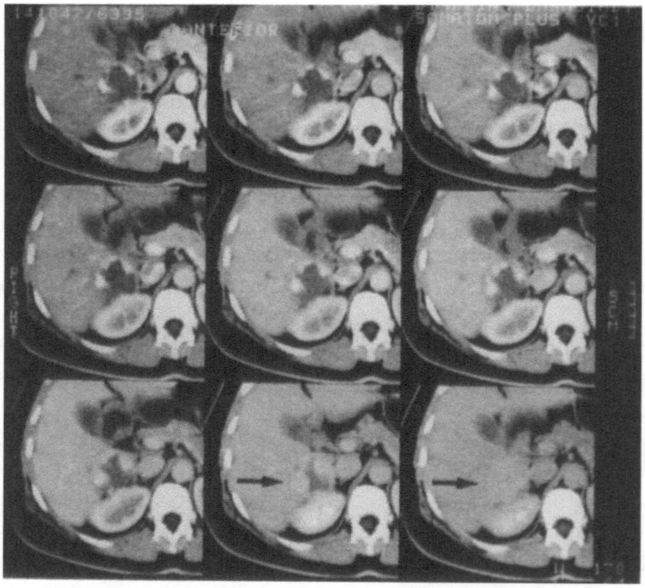

Fig. 2. Hepatic hemangioma on fast angio-CT (first image at 12 s). During the arterial phase there is strong nodular edge enhancement, and progressive enhancement toward the center during the portal phase. Fill-in pattern is observed on delayed images *(arrows)* after 1 and 3 min

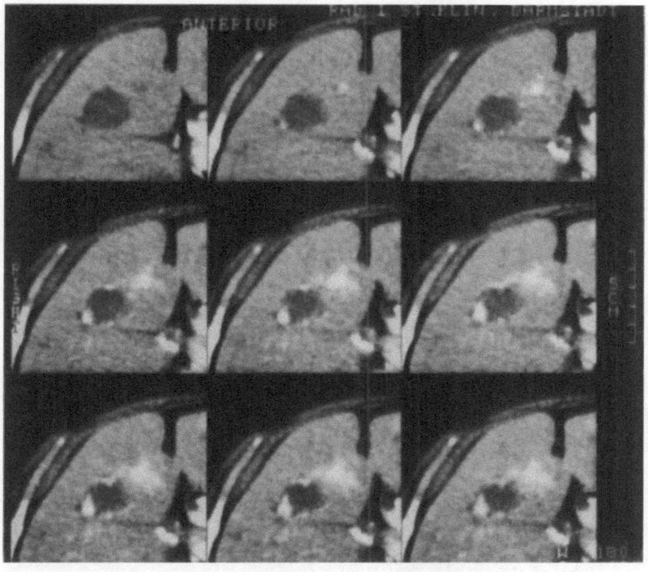

Fig. 3. Two hepatic hemangiomas with a diameter of 2.5 cm and 0.8 mm. In contrast to the characteristic nodular edge enhancement of the larger lesion, the smaller hemangioma shows a homogenous, hyperdense enhancement without evidence of nodular regions. Despite the small size of the lesion, no slice misregistration is seen

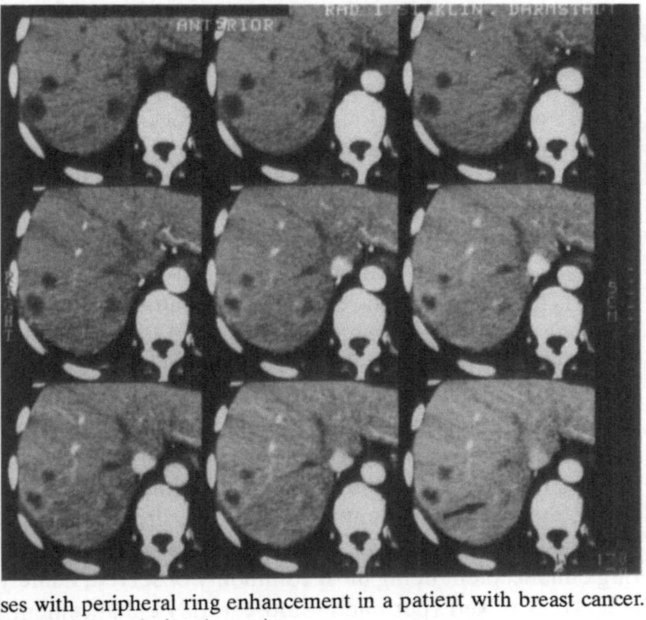

Fig. 4. Multiple liver metastases with peripheral ring enhancement in a patient with breast cancer. Note almost complete isodense fill-in of one lesion *(arrow)*

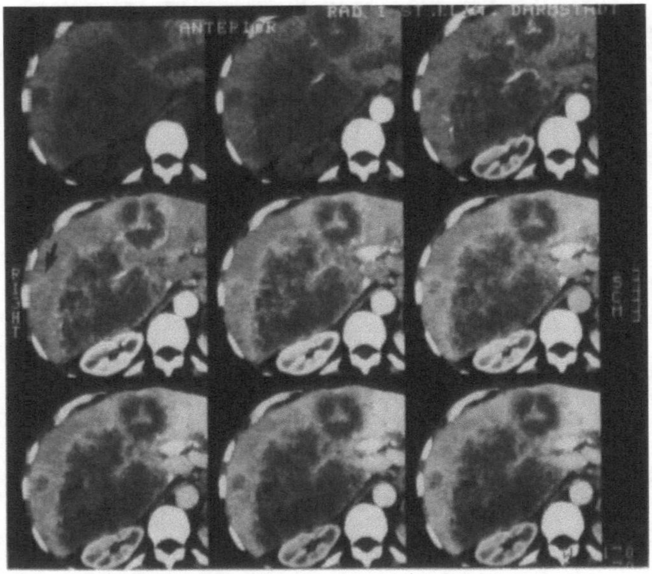

Fig. 5. Mixed enhancement pattern of liver metastases in a patient with rectal cancer. The smaller lesion becomes transiently isodense during the arterial phase *(arrow)*

Results

During the arterial phase of liver enhancement, 31 (89%) of 35 hemangiomas between 1.3 and 12 cm in size showed an especially intense, sharply circumscribed, nodular enhancement along the mural edge of the tumor (Fig. 1). The density of these mural nodules was similar to that in the aorta and hepatic arteries. While the density of the abdominal aorta diminished rapidly, the enhancing mural nodules were characterized by a persistent contrast medium pooling with a relatively slower fall in density. At the same time, there was a slow centripetal increase in size of the nodular areas, which eventually led to fill-in of the hemangioma on delayed scans (Fig. 2). This characteristic enhancement pattern was not observed in four hemangiomas: one thrombosed hemangioma (2.5 cm in diameter) showed no mural edge enhancement on fast angio-CT and remained hypodense on delayed scans. All three subcentimeter hemangiomas demonstrated an intense, homogeneous, hyperdense contrast accumulation with peak enhancement during the arterial phase (Fig. 3). In contrast, the typical CT criteria to establish a diagnosis of liver hemangioma as defined by Freeny and Marks [4] were found in 23 (69%) of 35 hemangiomas since only 23 hemangiomas showed isodense fill-in on delayed scans.

Metastases showed various patterns of contrast enhancement, with peripheral ring enhancement being most commonly observed, namely in 31 (72%) of 43 lesions (Fig. 4). A mixed (peripheral and central) enhancement pattern was seen in nine (21%) lesions. While one (2%) lesion showed only central enhancement, no enhancement was observed in two (5%) subcentimeter metastases. A total of seven

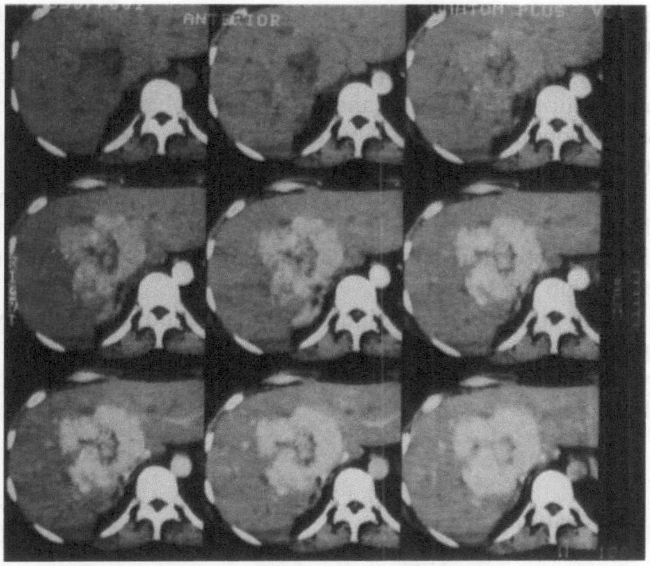

Fig. 6. Large focal nodular hyperplasia showing considerable contrast enhancement during the arterial and early portal phases with hypodense curvilinear areas corresponding to central fibrous scar.

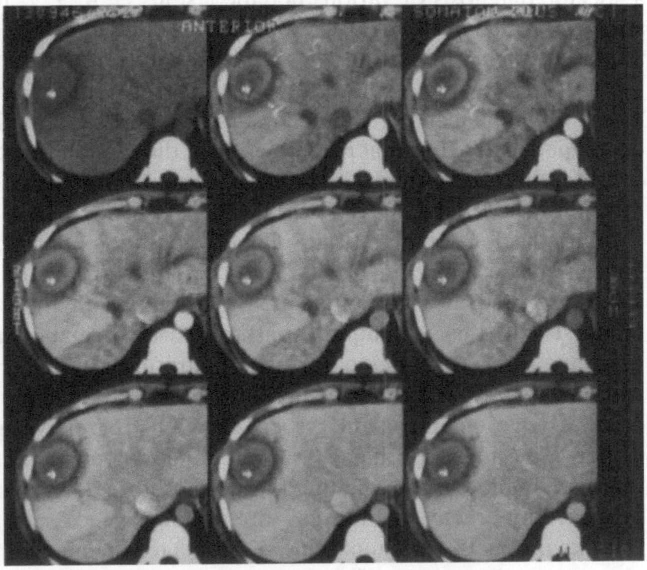

Fig. 7. Pyogenic liver abscess showing characteristic "double-target sign" and marked enhancement of surrounding inflammatory hepatic parenchyma

metastases showed transient isodensity compared with the surrounding hepatic parenchyma during the arterial ($n = 3$) and portal ($n = 4$) phases (Figs. 4, 5).

All focal nodular hyperplasias demonstrated a considerable contrast enhancement during the arterial and early portal phases with hypodense curvilinear areas corresponding to central fibrous scar (Fig. 6). A reduction in density was seen during the mid- and late portal phases.

Two liver abscesses showed a characteristic "double-target sign" and marked enhancement of surrounding inflammatory hepatic parenchyma (Fig. 7). One clinically inactive abscess with large calcifications showed no contrast enhancement during the fast angio-CT sequence.

The high-speed injection of nonionic contrast material was well tolerated by all patients, and no side effects occurred. Even in small lesions no slice misregistrations were encountered since fast CT sequences were performed during a single breath-hold.

Discussion

Hemangiomas and metastases are the most common benign and malignant liver tumors. Thus, differentiation of these tumors is a common clinical problem. Perfusion characteristics during contrast-enhanced dynamic CT have been widely used to make a specific diagnosis of various hepatic lesions [1, 4, 5, 9, 10]. However, in a classic study published in 1986, Freeny and Marks found only 54% of hepatic hemangiomas to have "typical" enhancing characteristics, while a large proportion of hemangiomas (46%) and liver metastases (77%) displayed "atypical" enhancement patterns [4]. These CT enhancement characteristics of benign and malignant liver tumors were developed with CT scanners that had scan times and interscan delay times that were considerably longer than with modern scanners. Moreover, the technique of contrast infusion varied widely [1, 3, 5, 9, 10].

With the development of slip-ring CT units, new approaches to lesion contrast enhancement became possible [6,7]. In our study protocol a fast angio-CT sequence was performed in conjunction with a low-dose, high-rate contrast injection technique. Using this technique, nonthrombosed hemangiomas larger than 1 cm in diameter showed a unique perfusion pattern and could be reliably differentiated from metastases and other benign lesions. Based on these findings we believe that nodular edge enhancement associated with progressive enhancement toward the center is the most specific CT sign in hepatic hemangiomas regardless of whether there is complete isoattenuating fill-in. Therefore delayed scans of up to 30 min – as proposed by Freeny and Marks – are no longer necessary, resulting in a substantial time-saving in CT examinations of suspected hemangiomas. No definitive lesion characterization was possible in one thrombosed hemangioma and in two subcentimeter metastases, which showed no significant enhancement during the fast angio-CT sequence. Additionally, the differentiation of small hemangiomas (< 1 cm) from hypervascular metastases might be difficult since both may demonstrate a homogenous, hyperdense enhancement in the arterial phase of fast angio-CT [2]. Although no slice misregistrations were encountered even for small lesions, the specific characterization of subcentimeter lesions by fast angio-CT continues to be a critical problem which might be better solved by magnetic resonance imaging (MRI [8]). Another distinct advantage of MRI (in addition to the lack of ionizing radiation) over CT lies in the fact that angio-CT must be performed on a single anatomic plane so that temporal perfusion information can be obtained, whereas with MRI the imaging plane can be varied to portray one or more lesions at different levels.

In conclusion, fast angio-CT is a promising technique in the differentiation of benign and malignant liver tumors. The major advantage of this technique is that a larger number of scans can be obtained during the arterial and venous portal phase, resulting in a better appraisal of the perfusion patterns of various liver lesions. However, diagnostic difficulties still exist in the differentiation of subcentimeter lesions (e.g., metastases vs. hemangiomas). Further examinations with this technique are desirable to evaluate the perfusion patterns of other lesions (e.g., hepatocellular carcinomas, liver cell adenomas).

References

1. Araki T, Itai Y, Furui S, Tasaka A (1980) Dynamic CT densitometry of hepatic tumors. AJR 135: 1037–1043
2. Bressler EL, Alpern MB, Glazer GM, Francis IR, Ensminger WD (1987) Hypervascular hepatic metastases: CT evaluation. Radiology 162: 49–51
3. Burgener FA, Hamlin DJ (1983) Contrast enhancement of hepatic tumors in CT: comparision between bolus and infusion techniques. AJR 140: 291–295
4. Freeny PC, Marks WM (1986) Patterns of contrast enhancement of benign and malignant hepatic neoplasms during bolus dynamic and delayed CT. Radiology 160: 613–618
5. Freeny PC, Marks WM (1986) Hepatic hemangioma: dynamic bolus CT. AJR 147: 711–719
6. Fuchs WA (1990) Advances in CT: European scientific user conference SOMATOM PLUS. Springer, Berlin Heidelberg New York, pp 179–234
7. Gaa J, Saini S, Ferrucci JT (1991) Perfusion characteristics of hepatic cavernous hemangioma using intravenous CT angiography (IVCTA). Eur J Radiol 12: 228–233
8. Itoh K, Saini S, Hahn PF, Imam N, Ferrucci JT (1990) Differentiation between small hepatic hemangiomas and metastases on MR images: importance of size-specific quantitative criteria. AJR 155: 61–66
9. Itai Y, Araki T, Furui S, Tasaka A (1981) Differential diagnosis of hepatic masses on computed tomography; with special reference to hepatocellular carcinoma. J Comput Assist Tomogr 5: 834–842
10. Itai Y, Ohtomo K, Araki T, Furui S, Iio M, Atomi Y (1983) Computed tomography and sonography of cavernous hemangioma of the liver. AJR 141: 315–320

Three-Dimensional Imaging in CT

R. Hupke, J. Ezrielev, and R. Fisler

Introduction

When three-dimensional (3D) imaging was introduced in the early 1980s, it was offered as a simplified method of interpreting large-volume data sets, allowing better perception of large-scale spatial relationships. In the beginning, 3D imaging suffered because of problems such as poor image quality, long processing time, as well as high costs. These issues together with the lack of economic stimulus contributed to the radiologists' reluctance to accept 3D imaging as a routine tool in clinical practice.

At the end of the last decade, a typical computed tomography (CT) examination took about 5 s per slice, resulting in a high likelihood of slice-to-slice misregistration. A fast CT scanner combined with powerful computer hardware, like the Somatom Plus-S, as well as various new algorithms for 3D rendering have improved the current technical performance of 3D imaging.

However, will the integration of new technology be sufficient to gain widespread clinical acceptance of 3D imaging? The gold standard for diagnosis is the cross-sectional image, but it is not the gold standard in treatment planning. Therefore, the area of greatest potential benefit and the key to acceptance of 3D as a clinical tool may not be in diagnosis, but in its ability to improve dramatically the communication between diagnostics and therapy.

Overview of 3D Algorithms

There are two main types of 3D algorithms in medical imaging today: volume and surface rendering. The main difference between them is in the surface definition. In surface rendering, the surfaces must be explicity defined before they can be displayed. In volume rendering, the surfaces are not defined at all. Volume-rendering algorithms assign models, consisting of color and opacities [1, 2], to all the voxel elements (voxels) and project the voxels according to the models. The resulting images can display translucent masses overlapping each other, if little opacity is assigned to the voxels in the model. The images can also show solid surfaces if enough opacity is assigned to the voxels in the model.

One way to define surfaces is to assign polygon tiles to the surface. This method is standard in computer graphics. What is more common in medical imaging is to define the surface as the faces of voxels [3, 4]. The polygon method suffers from poor resolution, a more difficult surface formation process, and the need to use special purpose hardware. The voxel method does not have these disadvantages and is therefore more popular in medical imaging. Here, it is often necessary to interpolate between adjacent transaxial slices to create cubic voxels. Surface-rendering algorithms are able to preprocess this stack of interpolated data in the surface formation step. This produces a significant reduction in the amount of data, and subsequent views of the surface can be produced very quickly. It should be noted that there exist 3D systems that utilize special purpose hardware and are able to produce 3D images in real time without any preprocessing. Surface rendering is able to utilize various lighting models for shading. An important aspect of shading is computation of the surface normals, which are necessary for most lighting models. Image space shading [5] computes the normal based on the orientation of the projected surface. Gray-level gradient shading [6] assigns the surface normal based on the gray-level gradients in the neighborhood of the surface voxel. Although the image space algorithms are slightly less computationally intensive, the gray-level gradient algorithms produce images of superior quality [7].

The process of extracting objects of interest from original slices is called segmentation. Segmentation is an important preprocessing step for both surface and volume rendering. The segmentation problem is trivial for the display of bone or skin tissues in CT, where a gray-level threshold can be used. However, segmentation necessary for the display of soft tissues or joint disarticulation is much more complex. Automated computer solutions for soft tissue segmentation fail in many cases because the signal to noise ratio in the original images is often too small to result in reproducible segmentations. Therefore, user interaction is still often necessary [8, 9].

The volume-rendering method has several advantages over its surface counterpart. It is a much more general model. Surface rendering may be considered a special case of volume rendering. Volume 3D rendering may be more effective at displaying soft tissues and several different tissues at the same time. Volume rendering also does not suffer from the false holes artifact present in some surface-rendered images. This occurs with tissues, such as thin bones, where the pixel value is too low to be detected by a gray-level threshold. On the other hand, volume rendering is much more computationally intensive than surface rendering because of the large amount of data that must be examined for every view produced. It is also not possible to reduce the image generation time by preprocessing data like it is in surface rendering. Therefore, images can be produced much faster with the surface algorithms.

It is important in medical imaging not just to produce 3D images, but also to evaluate and manipulate them. Physicians often want to measure 3D distances and volumes and to simulate cuts of the tissues to reveal internal structures. Some surgeons may even perform surgical simulation on the tissues to generate a better surgical plan [10]. The surface model has here an advantage since surfaces to be measured or cut are readily available.

Another 3D technique that has found uses in medicine is maximum intensity projection (MIP). The MIP technique projects the maximum intensity voxel along a ray onto a 2D plane. Although it does not fully fit either the surface or the volume model, it is more similar to the volume model. The advantages of MIP-rendered images are mostly appreciated when a range of them is rapidly rotating around a fixed axis. Its main use originates in displaying intracranial vessels measured with magnetic resonance imaging (MRI). However, the interest in MIP applications is increasing also in CT.

Clinical Applications of 3D Algorithms

The 3D CT has found many clinical applications so far [11]; however, its acceptance in diagnosis is still limited. In contrast to the reconstruction of 2D images, which is dominated by one algorithm, the variety of existing 3D reconstructions appears more confusing to the potential user. The debate over surface versus volume-rendering methods continues. We do not see any evidence that one rendering technique is superior to another in all cases. Validation of rendering methods for specific applications is required.

Surface rendering established its first application in orthopedics [12, 13], because the contrast between bone and soft tissue is high, so the required segmentation is trivial. Straight software implementations today feature the real-time rotation of full data sets, and a full resolution, high quality image will be rendered in a few seconds. A typical result is shown in Fig. 1 with an example of a huge sarcoma of the hip viewed posteriorly. About 100 transaxial slices were measured in this case. Each 2D image demonstrates the sarcoma by some bone-like fragments. Only a 3D image like in Fig. 1 offers a quick and comprehensive overview of the spatial extent of the disease. Orthopedic problems often require an integrated 2D and 3D approach. This can be realized by a surface-rendered image acting as a reference image for multiplanar reconstructions (MPR). The user gains the direct relationship between surface overview and detailed cross-sectional images, as indicated in Fig. 2. This offers easy access to standard views ("sag, cor" in Fig. 2) and to complicated, oblique ("obl" in Fig. 2) MPRs, as well as the opportunity for exact measurements of these MPR images. In the 3D image in the top left part of Fig. 2, the problem of artificial holes becomes obvious. The scans of this study were taken with the thin slice technique, and the 2D images were recon-

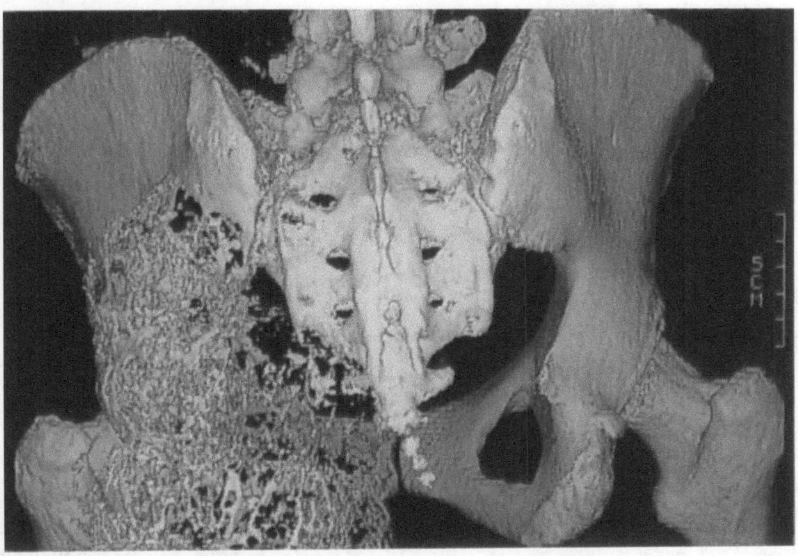

Fig. 1. 3D Surface rendering of a hip

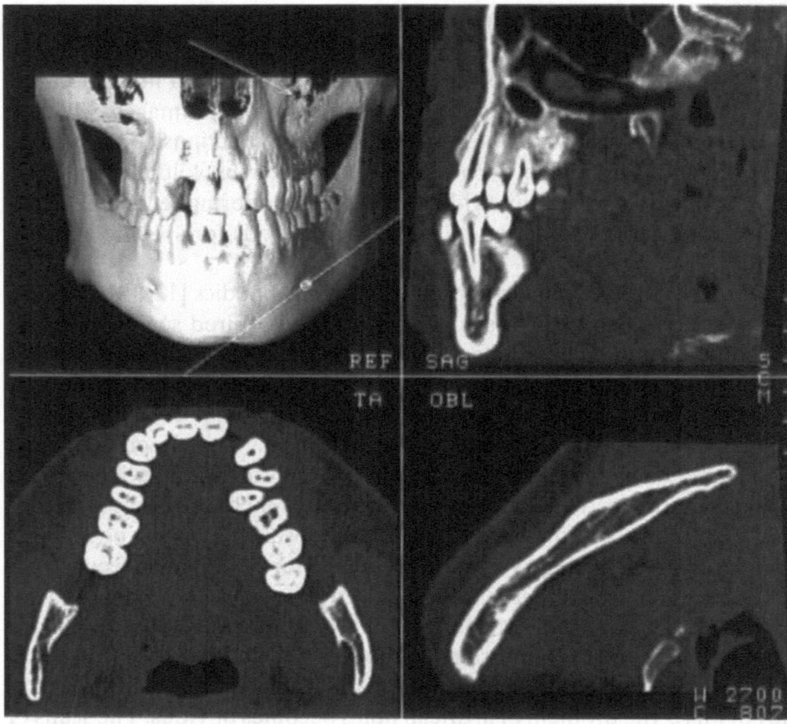

Fig. 2. High-resolution surface rendering and concurrent MPR of the lower skull

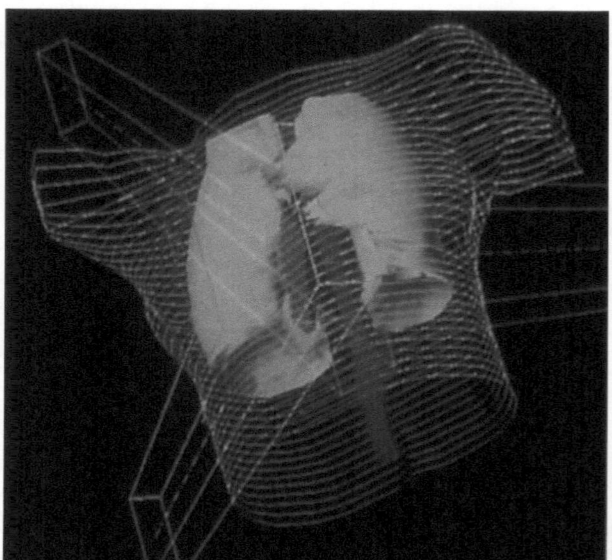

Fig. 3. 3D therapy planing utilizing the Siemens Axiom RTP system and spiral CT images

structed with a high resolution kernel, introducing a relative high level of pixel noise to the transaxial images. This requires a high threshold for the binary segmentation, resulting in holes in the 3D image wherever the bone is thin in the object.

Another application of surface-rendered 3D images is radiation therapy planning [14]. The oncologist needs to merge anatomic information gained mostly with CT scanning and data of simulated radiation therapy planning to delineate those dose distributions to both tumor and normal tissue. Results like those presented in Fig. 3 may help the oncologist towards more efficient treatment planning and improved design of customized beam filters. Thus, 3D imaging has the potential to reduce the radiation exposure of healthy tissue during the treatment.

High quality surface renderings of high-contrast structures like bones or the lung bronchial tree are feasible. After successful segmentation, it will even be possible to display a low-contrast object like the liver by this 3D technique. However, this appears to be without clinical interest; the presentation of the liver together with its vascularity would receive more attention. For this class of applications the volumetric approach for 3D imaging is advantageous. The anatomy can be demonstrated by a more or less transparent volume, showing overlapping structures and providing the user with the full spatial relationship between two or more 3D objects. Since the introduction of spiral CT [15, 16], the range of potential applications for volume-rendered 3D has strongly increased [11]. By using spiral CT, a large number of contiguous slices can be obtained without any interscan delay, minimizing motion degradation and optimizing the utilization of contrast agents, thus resultung in an excellent enhancement of the vascularity. This provides an appropriate input for the volume or MIP imaging methods. Its applications include the staging of mediastinal disease or the rapidly growing field of surgical planning. The importance of a well balanced synergy between data acquisition and image presentation is illustrated in Fig. 4. With this picture, we demonstrate our most recent results with the MIP technique applied to spiral images. This neck case offers an excellent view of the carotid artery as well as the hypervascular tumor. This measurement of data took only 24 s, compared with approximately 5–7 min used for an equivalent MRI study. The combination of thin-slice spiral CT and MIP imaging opens the way for a fast, non invasive screening tool for patients with suspected vascular disease. Some further technical improvements will likewise support CT angiography.

Future Directions of 3D-Imaging in CT

The development of all 3D methods was driven by the need to visualize difficult diagnostic problems. However, these advantages have not been dramatic enough to justify additional 3D systems and evaluations. The golden standard for diagnosis today is still the cross-sectional image. This is no longer true in the general field of therapy, running from surgery to radiation treatment planning. There seems to be a consensus among the radiologists that the utility of 3D in diagnosis is limited. According to this fact, the key to the acceptance of 3D imaging as a clinical tool may not be in diagnosis, but in its ability to improve dramatically the communication between radiologists and referring physicians. Up to now, it was relatively difficult for CT

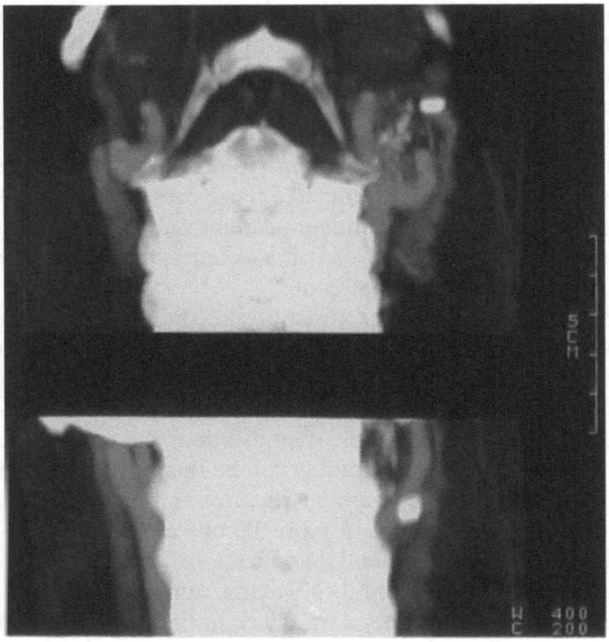

Fig. 4. MIP representation of a carotid artery. 2D images were acquired by spiral CT

users to justify the purchase of a 3D system. To bridge the gap between diagnosis and therapy, clinical practice has to reach a point at which it requires 3D imaging.

At least for CT, this step has already been reached with the introduction of fast and ultrafast scanners along with spiral CT. Today, the Somatom Plus-S allows an acquisition of a volume up to 30 cm in lenght in only 30 s. A 3D reconstruction should result in high image quality, since the slice misregistration is minimized. An even more important aspect to understand 3D as a clinical tool is that a single spiral scan, as described above, can provide the radiologist with up to approximately 300 images, containing 150 Mbytes of information (corresponding to roughly 30000 typed book pages). This is the point at which 3D, or in a more general sense volumetric imaging, will find its key for acceptance as a clinical tool by improving the handling of this large amount of information. Obviously, not all of the information is necessary for, e.g., the surgeon. For example, it will not be very productive to face the surgeon with 50 standard-sized sheets of radiography film. He might be interested in the spatial relationship between tumor and healthy tissue, which will be demonstrated by a volume-rendered 3D or MIP image, rather than in each pixel of the whole volume. Future developments of volumetric imaging, therefore, have to concentrate on improvements of information management. This will contribute to health care by improving patient management.

Because of the production of hundreds of Mbytes of information per patient examination, in the future new concepts in imaging will be required in which 3D will play its role as well as the normal 2D transaxial image of today. The scanner will act only as a pure image generator. Several workstations, perhaps with various imaging capabilities, are networked to the scanner. Before the measurement takes place, the destination of the images is allocated to a specific workstation, belonging to a group of physicians. Smart control of the image transfer and fast special purpose hardware will allow instant access to prepared 3D/MPR data at the specific workstation, as well as very fast roaming through the original image stack (cine-loop). However, to fulfill all practical needs, it will also be necessary to pull out of this 3D representation of the measured volume 2D images of interest: transaxial as well as sagittal, or even arbitrarily shaped ones. The connection between 3D and so-called MPR is needed (see Fig. 2). In general, this implies that the user has to be enabled to work with this image dataset of the measured volume of interest. A 3D surface rendering is within this concept only one out of multiple display modes.

All applications should be tailored for the specific need of the individual physician: 3D-surface images for the orthopedist (Fig. 1) and 3D volume or MIP images (Fig. 4) for the liver surgeon. No user should be bothered with the problem of segmentation or the type of slice-interpolation utilized. Not only does the CPU time of the algorithms implemented have to be minimal, the man-machine interface also has to be as easy and as fast as possible. If not, this will reduce again the acceptance of post diagnosis imaging dramatically. The final goal should be to concentrate the information content of the acquired images to the amount necessary for optimal communcation between diagnostics and therapy in order to enhance patient care and management.

Conclusion

The acceptance of volumetric imaging, especially 3D, is grounded on three major supports. First, the knowledge of the various algorithms and its implementation on fast, mostly special purpose hardware, should assure good image quality and practical cycle times. This is today mostly accomplished. The second is to select a proper algorithm for a specific clinical problem. Up to now, this has not really been solved, although, the request for specific applications of volumentric imaging is increasing. Examples are dental CT or interventional imaging. Unfortunately, the third and most important support, the clinical request for 3D imaging, is not yet evident enough to bear the extant external administrative pressure. However, the rapidly increasing amount of information gathered with today's and tomorrow's CT scanners will stabilize this situation toward a general acceptance of 3D methods. Therefore, radiologists offering a 3D service will take on a more collaborative role in medicine, and they will consult with surgeons and therapists to create computer-assisted surgery or therapy. The evolution of 3D imaging will present the radiologists with opportunities to become more involved with therapy and patient care.

References

1. Levoy M (1988) Display of surfaces from volume data. IEEE Comput Graph Appl 8 (3): 29–37
2. Ney DE, Fishman E, Magid D, Drebin R (1990) Volumetric rendering of computed tomography data: principles and techniques. IEEE Comput Graph Appl 3: 24–32

3. Cline HE et al. (1988) Two algorithms for the three-dimensional reconstruction of tomograms. Med Phys 15 (3): 320–327
4. Tiede U et al. (1990) Investigation of medical 3D-rendering algorithms. IEEE Comput Graph Appl 3: 41–53
5. Gordon D, Reynolds RA (1985) Image space shading of three-dimensional objects. Comput Vis Graph Image Proc 9: 361–376
6. Hoehne KH, Bernstein R (1986) Shading 3D-images from CT using gray-level gradients. IEEE Trans Med Imaging 5 (1): 45–47
7. Tiede U et al. (1987) Comparison of surface rendering techniques for 3D tomographic objects. Proc CAR, pp 610–614
8. Ezrielev J, Dzik S (1990) An image editor for a 3D-CT reconstruction system. Proc SPIE Med Imaging IV: Image Proc 1233: 67–76
9. Ney D, Fishman E (1991) Editing tools for 3D medical imaging. IEEE Comput Graph Appl 11: 63–71
10. Yokoi S et al. (1990) A simulation system for craniofacial surgeries bases on 3D image processing. IEEE Eng Med Biol 9 (4): 29–32
11. Fishman E et al. (1991) Three-dimensional imaging. Radiology 181: 321–337
12. Magid D, Fishman E (1989) Imaging of musculoskeletal trauma in three dimensions. Radiol Clin North Am 27: 945–956
13. Vannier MW, Totty WG (1985) Musculoskeletal applications of three dimensional surface reconstructions. Orthop Clin North Am 16: 543–555
14. Goitein M (1979) The utility of computed tomography in radiation therapy: an estimate of outcome. Int J Radiat Oncol Biol Phys 5: 1799–1807
15. Kalender W, Seissler W, Klotz E, Vock P (1990) Spiral volumetric CT with single-breathhold technique, continuous transport and continuous scanner rotation. Radiology 176: 181–183
16. Rigauts H, Marchal G, Baert AL, Hupke R (1990) Initial experience with volume CT scanning. J Comput Assist Tomogr 14 (4): 675–682

Optimized Scan Modes and Reconstruction Techniques for Three-Dimensional Display of Bone Structures

T. Fleiter, A. Rieber, P. Wakat, H. J. Brambs, and C. D. Claussen

Introduction

The high quality three-dimensional (3D) presentation of computed tomography (CT) data has become a common technique since fast imaging systems and 3D software became widely available at the beginning of the 1980s. Unfortunately, the quality of the 3D images produced by standard 3D packages depends not only on several basic scanning parameters like voltage, amperage, slice, and imcrement, but also on the primary reconstruction algorithm, image separation, and 3D reconstruction and shading method. Therefore, no standard 3D scanning method providing a high quality 3D display combined with an acceptable acquisition and reconstruction time has been established. New volume scanning methods such as the spiral CT offer additional methods to shorten the examination time. There are some problems for 3D imaging in the use of spiral CT. The aim of our study was to compare different scanning – and 3D – reconstruction methods in order to develop standard scanning sequences for routine 3D CT imaging.

The 3D display of CT images has been described as a useful tool in preoperative studies and different areas of investigation [1–4]. Many reports have been published about the principles of 3D display and the different reconstruction techniques [5–9], but only a few about basic scanning methods for fidelity 3D images [10–13]. Compared with 2D images, the settings of voltage, amperage, slice, and increment as well as the primary algorithm used have – in our experience – a dramatic infuence on the quality of the secondarily reconstructed 3D images. The aim of our study was to demonstrate the influence of the scanning and reconstruction mode and to optimize the standard scan parameters by studying the same object with varying scan mode, scan time, mA s, algorithm, and kernel.

The review was done by experienced radiologists who judged the image quality, accuracy, and spatial impression.

Material and Method

Two bone phantoms of the pelvis and lumbar region (pelvis phantom by 3M – X-ray products and Anderson Man) were used for conventional axial scans. Both phantoms are composed of a skeleton and soft tissue equivalent epoxy materials. The phantoms were examined using a Somatom Plus with a Somaris software version VD 1A installed. For all scans, the phantoms were fixed in the middle of the patient table, and the scan orientation was exactly axial to the lumbar joint L2/L3. The slice thickness and increment were set to 2 mm, and in all modes 120 kV and standard algorithm were used. For each parameter setting, two scan sets were acquired: from L3 to the upper femoral shaft with 99 scans and from L3 to the iliosacral joint with 45 scans. A 1.8 and 4.3 zoom factor was used for the acquisitions. Subsequently, mA s was changed between 60 and 420 mAs. The scan time was varied from 0.7 to 2*2 s, and two reconstructions with a kernel of 3 and 7 were performed on each raw data set. In spiral mode, a slice thickness of 2 mm was combined with a 2-mm increment, 120 kV, 165 mAs and kernel 3. To acquire the whole volume, nine continuous, 12-s spiral scans were needed. All images were 3D reconstructed using the standard 3D Somaton Plus software package and printed by a 3M Laserimager. To eliminate reconstruction artifacts, all 3D images were filtered three times by the standard smoothing filter. Original and smoothed images were printed on different films. In case of the Alderson Man phantom, the images were transferred via Pacsnet/Isonet to a remote imaging station (Kontron Mirpon with MIP3D software) and reconstructed from 36 viewpoint angles in X-orientation and a step width of 10°. These images were replayed in a movie mode and compared with the standard projections of the Somatom Plus software. For the binary separation, the threshold was varied to minimize separation artifacts. All images were displayed and printed with equal window and center settings. Of all studies, two images of equal scan positions were printed by a 3M Laserimager on a separate film. The reviewers did not know the scanning parameters, and they could compare the transparent pelvis phantom with the reconstructions, as well as the 3D images in movie-mode on the imaging system with the standard projections of the Alderson Man studies.

Results

All reviewers preferred the 2*2 s/420 mAs/kernel 3 axial images, but the quality of the 0.7 s/175 mAs/kernel 3 images was thought to be comparable and of satisfying quality. Kernel 7 images gave a soft impression, whereas the quality of the 0.7/60 mAs could be improved by using kernel 7 (Fig. 1 a–d).

The reconstruction quality of the Somatom Plus software and of the remote imaging system was comparable, although the differences between the volumetric rendering of the Kontron and the binary separation of the Somaris 3D option were clearly detectable in increased surface artifacts and sharpened edges in the case of Somaris 3D images. All reviewers mentioned no diagnosis-relevant artifacts on both image types.

Due to large artifacts, the 3D images of the low dose 120 kV/60 mAs/kernel 3 scans were absolutely unusable. However, the same images were dramatically improved by changing the kernel from 3 to 7 (Figs. 2, 3). Unlike on axial 2D scans, the 2*2 s/420 mAs-based 3D images were not superior. In fact, the 3D images using this mode were thought to be inferior to those scanned by 0.7 s/175 mAs/kernels 3 and 7 (Figs. 4–6). The low dose/kernel 7 3D images were again comparable for the lumbar region in primary magnified studies. Although acquired with contiguous scans, there are some visible axial gaps on the spiral CT images (Figs. 7, 8). The secondary

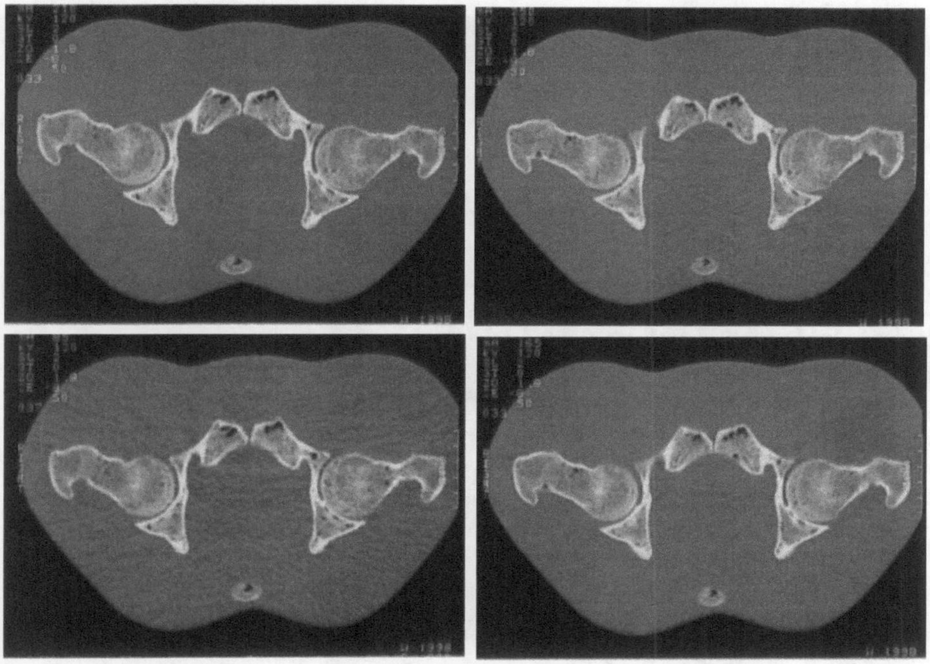

Fig. 1. **a** Frontal view of the pelvis, scanned using 2*2 s/420 mAs/kernel 3 mode. **b** Standard 0.7 sec/175 mAs/kernel 3 axial scan. **c** Low dose 0.7 s/60 mAs/kernel 7 axial scan. **d** Axial scan spiral mode

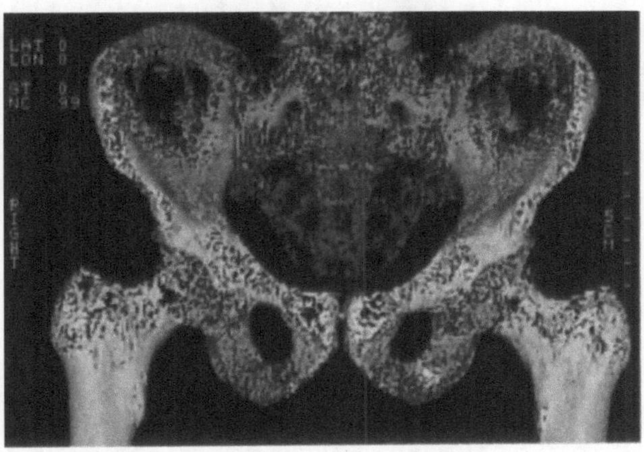

Fig. 2. Unusable, disturbed 3D frontal view of pelvis by 0.7 s/60 mAs/kernel 3 scan

smoothed images did not have any advantage for the whole pelvis display, but in detailed reconstructions of the lumbar spine, crisp and sharp edges, disturbing the spatial impression, could be reduced by the smoothing filter (fig. 9 a, b). Overall the reviewers preferred the 3D reconstructions of the 0.7 s/175 mAs/kernels 3 and 7 images.

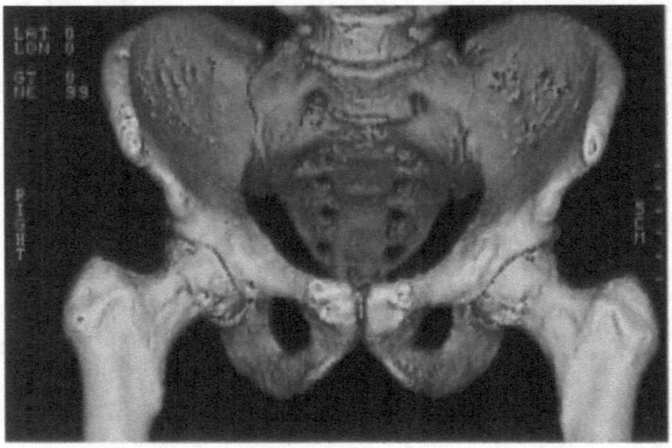

Fig. 3. Same dataset as Fig. 5, reconstructed with kernel 7

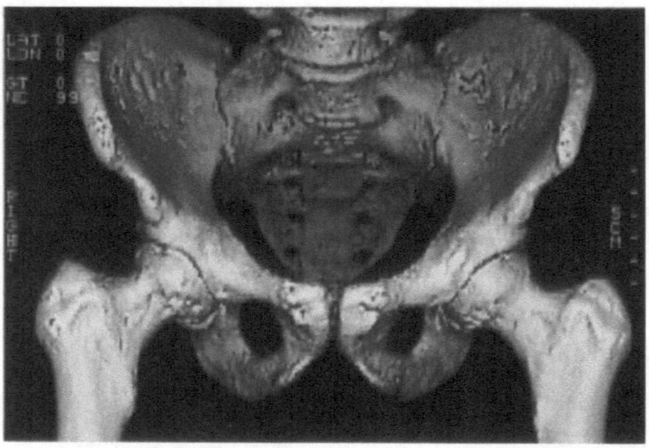

Fig. 4. Frontal view of pelvis, standard 2*2 s/420 mAs mode

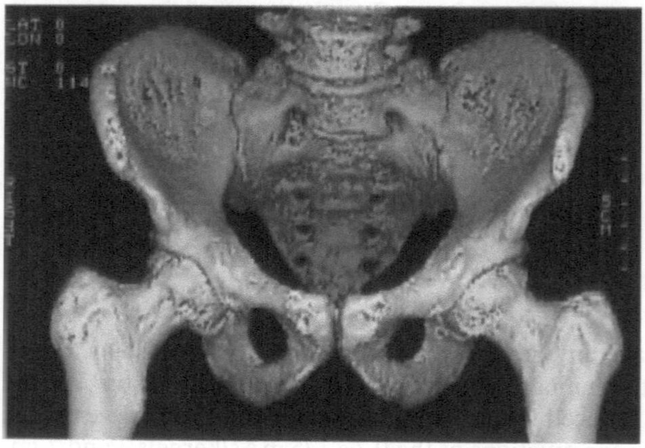

Fig. 5. A scan in 0.7 s/175 mAs/kernel 3 mode

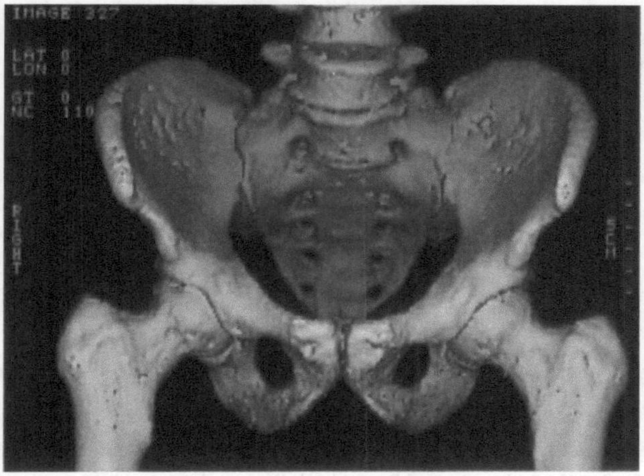

Fig. 6. A scan in 0.7 s/175 mAs/kernel 7 mode

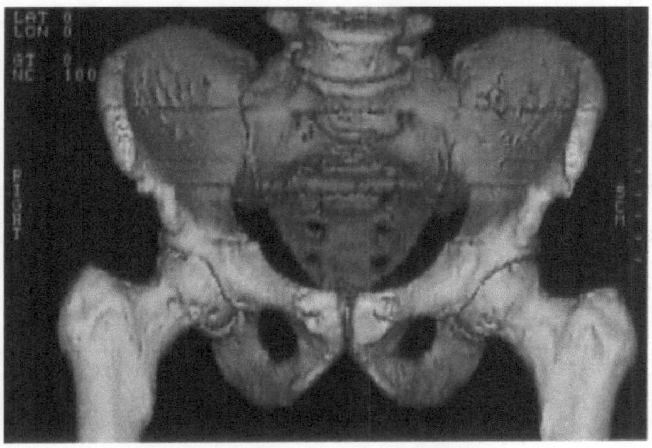

Fig. 7. Frontal view of pelvis with visible spiral CT horizontal scan margins

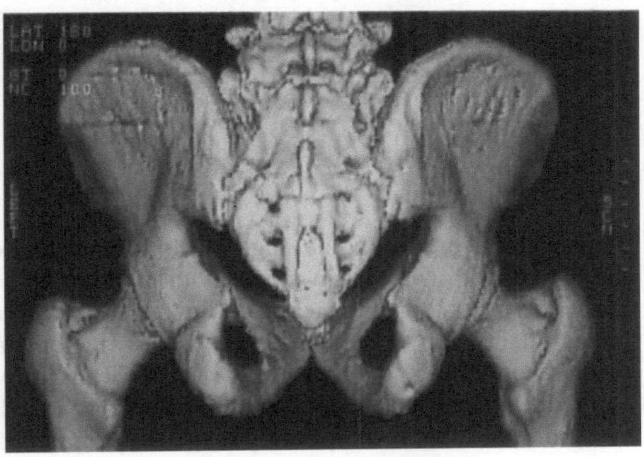

Fig. 8. Dorsal view of pelvis, whole data set consisting of nine 2/2 mm/165 mAs spiral scans

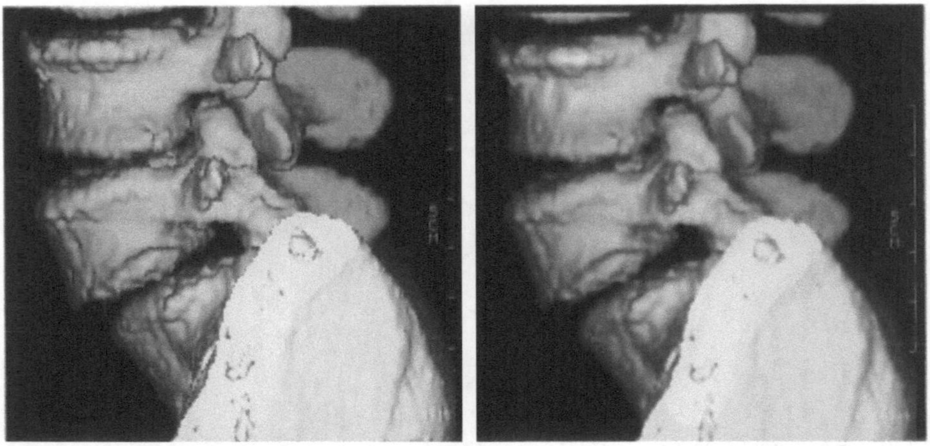

a b

Fig. 9. a Low dose/kernel 7 standard displayed image, **b** after smoothing by standard smoothing filter

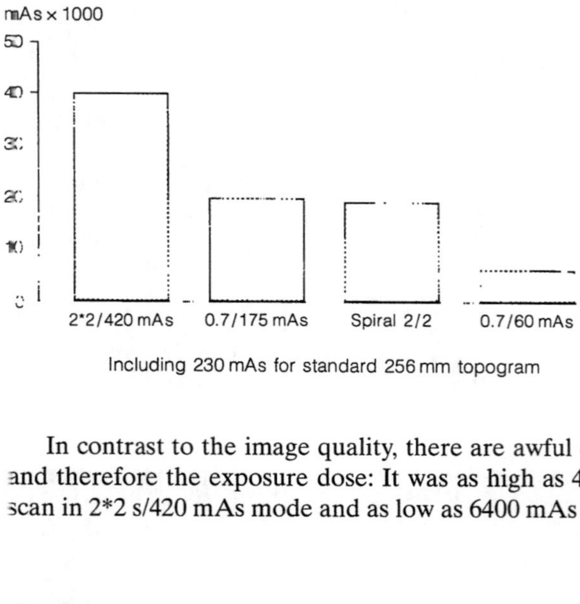

Fig. 10. Scan mode and corresponding mAs product

In contrast to the image quality, there are awful differences in the mAs product and therefore the exposure dose: It was as high as 41 810 mAs for the whole pelvis scan in 2*2 s/420 mAs mode and as low as 6400 mAs in the low dose mode (Fig. 10).

Discussion

Our results clearly show that high resolution imaging does not necessarily improve the 3D image quality. Scan modes with medium mA and standard algorithm, and kernel offer good diagnostic resolution on axial scans and provide a reasonable 3D image quality. Up to now, most 3D reconstructions in our department have been made secondarily, and only a few special 3D scans for preoperative studies were performed. Especially in these cases, low dose scans are adequate for reliable 3D reconstructions, as long as the primary diagnosis is made based on the original standard axial scans. In agreement with other published results [10, 11], we recommend a 120 kV/175 mAs/standard algorithm/kernel 3 scan to be the best compromise according to exposure dose (Fig. 10), scanning time, diagnostic accuracy, and 3D image quality. Due to axial gaps at the scan borders and unacceptably long examination times, spiral CT with comparable scan parameters and image quality is not an usuable alternative in 3D scans of large areas of the musculoskeletal system. On the other hand, scan modes with good quality for overall reconstructions such as of the entire pelvis are not the best solution for displaying small parts of detailed bone segments like the spine or the intervertebral regions. Edge-enhanced scans, as usually used in axial scans for spinal displays, lead to separation artifacts and sharpened edges in the resulting 3D images. Secondary smoothing by Gaussian filters improves – in our experience – the spatial impression of these images.

References

1. Vannier MW, Marsch JL, Warren JO (1984) Three dimensional CT reconstruction images for craniofacial surgical planning and evaluation. Radiology 150: 179–184
2. Burk DL, Mears DC, Kennedy WH, Cooperstein LA, Herbert DL (1985) Three-dimensional computed tomography of acetabular fractures. Radiology 155: 183–186
3. Wojcik WG, Edeiken-Monroe BS, Harris JH (1987) Three-dimensional computed tomography in acute cervical spine trauma: a preliminary report. Skeletal Radiol 16: 261–269
4. Soyer P, Roche A, Gad M et al. (1991) Preoperative segmental localization of hepatic metastases: utility of three-dimensional CT during arterial portography. Radiology 180: 653–658
5. Artzy E (1979) Display of three-dimensional information in computed tomography. Comput Graph Image Proc 9: 196–198
6. Marsh JL, Vannier MW (1983) Surface imaging from computerized tomographic scans. Surgery: 159–165
7. Totty WG, Vannier MW (1984) Complex musculoskeletal anatomy: analysis using three dimensional surface reconstruction. Radiology 150: 173–177
8. Herman GT (1988) three-dimensional imaging on a CT and MR scanner. J Comput Assist Tomogr 12 (3): 450–458
9. Wrazidlo W, Brambs HJ, Lederer W et al. (1991) An alternative method of three-dimensional reconstruction from two-dimensional CT and MR data sets. Eur J Radiol 12: 11–16
10. Ney DR, Fishman EK, Magid D et al. (1991) Three-dimensional volumetric display of CT-data: effect of scan parameters upon image quality. J Comput Assist Tomogr 15 (5): 875–885
11. Drebin RA, Magid D, Robertson DD et al. (1989) Fidelity of three-dimensional CT imaging for detecting facture gaps. J Comput Assist Tomogr 13 (3): 487–489
12. Howard JD, Elster ED, Max JS (1990) Temporal bone: three-dimensional CT, part I. Radiology 177: 421–425
13. Howard JD, Elster ED, May JS (1990) Temporal bone: three-dimensional CT, part II. Radiology 177: 427–430

Three-Dimensional Imaging of Thoracic and Abdominal Organs and Vessels from Spiral CT Data Sets

M. Lenz, J. Gmeinwieser, A. Wunderlich, W. Bautz, B. Kersting-Sommerhoff, and P. Gerhardt

Introduction

A prerequisite for the three-dimensional (3D) reconstruction of anatomical structures from computed tomography (CT) scans is contiguous scanning of the region of interest [8, 9, 23, 27]. Using CT scanners of the third generation with long scanning times, this was only possible in regions of the body not subjected to respiratory motion. Thus, 3D reconstruction was restricted to the CNS and musculoskeletal regions of the extremities [8, 9, 17, 23, 27, 28]. The recent development of CT scanners with continuously rotating scanners (first realized with the Somatom Plus from Siemens) offers the chance to measure a definite volume during a single breath hold by obtaining a spiral CT scan with continuous table movement [10–12]. From this CT data set, it is possible to calculate consecutive slices that were acquired during the same respiratory phase. The short measurement time (24 s) allows a specific and optimized vessel contrast. Spiral CT has been successfully used in two-dimensional imaging of thoracic and abdominal organs [1, 19, 24]. At the same time, organs subjected to respiratory motion become accessible for 3D reconstruction [7].

Methods

Spiral CT scans were acquired on a Somatom Plus (Siemens, Erlangen, FRG) using a slice thickness of 10 mm, a table speed of 10 mm/s, and 24 gantry rotations, permitting the scanning of a volume of 24 cm length during a single inspiratory breath hold of 24 s. From the spiral CT data set, 111 scans with a gap of 2 m (8 mm overlap) were reconstructed. Vessel contrast was enhanced with the application of iopàmidol (Solutrast, Byk Gulden, Constance, FRG) into a cubital vein using a motorized infusion pump (Ulrich, Ulm, FRG). In patients with aortic disease 150 ml (50 ml at 3 ml/s and 100 ml at 2 ml/s) and in those with liver disease 200 ml (50 ml at 3 ml/s and 150 ml at 1 ml/s) of contrast medium was given. The acquisition of the spiral CT started only after complete administration of the contrast medium. This technique resulted in good vessel contrast in aortic disease and scanning of the liver during the portal-venous phase (good contrast between the liver parenchyma and pathologic structures), while at the same time the liver veins and portal veins were well delineated.

The *3D reconstruction* was done using Mipron software (MIP-CT program) on a Kontron working station (Kontron, Eching near Munich, FRG). Data transfer was realized with CT-Net, reducing the 512 × 512 matrix of CT scans to a 256 × 256 matrix. The MIP-CT program allows the segmentation and depiction of up to four objects in different colors. In a first step, the structures of interest (vessel lumina, tumors, liver parenchyma, thrombus in aortic aneurysm) were delineated by segmentation. This was done on selected representative CT scans with the help of an upper and lower gray-scale threshold; afterwards, the system automatically recognized the marked objects and traced them on consecutive CT scans. Structures of the same density that did not belong to the structure of choice could be eliminated interactively. After coding the structures with the four different colors, 3D reconstruction was done from different angles. To improve the optical effect, a mathematical program to smooth the edges was applied. The spatial effect was optimized with additional brightness modulation. Anatomical or pathologic structures, e.g., the thrombus within an aortic aneurysm, could also be rendered in a transparent mode. The 3D reconstruction was documented either dynamically with a video sequence from different angles or statically in representative single images with a video color printer.

Results

The spiral CT imaging resulted in excellent to good quality images in 70 of 75 patients (93 %) who were examined during a single breath hold. Two patients (penetrating aortic aneurysm, spurious aneurysm) were scanned during shallow breathing. Only two examinations (2.6 %) were distorted by respiratory artifacts and unusable for 3D reconstruction. While vessels running perpendicular to the scanning plane were reconstructed virtually artifact-free, vessels running within the scanning plane were difficult to reconstruct. Due to the spiral movement of the scanners, the nominal slice thickness of 10 mm is broadened to 13 mm. This results in partial volume effects not be undone even with a maximum overlap of respective slices. If a vessel diameter is smaller than the slice thickness, its diameter is not reproduced correctly. The partial volume effect leads to diffuse borders of organs and vessels and a significant decrease in vessel density, which interferes with the automatic tracing. Intense pulsations of vessels lead to motion artifacts: In vessels running perpendicular to the scanning plane, the vessel diameter in 3D reconstruction was overestimated, and the borders appeared irregular (as in a kymogram).

Liver Lesions

A 3D reconstruction of upper abdominal lesions is reasonable only if a surgical procedure (e.g., resection of a liver metastasis) is planned. Lesions in question are either solitary (Fig. 1) or defined to a certain area (Fig. 2). For the surgeon, the exact location of a lesion within a certain segment of the liver, the presence of anatomical variations, and the spatial relationship to key structures (e.g., portal vein and its branches, choledochal duct, and liver veins) is important for the determination of a surgical approach. Localization of a lesion within a certain segment was demonstrated with 3D reconstruction much better than with consecutive CT scans. In con-

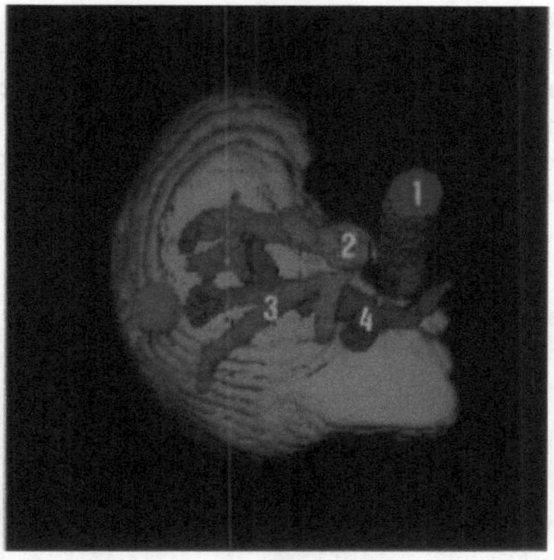

Fig. 1. Solitary metastasis of the liver (3D image): *1*, aorta *(red)*; *2*, vena cava inferior *(blue)*; *3*, vena mediana hepatic *(blue)*; *4*, vena portae *(red)*. Cranial view, metastasis *(green)* in segment 8 of the right liver lobe

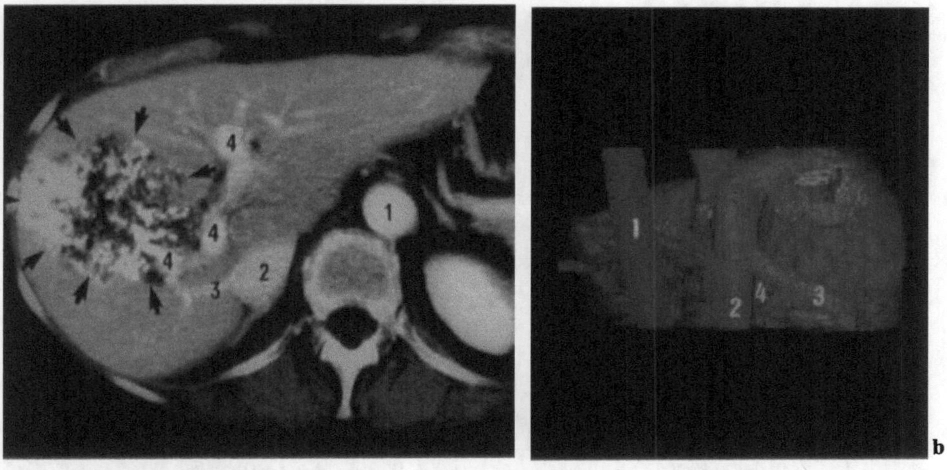

a b

Fig. 2a,b. Extended metastasis of the liver (colorectal carcinoma): *1*, aorta *(red)*; *2*, vena cava inferior; *3*, vena hepatis from segment 6 (anatomical variation); *4*, branches of vena portae. **a** Spiral CT scan, metastasis in segment 8 and 4 after embolization with Epirubicin and Lipiodol. Infiltration and obstruction of branches of the vena portae and liver veins. **b** A 3D image (dorsal view), topographical relationship between liver lesion and vessels are clearly demonstrated. Anatomical variation (here a liver vein of segment 6 running directly into the inferior caval vein) is easily detected

ventional CT scans, the portal veins are the dominant structures, while the liver veins, the actual determinants of segmental anatomy, can only be discerned in the cranial sections of the liver, where they run into the inferior caval vein. With 3D reconstruction, semi-automatic segmentation is able to trace the liver veins into the caudal parts of the liver and differentiate them from the portal veins, which is important especially in patients with anatomical variations. In one patient, a liver vein of segment 6 running directly into the inferior caval vein was only detected with 3D reconstruction (Fig. 2). In addition to conventional CT scans, 3D reconstruction facilitated the demonstration of the topographical relationship between the liver lesions and key structures in all cases. Details, however, were better seen in the original data set (e.g., tumor infiltration of vessels, relation of lesions, and hepatic artery in the liver hilus; Fig. 2 a). This deficit of 3D reconstruction was mainly due to partial volume effects, matrix reduction, and the segmentation process, which equals a diagnostic selection of pertinent information with simultaneous exclusion of unnecessary details.

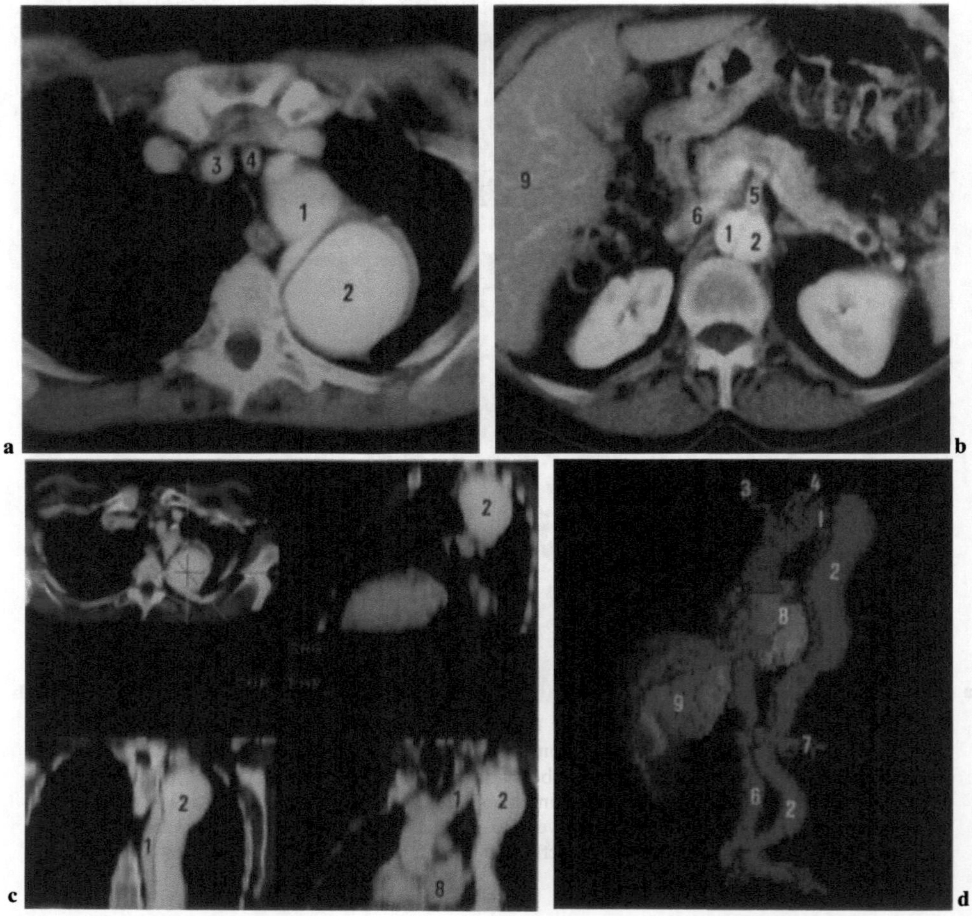

Fig. 3 a–d. Dissecting aneurysm of the whole aorta: *1,* true lumen of the aorta; *2,* false lumen of the aorta; *3,* truncus brachiocephalicus; *4,* arteria carotis communis sinistra; *5,* arteria mesenterica superior; *6,* vena cava inferior; *7,* a. et v. renalis sinistra; *8,* heart; *9,* liver. **a** Spiral CT scan (upper thorax), good vessel contrast in the spiral CT scan showing the dissection membrane, the true lumen, and the sack of the false lumen. **b** Spiral CT scan (upper abdomen), good vessel contrast showing the superior mesenteric artery comming out of the true lumen. **c** A 2D reconstruction (sagittal, coronal, paraxial view); spiral CT scans are the ideal basis for consecutive 2D reconstruction without artifacts caused by respiratory motion. **d** A 3D image (ventral view), reconstructed out of two spiral CT data sets (notice the gap caused by respiratory motion). The topographical relationship between aneurysm and branching vessels is well demonstrated

Vessel Lesions

Forty patients with vessel lesions (32 patients with an aortic aneurysm, two patients with a tumor thrombus within the renal and inferior caval vein caused by hypernephroma, and six patients with anatomical variants) were examined. In patients with an aortic aneurysm, the major interest is in its location, size, extent, and especially relationship to the branching vessels. Important additional information like the degree of parietal thrombosis or the detection of penetration with hemorrhage and the exact location of the intimal lesion in dissecting aneurysm with definition of true and false lumen are essential for the diagnosis, prognosis, and surgery planning. Generally, all this information can be obtained with conventional contrast-enhanced CT scans. Compared with conventional CT, spiral CT significantly improves the demonstration of these lesions due to a better timing of contrast application throughout the examination (Figs. 3, 4). However, a presurgical angiography is almost always requested by clinicians, who have difficulties transferring the CT information into a topographical view. Spiral CT and consecutive 3D reconstruction excels with exquisite image quality (good vessel contrast), a fast imaging mode that is tolerable even for very sick patients, and graphic presentation of the topographical information needed by clinicians. The dynamic presentation of a 3D reconstruction, via a video sequence is especially instructive. The size and extent of the false lumen in dissecting aneurysms were demonstrated reliably using two consecutive spiral CT scans covering the thoracic and abdominal aorta including the iliac vessels (Fig. 3). In true aortic aneurysms, spiral CT was definitely superior to angiography in depicting simultaneously the vessel lumen and parietal thrombosis (that may be shown in a semitransparent mode; Fig. 4). Branching vessels were demonstrated in all cases, although the lumina of renal arteries running in the scanning plane were not assessed reliably (see above

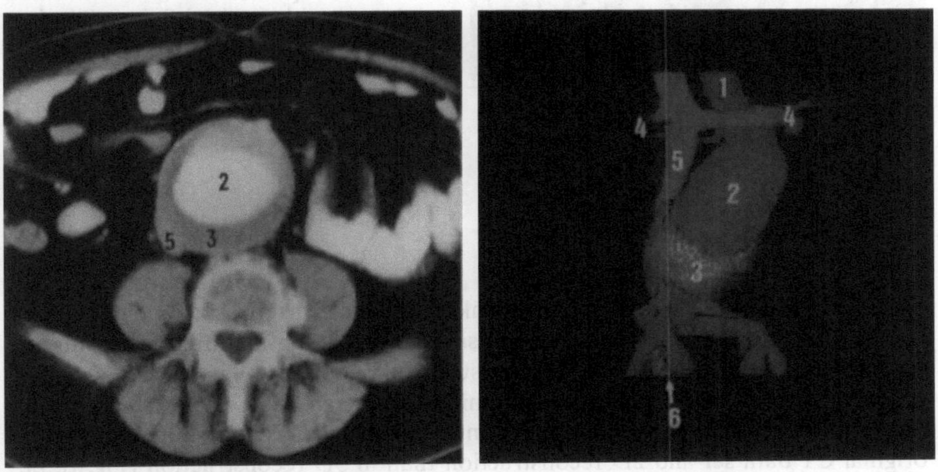

a b

Fig. 4a,b. True aortic aneurysm and aneurysm of the iliac artery: *1,* aorta; *2,* aortic aneurysm; *3,* thrombus; *4,* renal vessels; *5,* vena cava inferior; *6,* iliac aneurysm with thrombus. **a** Spiral CT scan (lower abdomen), good contrast between lumen and parietal thrombus. **b** 3D image (ventral view), the topographical relationship between aneurysm, thrombus, and branching vessels (e.g., renal vessels) is clearly shown

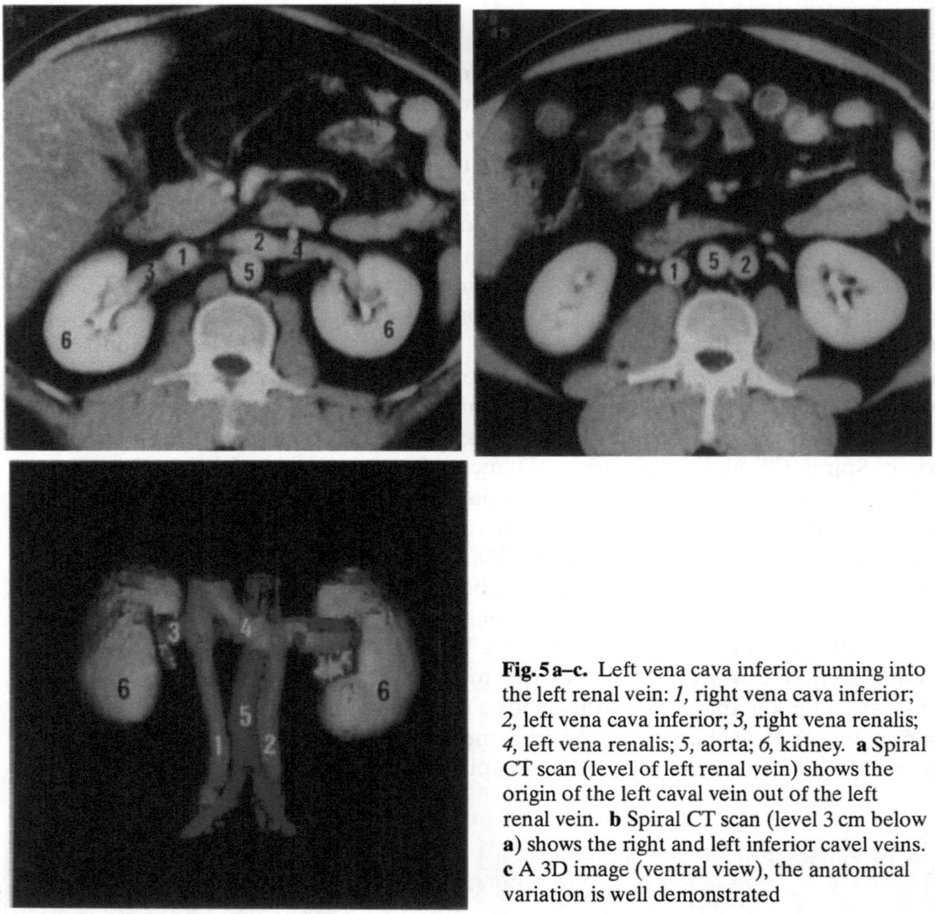

Fig. 5 a–c. Left vena cava inferior running into the left renal vein: *1,* right vena cava inferior; *2,* left vena cava inferior; *3,* right vena renalis; *4,* left vena renalis; *5,* aorta; *6,* kidney. **a** Spiral CT scan (level of left renal vein) shows the origin of the left caval vein out of the left renal vein. **b** Spiral CT scan (level 3 cm below **a**) shows the right and left inferior cavel veins. **c** A 3D image (ventral view), the anatomical variation is well demonstrated

reasons), and vessels with pronounced kinking produced artefacts. Angiography was always essential when, besides an aneurysm, vascular stenosis (thrombus or atherosclerosis) had to be analyzed. A 3D reconstruction is most useful in the assessment of simple aneurysms and in complex anatomical variants of the venous system (Fig. 5). The depiction of tumor thrombus in the inferior caval vein is more impressive in the original CT data set and 2D reconstruction than in 3D reconstruction (Fig. 6), because of difficulties during segmentation to differentiate thrombus from flow or contrast media dilution phenomena and again due to the fact that the left renal vein runs within the scanning plane. Angiography remains the method of choice in these cases.

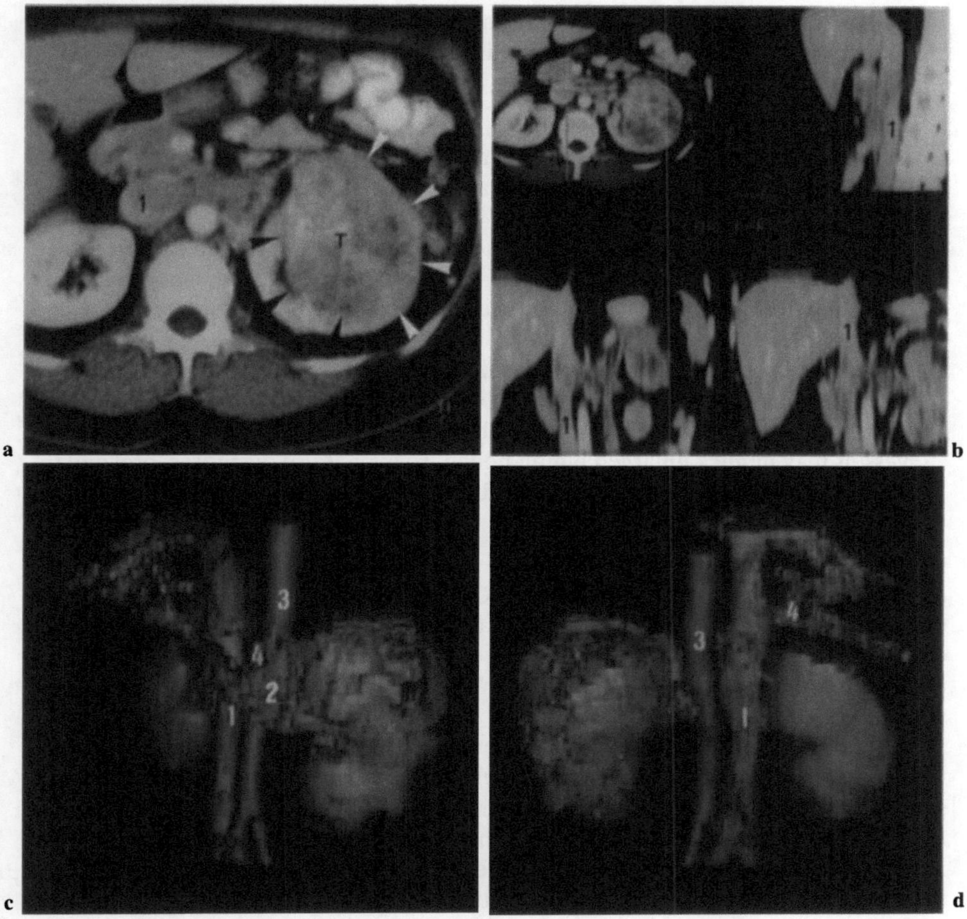

Fig. 6a–d. Tumor of the kidney with tumor thrombus of the caval vein: *1*, vena cava inferior (with tumor thrombus); *2*, left renal vein (with tumor thrombus); *3*, aorta; *4*, truncus coeliacus; *T*, tumor. **a** Spiral CT scan (level of left renal vein), good contrast of the vessels and the renal parenchyma with good delineation of the tumor and the tumor thrombus. **b** A 2D reconstruction (sagittal, coronal, paraxial view) without artifacts caused by respiratory motion showing the tumor thrombus within the renal and inferior caval vein. **c** A 3D image, ventral view; **d** dorsal view

Discussion

After 20 years of technical development mainly focussed on shortening the measurement time (now 1 s or less) and on improving the spatial resolution (slice thickness 1 mm, image matrix 512 × 512, with a display matrix of 1024 × 1024), state-of-the-art CT today offers high resolution and superimposition-free scans with high detail recognition that are further improved by the application of intravenous or even intra-arterial contrast media. As it contains a wealth of information combined with a low risk for the patient, CT has become one of the most important imaging techniques.

However, there are three major drawbacks that should be taken into account if a CT finding has to be demonstrated to a clinician, who is not experienced in reading CT films:

1. CT scans are usually obtained in the transverse plane, resulting in axial slices that are not primarily understandable for a clinician (who is used to images in the anterioposterior or sagittal projection, as this is what he is confronted with during surgery).
2. CT offers only slice images that have to be mentally combined and postprocessed to render a spatial picture of the actual situs and thus lead to a diagnosis. The 3D view, however, is what is needed by the surgeon to picture the surgical situs and plan operative strategies.
3. CT images contain redundant information that is of minor importance for the respective diagnosis but may preoccupy or confuse the observer and even lead to wrong diagnoses. Bowel loops in the abdomen may be interpreted as tumors, or vessels may mimick enlarged lymph nodes. To avoid false diagnoses, oral and intravenous contrast media are used to differentiate anatomical from pathological structures.

For the experienced reviewer, who knows about these pitfalls, it is fairly easy to deduce a correct diagnosis. The transfer of CT findings to a nonradiologist, however, may be difficult. The process can be facilitated by offering (a) a reconstruction in another plane, (b) a 3D reconstructed image, or (c) a picture that contains only relevant information pertaining to the specific clinical problem in addition to conventional scans.

Even in the early stages of CT, 3D reconstructions from CT data sets were recognized as desirable [6] and have been postulated for years [2, 8, 9, 13, 16, 17, 23]. The same holds true for magnetic resonance imaging (MRI) [14, 15, 18]. Easy-to-handle 3D software that is based on a gray-scale threshold is implemented in many CT scanners and offers a 3D reconstruction of skeletal structures within a reasonable time frame. Reconstruction of soft tissue structures is more time consuming, as for each structure two gray-scale thresholds have to be selected, and usually more than one structure has to be reconstructed.

The 3D reconstruction with the MIP-CT program on a Kontron work-station offers semiautomatic, interactive segmentation of up to four different soft tissue structures with specific color coding [7]. Until now, organs subjected to respiratory motion were not assessed faithfully for their actual size and location. The new spiral CT technique, however, permits the scanning of a volume of 24 cm in length within a single breath hold [1, 11, 12, 19, 23]. In addition to the many advantages of this technique (fast measurement time, less exposure to radiation, better and more specific vessel contrast), spiral CT finally offers a basis for the 3D reconstruction of organs subjected to respiratory motion [7, 24].

The role of conventional CT in the diagnosis of liver lesions has long been established. Color-coded 3D reconstruction finally permits the transfer of important topographical information that is immediately usable. However, compared with conventional scans, the 3D image contains less information and offers fewer details. It cannot and should not replace the original CT scan but rather illustrate topographical information that is otherwise hard to understand [7, 20, 21].

Great vessel lesions, especially those of the aorta, are another stronghold of contrast-enhanced CT [3, 22, 25, 26]. This is also true for abdominal vessels like the inferior caval or renal vein containing a tumor thrombus in patients with hypernephroma [5]. In patients with an aortic aneurysm, CT is superior to angiography in depicting not only the dilated true lumen delineated by flowing blood, but also the real borders of the aneurysmal vessel, so a parietal thrombus can be differentiated from the perfused true lumen. In penetrating or dissecting aneurysms, CT depicts the localization and extent of hemorrhage and intimal lesions as well as angiographic studies and with significantly less risk for the patient. Of course, optimal vessel contrast is mandatory. Demonstration of the topographical relationship between the aneurysm and branching vessels of the aorta relies on contiguous scanning and acquisition of CT scans that are not distorted by respiratory motion or pulsation artifacts [4]. Spiral CT meets these conditions. The entire volume of interest is scanned during a single breath hold of 24 s. Optimal vessel contrast during the measurement time is maintained by predefined intravenous contrast media application. The reconstruction of transverse slices from the original spiral data set with a 2-mm increment in contiguous scanning without respiratory movement allows the reliable identification of the large thoracic and abdominal vessels. The absence of respiratory artifacts makes spiral CT the ideal basis for consecutive coronal, sagittal, or paraxial 2D reconstruction or color-coded 3D reconstruction. The postprocessed and reconstructed image necessarily contains only relevant topographical information. Since it does not depict all the gray-scale coded details of the original scan, the specific information that has been deduced by segmentation is especially emphasized by the elimination of redundant information. A 3D reconstruction illustrates complex topographical relationships better than projectional angiographic images or even the paraxial MR images (that remain slice images). Patient exposure to radiation, examination time, and risk of invasive procedure are significantly less with spiral CT than with angiography.

References

1. Bautz W, Skalej M, Thomas C (1990) New directions in CT diagnosis of the pancreas. In: Fuchs W (ed) Advances in CT. Springer, Berlin Heidelberg New York, pp 37–48
2. Baxter B, Hichner L, Anderson R (1982) Application of three-dimensional display in diagnostic imaging. J Comput Assist Tomogr 6: 1000–1005
3. Blair RH, Resnik MD, Polga JP (1989) CT appearance of mycotic abdominal aortic aneurysms. J Comput Assist Tomogr 13: 101–104
4. Burns M, Molina P, Gutierrez F, Sagel S (1991) Motion artifact simulating aortic dissection on CT. AJR 157: 465–467
5. Didier D, Racle A, Etievent JP, Weill F (1987) Tumor thrombus of the inferior vena cava secondary to malignant abdominal neoplasms: US and CT evaluation. Radiology 162: 83–89
6. Glenn W, Johnston R, Morton P, Dwyer S (1975) Image generation and display techniques for CT scan data. Invest Radiol 10: 403–416
7. Gmeinwieser J, Wunderlich A, Gerhardt P, Strotzer M (1991) Dreidimensionale Rekonstruktion von atemverschieblichen Organen und Gefäßstrukturen aus Spiral-CT-Datensätzen. Rontgenpraxis 44: 2–8
8. Hodler J, Kuoni W, Rodrigues M (1990) Three-dimensional imaging: technical aspects. In: Fuchs W (ed) Advances in CT. Springer, Berlin Heidelberg New York, pp 115–124
9. Imhof K (1989) Die dreidimensionale Darstellung von CT-Bildern: Methode und Möglichkeiten. Electromedica 57: 154–159

10. Kalender W, Seissler W, Klotz E, Vock P (1990) Spiral volumetric CT with single-breath-hold technique, continuous transport, and continuous scanner rotation. Radiology 176: 181–183
11. Kalender W, Vock P, Polacin A, Soucek M (1990) Spiral-CT: Eine neue Technik für Volumenaufnahmen. I. Grundlagen und Methodik. Rontgenpraxis 43: 323–330
12. Kalender W, Vock P, Seissler W (1990) Spiral CT scanning for fast and continuous volume data acquisition. In: Fuchs W (ed) Advances in CT. Springer, Berlin Heidelberg New York, pp 55–64
13. Kashiwagi T, Mitsutani N, Koizumi T, Kimura K (1988) Three-dimensional demonstration of liver and spleen by a computed graphics technique. Acta Radiol 29: 27–31
14. König H, Laub G (1988) The processing and display of three-dimensional data in magnetic resonance imaging. Electromedica 56: 42–49
15. Lang P, Genant H, Steiger P, Stoller D, Heuck A (1989) 3-D reformatting asserts clinical potential in MRI. Diagn Imaging 5: 32–36
16. Levinthal C, Macagno E, Tountas C (1974) Computed-aided reconstruction from serial sections. Fed Proc 33: 2336–2340
17. Pate D, Resnick D, Andre M, Satoris D (1986) Perspective: three-dimensional imaging of the musculoskeletal system. AJR 147: 545–551
18. Seiderer M, Bauer W, Villringer A, Einhäupl K (1990) 3D-MR-Angiographie mit Gd-DTPA. Fortschr Rontgenstr 152: 327–332
19. Soucek M, Vock P, Daepp M, Kalender W (1990) Spiral-CT: Eine neue Technik für Volumenaufnahmen. II. Klinische Anwendung. Rontgenpraxis 43: 365–375
20. Soyer P, Roche A, Gad M, Shapeero L, Breittmayer F, Elias D, Lasser P, Rougier P, Levesque M (1991) Preoperative segmental localization of hepatic metastases: utility of three-dimensional CT during arterial portography. Radiology 180: 653–658
21. Takemura M, Oguma S, Mori S, Ishii M, Starzl T, Demetris A, Takahasi T (1991) Peribiliary vascular diseases in rejected livers; computer-aided three-dimensional reconstruction and morphology. Transplant Proc 23: 1409–1412
22. Tobben PJ, Zajko AB, Sumkin JH, Bowen A, Fuhrman CR, Skolnick ML, Bron KM, Esquivel CO, Starzl TE (1988) Pseudoaneurysms complicating organ transplantation: roles of CT, duplex sonography, and angiograhy. Radiology 169: 65–70
23. Vannier M, Marsh J, Gado M, Totty H, Gilula L, Evens R (1983) Klinische Anwendung der dreidimensionalen Oberflächenrekonstruktion aus CT-Scans-Erfahrungen bei 250 Untersuchungen. Electromedica 51: 122–131
24. Vock P, Soucek M, Daepp M, Kalender W (1990) Single-breathhold spiral volumetric CT (SVCT) of the lung and hepatobiliary system. In: Fuchs W (ed) Advances in CT. Springer, Berlin Heidelberg New York, pp 77–84
25. Yamada T, Tada S, Harada J (1988) Aortic dissection without intimal rupture: diagnosis with MR imaging and CT. Radiology 168: 347–352
26. Yamaguchi T, Guthaner DF, Wexler L (1989) Natural history of the false channel of type A aortic dissection after surgical repair: CT study. Radiology 170: 743–747
27. Zonneveld F, van der Meulen J, von Akkerveeken P, Koorneef L, Vaandrager J, van der Horst C (1988) Dreidimensionale Bildgebung durch Verarbeitung von CT-Daten und klinische Anwendung in der Orthopädie und Chirurgie des Gesichtsschädels. Röntgenstrahlen 59: 28–29
28. Zwicker C, Langer M, Astinet F, Felix R (1990) Wertigkeit der 3D-CT in der kieferchirurgischen Diagnostik und Therapieplanung. Fortschr Rontgenstr 152: 393–397

Three-Dimensional Imaging: Preliminary Examinations and Experience with the Somatom Plus-S

M. Ozan Tanyü, B. Wimmer, and P. Vinée

Introduction

Conventional radiographs arise from the projection of a volume and, as a result, show superimpositions. The role of the radiologist is the extraction of normal and pathological details that can be interpreted in terms of three-dimensional structures. Superimposition was overcome by scanning. Translation of the scans in the third dimension requires a capacity of imagination only gained after extensive training. It is therefore not surprising that three-dimensional imaging encounters an enthusiastic response from surgeons.

We report our experience with three-dimensional (3-D) reconstructions made on the Somatom Plus-S available in our department since October 1991.

Material and methods

More than 1500 patients with usual indications were routinely examined in the University Hospital with the Somatom Plus-S between 21 October 1991 and 31 January 1992. In 60 cases, we performed 3-D reconstruction using the resident software, mostly for skeletal pathology (Table 1). The 3-D reconstruction was planned before the examination in only 20% of the patients. Transversal scanning was always continuous; the slice thickness and further parameters were adjusted for the examined region (e.g., for the calcaneus 2–3 mm, for the vertebra 3–5 mm).

The 3-D reconstructions were performed on a separate DSC console linked to the image computer, thus avoiding interference with patient examinations. A threshold definition of 150 HU for highlighting of the pixels was chosen with possible adjustments between 50 and 200 HU in individual cases. Image matrix was 512 × 512.

Table 1. Three-dimensional reconstructed regions ($n = 60$)

Region examined	Number
Skull	12
Spine	18
Shoulder	9
Ankle	5
Calcaneus	8
Pelvis	6
Other	2

Knowing the diagnosis from the CT scans we interactively manipulated the calculated 3-D image (in terms of rotation, tilting, lighting or shadowing effects, and especially cutting) to optimize the representation of the pathological details. The 3-D images obtained were submitted to five radiologists (with 1.5–24 months of CT experience) who were asked for therapeutically relevant image details.

Results

Technical Management

The calculation time on previous systems (Somatom DRH) lasted for 20–40 min. Furthermore, the lack of a separate console made concomitant patient examination impossible. The image computer and the resident software of the Somatom Plus-S allowed the reconstruction of a 3-D image within 3–5 min (from the very beginning of the procedure to the presentation of the first 3-D image). Supplementary reconstructions were possible within seconds using the interactive mouse-driven menu, while on the DRH a previous declaration of such manipulations was necessary. The ability to reconstruct 2-D images at any plane of the object while working in the 3-D program at the same time helped clarify structures that might have been hidden on an external view.

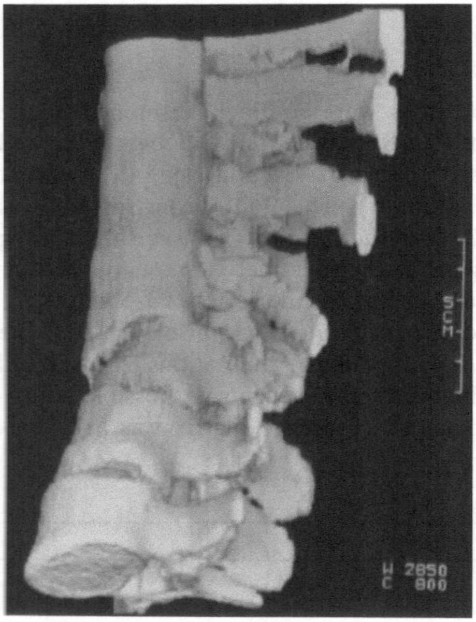

Fig. 1. A 28-year-old weight lifter was injured by the weights falling on his back. Clinically paraparesis. The CT showed thoracolumbar fracture dislocation. Contiguous 10-mm slices of the thoracal spine, 5 mm of the fractured lumbar spine. The smoothing effect on a 3-D image makes the intervertebral spaces of the thoracal spine seem to disappear, creating the appearance of Bechterew's syndrom

Diagnostic Value and Evaluation

The diagnostic value of 3-D imaging is definitely lower than the transversal scanning. To avoid steps in the 3-D image at the junction between the transversal scans we used a smoothing algorithm leading to a jointless aspect (Fig. 1). However, this caused a blurring of the fracture lines in some cases. The smoothing effect could be reduced by defining a higher threshold for the primary scans. Thinner and less dense structures like spongiosa or contrasted small vessels in the liver and lung were not demonstrated on the images so obtained. On the other hand, this led to defect simulation or artifical enlargement (Fig. 2).

In our experience, 3-D imaging was overvalued by surgeons. The reconstruction altered the planned therapeutic management in only 2 of 60 cases. In a case of a large traumatic defect of the frontal bone including the orbital arch, the 3-D image facilitated planning of the size and shape of the bone transplant. In the second case, the 3-D image showed complete reconstruction of the hemi-pelvis (including the acetabulum) to be impossible in Gorham-Stout syndrome (Fig. 3). A 3-D image cannot contain

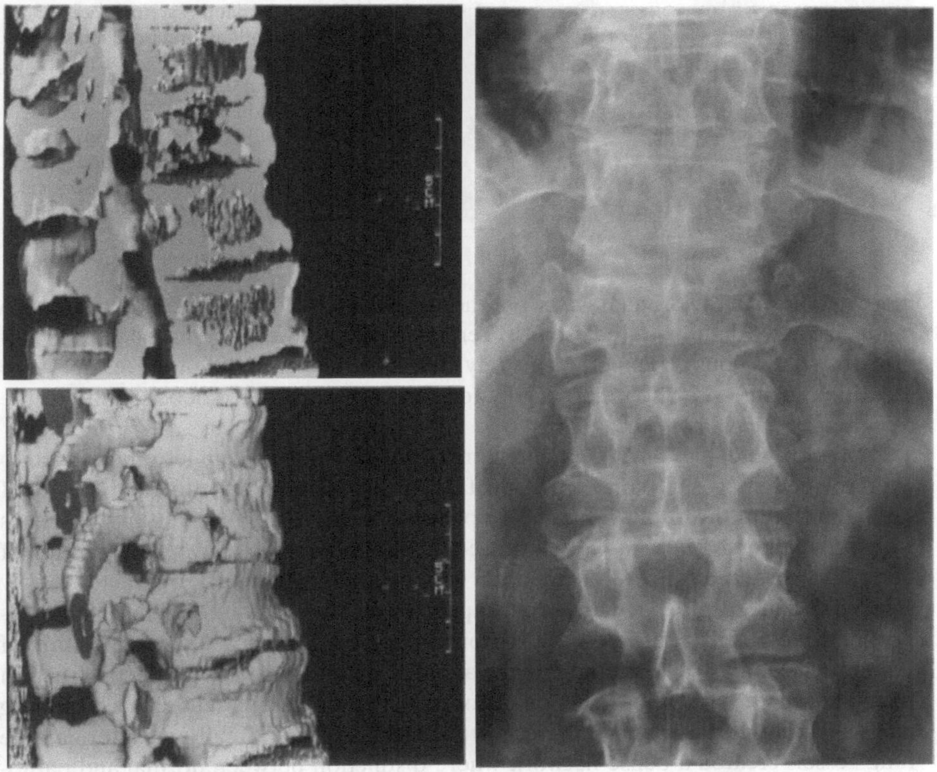

a b c

Fig. 2 **a** A 57-year-old patient with pheochromocytoma and metastatic osteolysis of T_{12}. Sagittal cut of the 3-D image shows metastatic defect of the spongiosa and the cortical bone of T_{12}. Thinner parts of the spongious bone of T_{11}, L_1 and L_2 have disappeared by subtraction, simulating further defects. **b, c** The defect seen on the 3-D reconstruction in the right lateral part of L_1 is simulated as there is no evidence of such a lesion on the plain X-ray or on the primary scans (not shown)

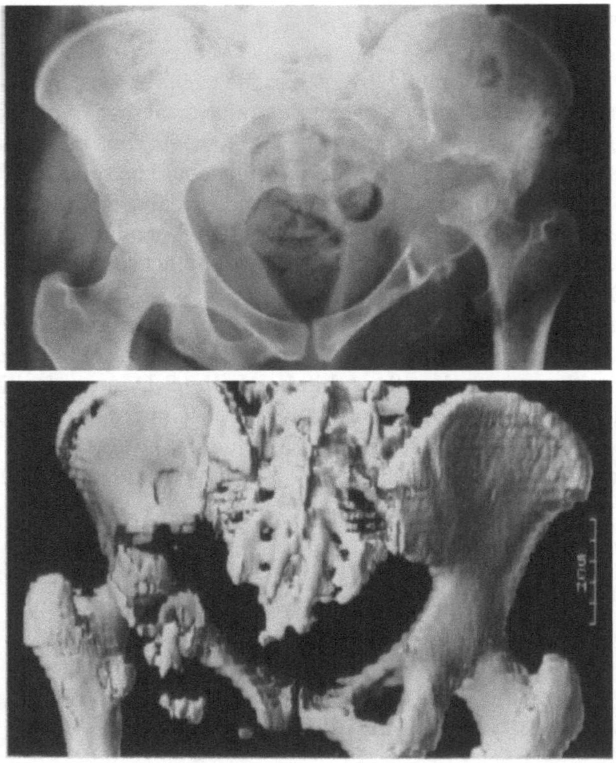

a

b

Fig. 3 a, b. A 48-year-old patient with Gorham-Stout syndrome (vanishing bone). **a** Osteolytic destructions in os ileum, sacrum, acetabulum and femoral head are shown on the plain X-ray **b** Perhaps more impressive demonstration on the 3-D reconstruction (5 mm scans, posterior view), giving our surgeons the impression that surgical repairement was impossible

more details than the original scans, but those details proved to be definitely harder to recognize as we demonstrated in a test. Ten selected cases were submitted to five radiologists with various CT experience. Only 10%–30% (mean 16%) of the lesions were identified, with a poor score especially for complex fractures, independently of the thickness of the primary slices (Fig. 4).

Attempts to depict the 3-D architecture of vessels and adjacent lesions only led to overcrowded images. Despite arterioportal contrast medium injection and the use of several different threshold values, clear pictures of the vena portae and its branches were not obtained. The same conclusion could be applied to the 3-D reconstruction of the biliary system after contrast medium application through a PTD catheter. A low threshold value resulted in many superimposed structures making the image nondiagnostic, while a high threshold only demonstrated vessel stumps. Superimposition of the thoracic bony structure could not be avoided. Even worse was the reconstruction from a spiral CT with bolus injection of contrast medium in a patient with a dissecting and rupturing aortic aneurysm and aortobronchial fistula. Small and intermediate lung vessels created a dense network where distinction between normal and pathological details was not possible. Moreover, cardiac and skeletal structures hindered exposition of the region of interest.

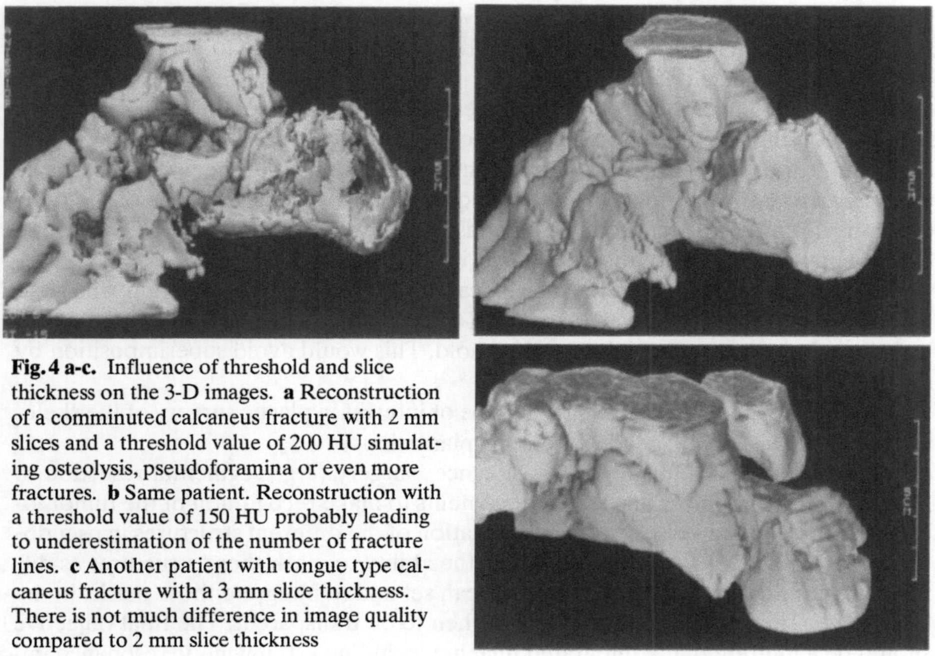

a b c

Fig. 4 a-c. Influence of threshold and slice thickness on the 3-D images. **a** Reconstruction of a comminuted calcaneus fracture with 2 mm slices and a threshold value of 200 HU simulating osteolysis, pseudoforamina or even more fractures. **b** Same patient. Reconstruction with a threshold value of 150 HU probably leading to underestimation of the number of fracture lines. **c** Another patient with tongue type calcaneus fracture with a 3 mm slice thickness. There is not much difference in image quality compared to 2 mm slice thickness

Discussion

In recent years, 3-D CT has gained increased popularity [3], and further efforts are being made by physicians and software specialists to improve this method. The 3-D imaging of luxations and dislocated fragments have proven to be helpful in surgical planning [4, 9, 10]. The therapeutic planning in orthopedics cases was affected by the results of 3-D imaging in 20%–30% in Fishman's studies [1, 2]. In assessing a pelvic pathology, suboptimal conventional exposures, difficult positioning of patients, and bowel artifacts might be troublesome. In those cases, 3-D imaging can eliminate such difficulties and even decrease the radiation dose to the patient [7]. The utility of imaging in 3-D can also be documented in the planning of radiation therapy, in which the calculation of the 3-D dose distributions enables a tumor-tailored radiotherapy of localized target volumes with increased radiation doses and improved sparing of organs at risk [6].

With the Somatom Plus-S, due to a faster image computer and interactive possibilities, the clinical use of 3-D imaging has been improved. The primary scans contain more details relevant for surgical planning, so that 3-D imaging is not yet a first-line diagnostic tool. The most important example in our report was the calcaneus fracture, mostly a multifragment fracture involving multiple articular surfaces. Most of the fracture lines or small fragments within a joints or fracture space were overlapped and not to be seen without selective cuts, relying on the information gained on the primary scans.

The 3-D representation of the spine may be helpful to surgeons in the cases where 2-D reconstructions show only part of the region of interest due to natural, acquired or positioning-related deformation.

The 3-D imaging of small bony structures like the foramina of the skull base, bony septa (e.g., cellulae ethmoidales) or spongiosa is strongly dependent upon the chosen threshold value (see Fig. 4a, b). Without this information from the primary scans, it would lead to misinterpretation and consequently false results. The role of the radiologist is not only restricted to the demonstration and estimation of the pathology but also includes the prevention of an overinterpretation of the image.

In our opinion, further relevant clinical applications of 3-D imaging will arise from improvements of the skeletal and soft tissue details, which can only be achieved by using a low-pass and a high-pass threshold. This would avoid superimposition by soft tissue details or skeletal parts.

Interactive operative planning would be of interest in plastic surgery of the skeleton or soft tissues (skull, pelvis, face, transplantations).

A practicable 3-D imaging to assist cancer surgery (e.g., segmental resection in liver metastasis) requires further improvements to make recognition of the tumor location relative to the vessels and representation of the different structures in pseudocolors possible [5, 8]. This again requires the ability to mark those structures as different regions of interest on the original scan set and to integrate those marks in the 3-D image. The surface of the organ has then to be transparent. The final objective should be a multimodality integrated imaging including CT, magnetic resonance imaging, sonography, and nuclear medicine.

References

1. Fishman EK, Drebin B, Magid D, Scott WW, Ney DR, Brooker AF, Riley LH, Ville JA, Zerhouni EA, Siegelmann SS (1987) Volumetric rendering techniques: applications for three-dimensional imaging of the hip. Radiology 163: 737–738
2. Fishman EK, Magid D, Mey DR, Chaney EL, Pizer SM, Rosenman JG, Levin GM, Vannier MW, Kuhlman JE, Robertson DD (1991) Three-dimensional imaging. Radiology 181: 321–337
3. Kern A, Waggershauser T, Zendel W, Astinet A, Hansen K, Lanksch WR, Felix R (1991) Dreidimensionale Rekonstruktionsverfahren in der lumbalen Computertomographie. Fortschr Röntgenstr 155 (2): 179–186
4. Kuner EH, Kuner A, Schlickewei W, Wimmer B (1992) Die Bedeutung der Ligamentotaxis für die Fixateur-interne-Osteosynthese bei Frakturen der Brust- und Lendenwirbelsäule. Chirurg 63: 50–55
5. Moyses B, Muller JN, Hollaender C, Methlin G (1991) Intérêt de la reconstruction scanographique tridimensionnelle abdominale. Rev Im Med 3: 751–754
6. Schlegel W (1991) 3 D Rekonstruktionen in der Bestrahlungsplanung. Radiologe 31: 457–466
7. Scott WW, Fishman EK, Magid D (1987) Acetabular fractures: optimal imaging. Radiology 165: 537–539
8. Soyer P, Breittmayer F, Gad M, Levesque M, Roche A (1991) Imagerie tridimensionnelle de la segmentation hépatique: anatomie et volumétrie. Rev Im Med 3: 741–745
9. Uhrmeister P, Langer M, Zwicker C, Astinet F, Felix R (1991) Dreidimensionale Computertomographie von Frakturen. Akt Traumatol 21: 129–134
10. Zinreich J, Wang H, Abdo F, Bryan RN (1990) 3-D CT improves accuracy of spinal trauma studies. Diagn Imaging Int July/August: 24–29

Multiplanar CT of the Lumbar Herniated Nucleus Pulposus

R. Dore, G. Monzillo, L. Cicuttini, P. Lolli, and L. Storti

Introduction

Usually, the lumbar spine computed tomography (CT) examinations for herniated disk evaluation involve just transverse scans. The diagnosis of herniated nucleus pulposus (HNP) made by CT in the past years has been very accurate, from 86.4% to 96.6% in overall accuracy (Table 1). We cannot in all certainty distinguish the extruded HNP from the not extruded one only on transverse images; moreover, it is difficult to evaluate correctly the intervertebral foramina and their normal or atypical contents based on transverse images. With past scanners, multiplanar reconstructions (MPR) were expensive in time and in radiation dose, and the obtained images were not so good.

Since we have been using the Somatom Plus, thanks to the rapidity of the examination and of the reconstruction, we have increased MPR use not just in presence of alterations already discovered on transverse images, but even for axial CT results which did not match the clinical presentation.

Our purpose is to verify the usefulness of MPR in the evaluation of HNP in a surgically proved series.

Patients

From September 1989 to January 1992, 507 lumbar spine CT exams were done at Sacra Famiglia Hospital in Erba (Italy). We have considered only 59 patients (11.6%) with surgically verified CT results. Their medium age was 46 years; 21 patients were women, 38 were men. The surgical results are summarized in Table 2: four patients had a narrow lumbar canal or posterior articular joints arthrosis; one patient

Table 1. CT diagnostic accuracy in lumbar herniated disc

Reference	Year	No. of cases	Accuracy
Livingston and Grayson [7]	1978	38	68.4%
Drovillard et al. [5]	1983		86.4%
Di Guglielmo et al. [3]	1982	81	90.1%
Di Guglielmo et al. [4]	1984	358	96.6%
Bonanni et al. [1]	1984	100	87.7%
Qui and Ge [10]	1990	47	90.4%
This study	1992	59	93.2%

Table 2. Surgical results in 59 patients

	No. of patients
Neurofibroma	1
Narrow lumbar canal	2
Narrow intervertebral foramina	2
Posterior HNP in L5-S1	17
Posterior HNP in L4–L5	23
Posterior HNP in L3–L4	6
Intraforaminal HNP	6
Lateral extraforamina HNP	2

had a small neurofibroma near the disc margin. In all, 54 HNP had been surgically treated.

Method

We used a continuously rotating scanner (Somatom Plus, Siemens) without spiral CT device. MPR were obtained on the basis of 12–15 single adjacent transverse scans at 137 Vp, 145 mA s, 2 mm slice thickness, and 2×2 multiscan cycle time for each intervertebral space. MPR were performed in 32/59 patients who were subsequently surgically treated:

- Sagittal recontructions (SR) were performed to examine central HNP
- Paraaxial (or oblique) ones to examine lateral and intraforaminal HNP
- Coronal ones to evaluate the relations of the HNP to the neural roots emergence and to examine the intraforaminal HNP

In the surgical findings, we considered "protrusive disc" the deformity of the disc border without an interruption of the superficial fibers of the anulus. "Not extruded" hernia was considered when the nucleus pulposus wanders through a completely ruptured anulus but remains limited by the posterior longitudinal ligament. Finally, in "extruded" hernia, the disc material escapes posterior to the longitudinal ligament.

Results

In 57/59 patients the CT findings diagnosed HNP. The true-positive CT diagnosis was confirmed at surgery in 55 patients, with an overall accuracy of 93.2%.

In Table 3 are shown the different types of HNP surgically demonstrated. CT had been correct in the not extruded diagnosis in 22/23 cases. The SR had been done in 11 cases of not extruded HNP: In nine cases, they confirmed the transverse scans, while in two cases they corrected the extruded HNP diagnosis made by the transverse images (Fig. 1).

In the 17 HNP extruded cases surgically recognized, CT was right in 13 cases; in three patients, it showed a not extruded type and in one case, an intraforaminal HNP. In this group, SR had been done in 10 cases; in four patients they showed more signs

Table 3. Surgical confirmation of herniated discs

	No. of cases
Non extruded HNP	23
Extruded HNP	17
Extruded with fragments HNP	6
Intraforaminal HNP	6
Extraforaminal HNP	2
Total	54

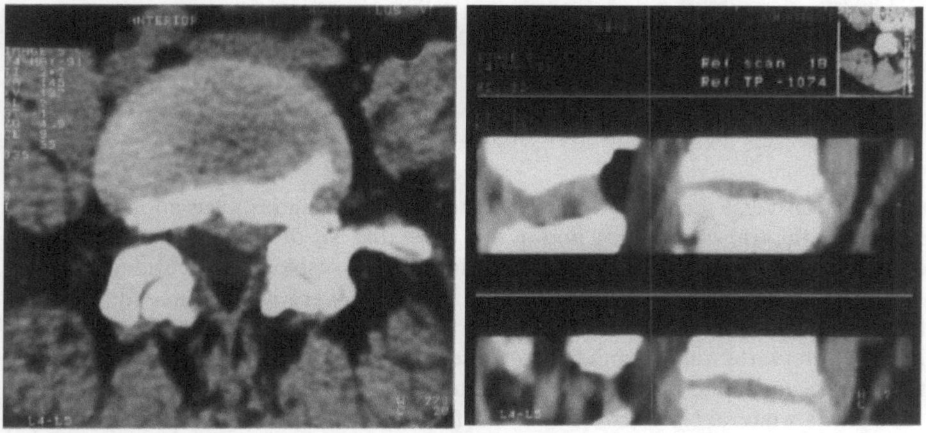

Fig. 1. L4–L5. Surgery revealed not extruded HNP; CT transverse scan showed suspected extrusion; CT sagittal plane had no evidence of extrusion

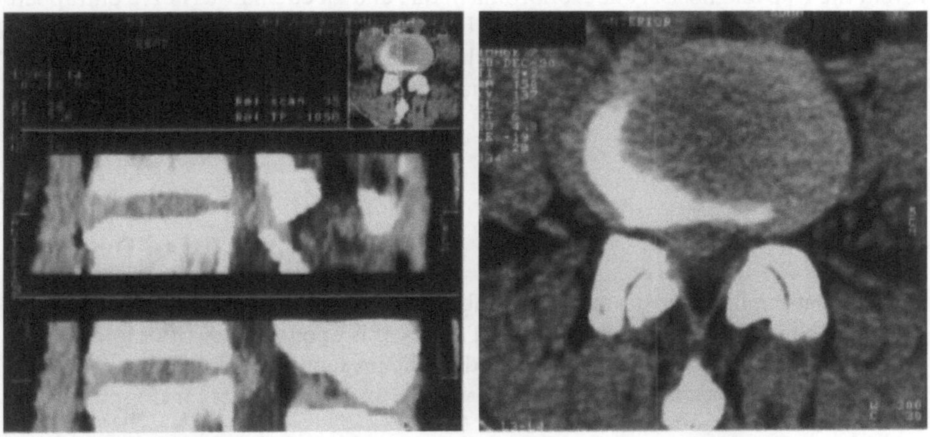

Fig. 2. L3–L4. Surgery revealed extruded HNP; CT sagittal plane showed PLL near body wall

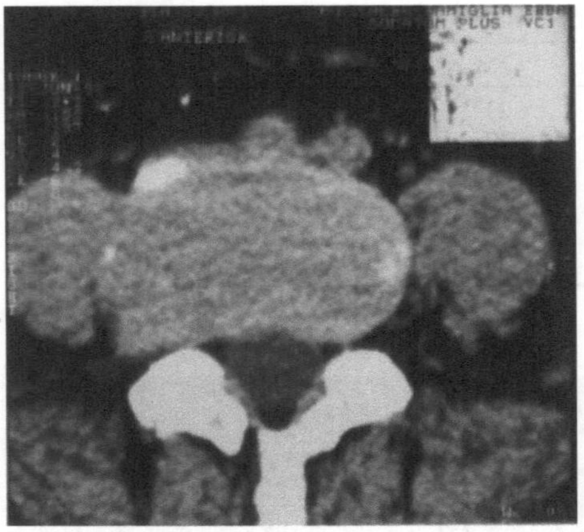

Fig. 3. L4–L5. At surgery, a large and edematous spinal nerve without any HNP is revealed

than the transverse scans (Fig. 2); in the other four, the diagnosis was already demonstrated by the transverse ones; and in two cases, the SR did not correctly show any extruded signs, while the transverse study indicated a suspicion of extruded HNP.

Six of seven extruded HNP with free fragments were well estimated: The one false result had been considered an intraforaminal hernia. The fragment had escaped into the intervertebral foramina in five cases; the MPR were helpful in representing the free fragment and the original side better.

In the six lateral HNP (two extra- and four intraforaminal), oblique and coronal comparative reconstructions had been useful in five cases. The overall accuracy in recognizing the type of HNP was 88.6%, but without MPR, it is reduced to 59.4%.

The CT diagnosis was not confirmed by surgery in four cases. In two, CT failed to reveal the true diagnosis: A neurofibroma in one and an edematous nerve entrapped between hypertrophic bone formation in the other were found during surgery (Fig. 3). In these cases, MPR would not have helped to correct the diagnosis. The other two cases were false-positive CT diagnoses of intraforaminal HNP, and MPR had not been performed.

Discussion

Thanks to its high diagnostic accuracy (Table 1), CT is the exam of first choice for the lumbar HNP diagnosis; in many cases CT by itself is enough to institute the correct therapy. Recently, no new results obtained by the present CT technology were noted in the literature; certainly the use of RM, with its excellent results for this pathology, has turned many practitioners away from CT.

Our results (93.2% overall accuracy) are among the best yet reported. Current technologies have made just a little improvement in HNP research compared with the great results published up to 1985. There are few data concerning the CT diagnosis of different HNP types (extruded, not extruded, and fragmented) requiring different treatments. Some authors have considered that is difficult or nearly impossible to distinguish the anulus protrusion only using CT [6]; others have categorically divided different findings [8]. At least it is recognized that a certain difficulty in the evaluation of intraforaminal HNP by CT exists. Recently, the use of reconstructions was suggested [2, 11]. At first, it seemed that just the use of SR could not improve the diagnostic results [9], but thanks to MPR CT studies of deep-frozen human cadavers, a 80% sensitivity and 100% specificity of intraforaminal HNP diagnosis have been demonstrated [11].

Diagnosis

In our series, MPR were never decisive for the posterior central HNP diagnosis, nor could they distinguish the not extruded HNP from the anulus protrusion. With SR, most of the not extruded HNP had the same aspect of the protrusion proved by

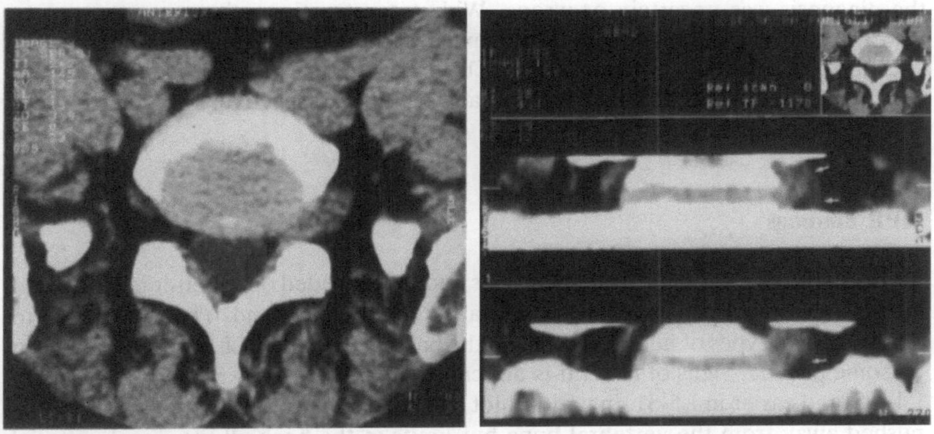

Fig. 4. L5-S1. Surgery revealed lateral intra- and extraforamina HNP; CT transverse scan showed mass is less dense than disc; CT coronal plane indicated nervous root *(arrows)* displaced by mass

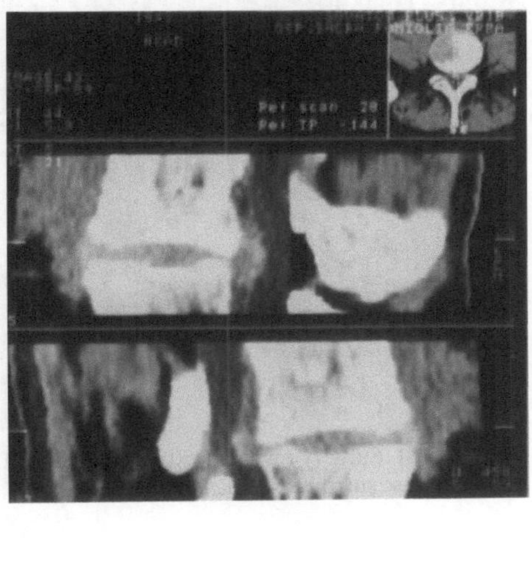

Fig. 5. L4–L5. Surgery revealed not extruded HNP; CT sagittal plane showed PLL pushed away from vertebral bone

surgery, that is, bulging of the disc margin without any caudal or cephalic expansion, which is more peculiar to not extruded HNP.

Instead, MPR have been more useful in recognizing lateral intra- und extraforaminal hernias (sensitivity 100%). MPR gave more data for transverse scans; even on coronal and oblique reconstructions, it was sometimes less difficult to evaluate the relations between nervous structure and mass and continuity between mass and disc that are the most important elements for the differential diagnosis between hernia and other masses (Fig. 4). The 75% CT false-positive results concerned intervertebral foramina; in two cases, no MPR were executed, in another case transverse and MPR abnormalities were due to a surgically proved edematous nerve.

Type

Without using MPR, the HNP type was diagnosed in just 58.4%; in the other cases, the diagnosis was uncertain or wrong. With reconstructions, the accuracy rose to 88.6%. The best results involved the not extruded hernia; 95% of them were correctly estimated, and 100% when using SR. The extruded type was more difficult to recognize; 76% and 80% accuracy without and with SR, respectively, so that SR were less helpful in this case.

MPR Findings

SR distinguished the not extruded hernias and the extruded ones better in L5-S1 and in the wide spinal canals where peridural fat ist largely found. They were able to divide the two types of hernia not just on the basis of disc and PLL relations, but even on some peculiar signs of HNP. It is difficult to identify PLL by SR in L3–L4 and in L4–L5, and easier in L5-S1. In various not extruded HNP the PLL, if recognizable, is pushed away from the vertebral bone but limits in the back all the discal material

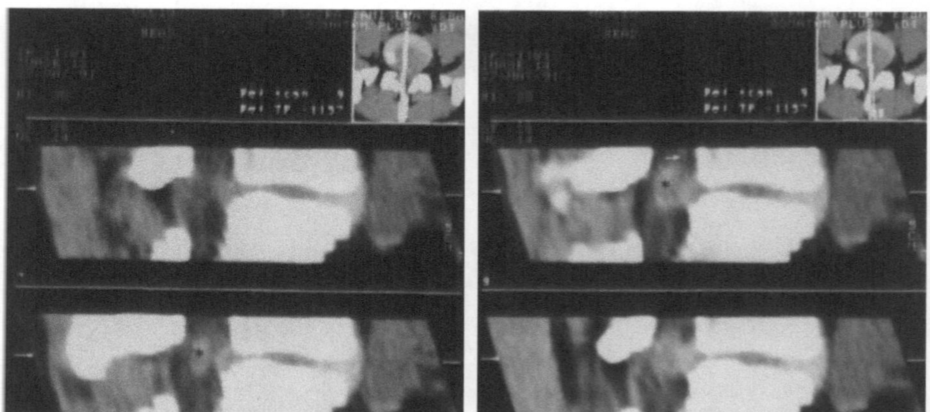

Fig. 6. L5-S1. Surgery revealed extruded HNP; CT sagittal plane showed the posterior (*) portion of herniated disc surrounds PLL *(arrows)*

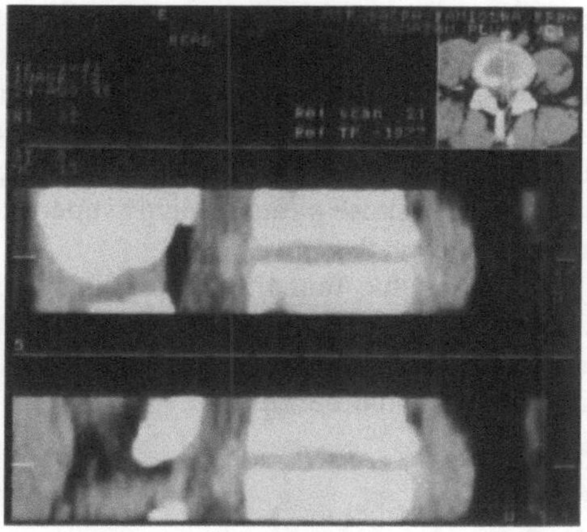

Fig. 7. L4–L5. Surgery revealed extruded and intradural HNP; CT sagittal plane showed type 3 extruded HNP finding; in the central sagittal plane, herniated mass seems separated from disc

(Fig. 5); the bulging discal margin can be symmetrical or more often spread down more than up.

We have observed differents findings of HNP:

1. PLL is more difficult to identify than in the not extruded HNP
2. If PLL is recognizable, it never moves away from body wall and is sheltered by the discal material that surrounds it anteriorly and posteriorly
3. In some extruded HNP we could observe in the spinal canal two discal density images: One anterior and contiguous with the disc, posteriorly defined or not by PLL; the other more posterior, distinguished and separate, ovoid, and with a vertical principal diameter (Figs. 6, 7). We think that this second image could be the discal extruded portion wandering around the PLL.

We believe the third sign observed, represented in one third of cases of extruded HNP, is the most certain sagittal finding, because it was not seen in not extruded HNP; it has never been described by other authors. We call it the "binocular" image. The second sign is not so frequent an observation; the first one cannot be used to distinguish between not extruded and extruded HNP.

Conclusions

Surgical results have proved the accuracy of axial and MPR CT findings. CT results in HNP diagnosis are a little bit better compared with the ones obtained with older, less sophisticated and expensive equipment, but there still remain some differential diagnosis problems.

Our data shown that MPR technical improvements can increase the capacity of distinguishing different types of hernia; sometimes, this will be useful to improve the selection of patients undergoing a further invasive check (discography) or surgical treatment. The sagittal evaluation has helped to estimate the HNP volume and the compression on nervous structures, to select patients for surgical treatment. Surgical results have allowed us to define better the findings we must research by MPR. We expect that especially SR images can help to search for or exclude further signs of extruded hernia suspected from transverse scans. A displacement of PLL is more easily seen with not extruded HNP, while the extruded hernia is better defined thanks to the "binocular" sign. Our findings encourage us to carry out lumbar CT examinations with MPR in those patients highly supected of suffering HNP (lumboischialgia resistant to medical therapy).

It is possible that the major diagnostic certainty and the further information about the hernia type obtained by MPR can justify the greater numbers of scans and radiation dose. Our data can be considered preliminary to the use of spiral CT examination of the lumbar disc.

References

1. Bonanni G, Recchioni F, Masciocchi C, Beomonte-Zobel B (1984) Accuratezza della TC nella patologia vertebrale lombo-sacrale: valutazione si 100 casi operati. In: APC: tomografia computerizzata della colonna vertebrale, delle articolazioni e dell'osso. Cortina, Verona, pp 89–93
2. Calabro A (1989) La tomografia computerizzata con ricostruzioni dell'ernia discale lombare. Riv Neuroradiol 2: 31–33
3. Di Guglielmo L, Garbagna GP, Cornalba GP, Vadala' G, Villa A, Ballarati P (1982) Valore della tomografia computerizzata nella diagnosi di ernia del disco lombare. Radiol Med 68: 51
4. Di Guglielmo L, Vadala' G, Garbagna GP, Dore R, Failoni S, Di Giulio G (1984) Ernia deldisco: valore diagnostico della tomografia computerizzata. Rassegna di 9000 casi. In: APC: TC della colonna vertebrale, delle articolazioni e dell'osso. Cortina, Verona, p 35
5. Drovillard J, Duperron P, Philippe JC (1983) La tomodensitometrie des sciaiques. Ann Radiol 26: 343
6. Gado M, Sartor K, Hodges FJ III (1989) The spine. In: Lee, Sagel, Stanley (eds) Computed body tomography. Raven, New York, pp 991–1061
7. Livingston LA, Grayson GV (1978) CT in the diagnosis of herniated disk in the lumbar spine. In: Post MJD (ed) Spine. Masson, Paris, p 308
8. Lange S, Grumme T, Kluge W, Ringel K (1989) Cerebral and spinal computerized tomography. Schering
9. Lutman M (1985) La tomografia computerizzata nella sciatica lombare. Cortina, Verona
10. Qiu YY, Ge BF (1990) Significance of CT scanning in diagnosis of herniated lumbar disc. Chung Hua Wai Ko Tsa Chih 28: 395–397
11. Volle E, Kern A, Stoltenburg G, Cloussen C (1988) CT reconstraction technique in lumbar intra-neuroforaminal disc herniation. Neuroradiology 30: 138–144

Multiplanar Imaging: A Comparison of Spiral CT and MRI

G. Marchal, R. Oyen, W. Kalender, A. Polacin, and A. L. Baert

Introduction

One of the main limitations of computed tomography (CT) is that for most of the body areas or organs only axial images can be obtained. Direct coronal image acquisition is almost limited to the skull and the foot, though in the past some techniques have been developed to acquire direct coronal scans of the pelvis and abdomen. With CT, coronal, sagittal, or oblique scans have to be reformatted from a stack of contiguous axial slices. Reformatted images have a limited anisotropic resolution; the resolution along the z-axis is largely determined by the slice thickness.

High quality reformatted images can only be calculated if the region of interest can be scanned with thin contiguous slices and if no misregistration nor data gaps occur during scanning. This means that no displacement of the object is allowed in between the consecutive scans.

The applications of image reformatting are therefore almost limited to the study of bony structures; it is useless in the abdomen and thoracic area where inconsistencies in the level of breath-holding and thus misregistration cannot be avoided. For this reason, multiplanar MRI is advocated whenever imaging in other than the axial plane is required today.

Spiral CT is a novel approach to CT, which was recently introduced [1–3]. Because of its capability to scan a continuous volume within a single-breath-hold period, it allows us to acquire a real three-dimensional (3D) data set. From this data set, multiple perfectly contiguous or overlapping slices can be calculated, thereby eliminating entirely the occurrence of data gaps. The advantage of this technique for the detection of small lesions in areas subject to respiratory motion has been established [4, 5]. The faster acquisition of a large body volume also permits a reduction in the amount of contrast agent used [6–9]. Improved visualization of the vascular anatomy has also been reported by several authors [10, 11]. The improved quality of image reformatting [11, 12] and 3D reconstruction [13] has been stressed.

The aim of the present study was to compare the diagnostic quality of reformatted images calculated from spiral CT with the results of direct multiplanar magnetic resonance (MR) image acquisition.

Material and Methods

Fifteen patients with upper abdominal lesions were imaged with both spiral CT and direct multiplanar MRI. The pathologies included tumoral pathology of the kidneys, adrenals, pancreas, and retroperitoneum.

Spiral CT was obtained with a Somatom Plus-S (Siemens, Erlangen, FRG). The entire body section of interest (between 15 and 24 cm) was acquired during a single-breath-hold period. Since the longest scan time available is 32 s, the scan parameters were adjusted to cover the area of interest within this time. Typical parameters used were a 5 mm slice thickness and table incrementation speed between 5 and 8 mm/s, 137 kV and 145 mAs.

Axial images were calculated with a 1-mm interval from the spiral data set after 180° data interpolation (see earlier chapter by Kalender et al.). Reformatting was done with the regular Recon software provided with the scanner.

Contrast enhancement (CE), when used, was obtained by an IV bolus injection of urographic contrast medium (Telebrix, Guerbet, France) at a rate of 4–6 ml/s for 15–30 seconds. Spiral scanning was started between 15 and 25 s after the beginning of the injection. MRI studies were realised in a 1.0-T Magneton SP system (Siemens, Erlangen, FRG). Besides regular axial T1- and T2-weighted spin-echo (SE) images, the upper abdomen was also imaged in the coronal plane with either a regular T1-weighted SE sequence (TR/TE = 500/15 ms) with a total acquisition time of 6.5 min or with a breath-held multislice T1-weighted FLASH sequence (TR/TE/α = 120/6/70) with a total acquisition time of 20 s. For both techniques, a slice thickness of 6–8 mm and an image matrix of 128–256 × 256 for a field-of-view of about 40 cm were selected. This provides images with a voxel size of about 2/2/6–8 mm. The image quality was subjectively evaluated by comparing MR and reformatted spiral CT images.

Since both techniques provide images with a different contrast which can either be beneficial or detrimental for the conspicuity of a particular lesion, we mainly focussed during this evaluation on the level of anatomical detail which could be visualized with both techniques. The following details were analyzed: the delineation of organs in both the lateral and craniocaudal direction; conspicuity of the larger abdominal vessels including the renal arteries, the coeliac trunk and splenic, hepatic, and superior mesenteric arteries; conspicuity of fine detail as evaluated by comparing the visibility of the perirenal fascias, the peritoneal layers, and the bowel detail.

Results

Both plain CT and T1-weighted images yield a high spontaneous contrast between fat, muscle, and soft tissues. Bone and calcifications are better seen on CT.

Regular coronal or sagittal T1-weighted SE images (Figs. 1a, 2a) suffer from respiratory and pulsatile motion. Blurring is obviously most accentuated in the craniocaudal direction, while pulsation artifacts and ghosting spread along the phase encoding direction. Blurring is visible as an overall lack of image sharpness and loss of conspicuity of the edges of organs perpendicular to the longitudinal axis of the body. This is particularly noticeable at the upper and lower poles of the kidney, the dia-

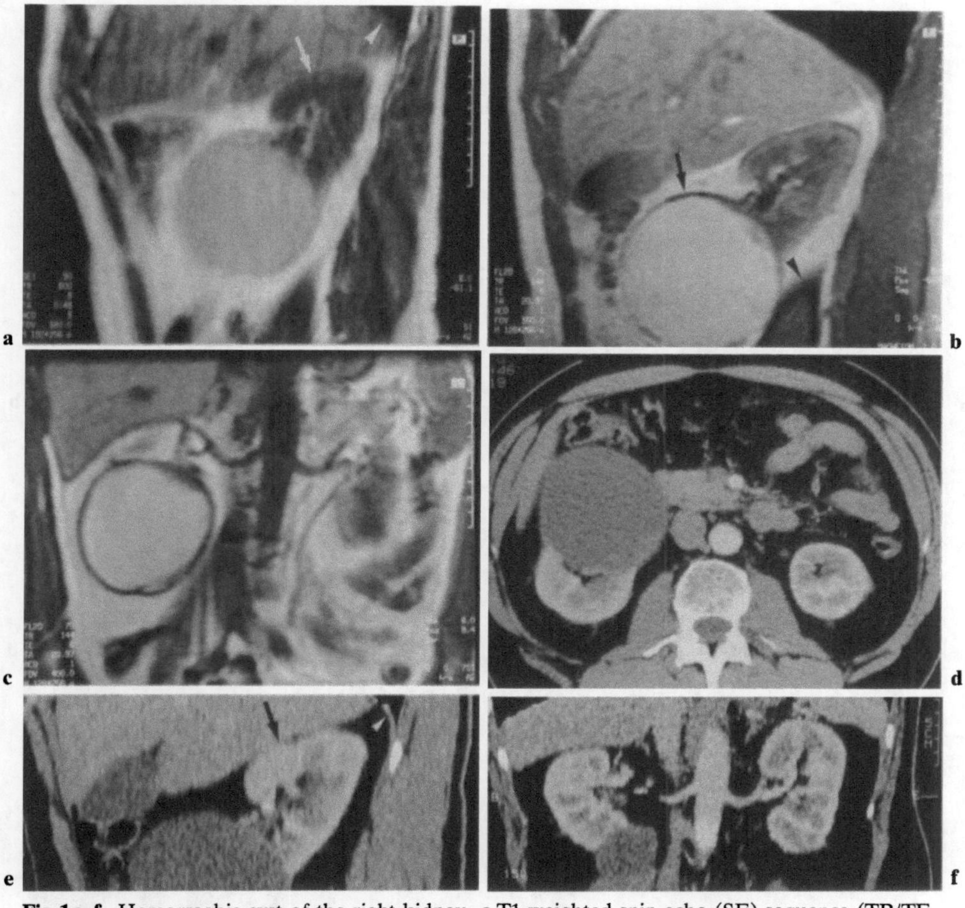

Fig. 1a–f. Hemorraghic cyst of the right kidney. **a** T1-weighted spin-echo (SE) sequence (TR/TE-600/8 ms). Sagittal scan, 3 acquisitions, total examination time 5.48 min. Large spontaneously intense mass in the lower pole. Note the overall blurring of the image due to respiratory motion, induced ghosting and volume averaging with, e.g., disappearance of the fat plane between kidney and liver *(arrow)* as well as the delineation of the muscular portion of the diaphragm *(arrowheads)*. **b, c** T1-weighted breathheld gradient-echo image (FLASH, TR/TE/α = 144/6/75), total acquisition time 21 s. **b** Dramatic improvement of the anatomical detail; however, some disturbing artifacts remain. Note the chemical shift artifacts suggesting a thick cyst wall *(arrow)* and the blurred contour of the psoas muscle *(arrowhead)* as the result of a combination of chemical shift and through plane volume averaging. **c** Coronal scan which shows the proximal segments of both renal arteries. **d** Spiral scan, slice thickness 5 mm, table incrementation speed 5 mm/s, higher order 180° data interpolation. Slightly noisy image, but with excellent anatomical detail. **e** Sagittal reformatted image. Note the well-preserved fat plane between the kidney and liver *(arrow)* (compare with **a** and **b**) and the clear delineation of the muscular part of the diaphragm *(arrowhead)*. Sharp demarcation of the psoas due to an absence of through plane volume averaging. **f** Reformatted image along the plane of the renal arteries. Note that the renal arteries are equally well shown as in the breath-held coronal MRI (**c**)

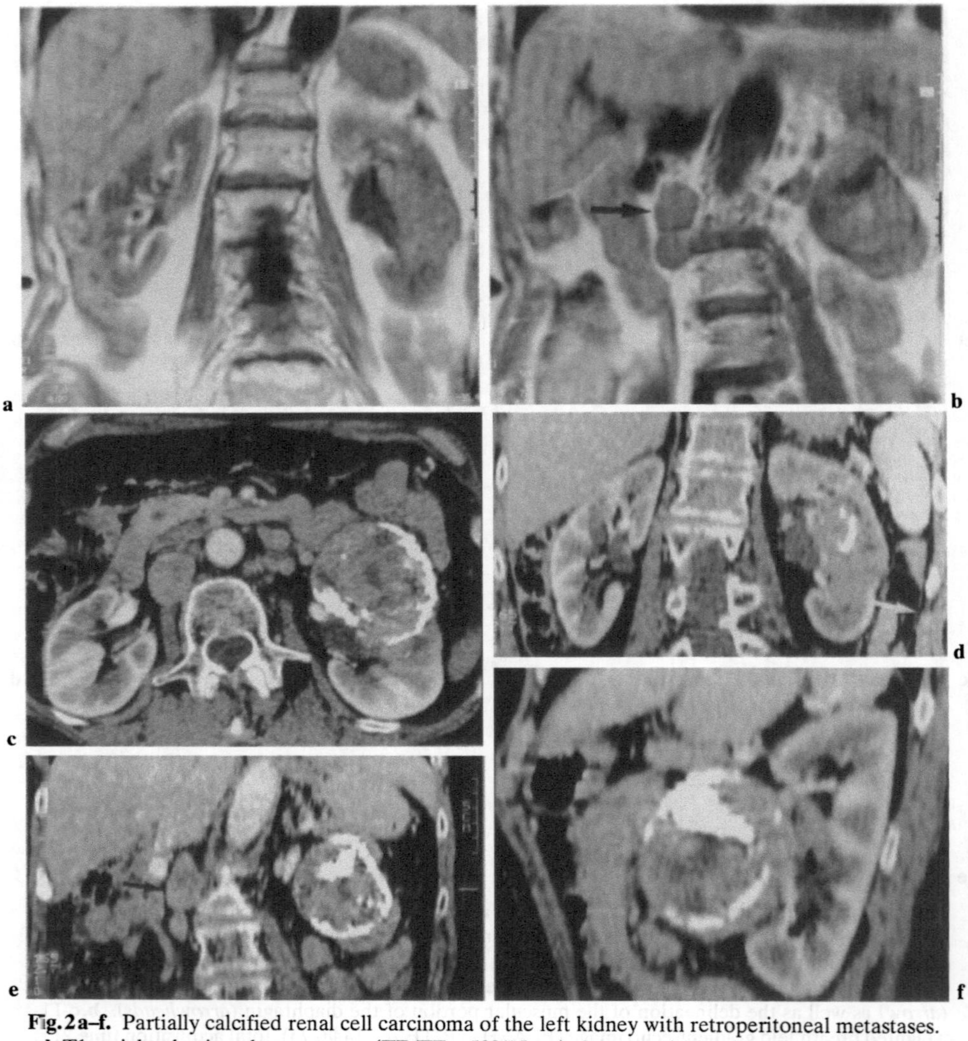

Fig. 2a–f. Partially calcified renal cell carcinoma of the left kidney with retroperitoneal metastases. **a, b** T1-weighted spin-echo sequence (TR/TE = 500/15 ms), four acquisitions, total acquisition time 627 s. **a** Tumoral changes in the left kidney, with loss of the normal cortical medullary differentiation. However, no calcification is visible. Note again blurring of the upper and lower edges of liver and kidney, due to respiratory-induced volume averaging. **b** Enlarged adenopathies *(arrow)* well shown because the retroperitoneal region is less subject to respiratory motion. **c** Spiral scanning, slice thickness 5 mm, table incrementation speed 7 mm/s, 180° higher order data interpolation. The large calcified tumor and the metastatic adenopathies are well shown. **d–f** Reformatted images. **d** The different viscera are shown with much greater detail than in the spin-echo images (**a**). Note the excellent visualization of the peritoneal layer (arrow). Minimal blurring in the craniocaudal direction. Clear tumoral calcification. **e** The retroperitoneal metastases (arrow) are shown as well as on the coronal MRI scan (**b**). **f** Sagittal reformation reveals almost extrarenal ventral development of the tumor

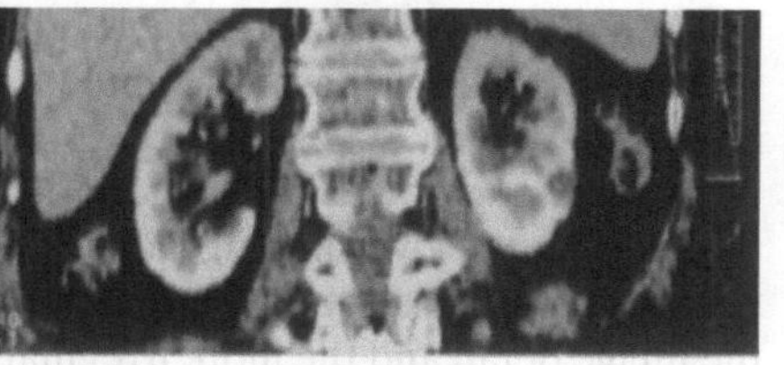

Fig. 3. Inproper timing of contrast injection and scanning. Spiral scanning 5 mm slice thickness, 7 mm/s incrementation speed, higher order 180° data interpolation. In this patient data were acquired during positive feed of the table (caudocranial table motion). The scan was started before the contrast bolus reached the level of the renal arteries. Therefore, only the last images show dense enhancement of the renal cortex. This explains the progressive increase in density from the upper to the lower pole in the reformatted images

phragm, and the lower edge of the liver. Only the proximal segments of the larger abdominal vessels are consistently identified, whereas the peripheral segments are completely smeared out. The perirenal fascias and peritoneal layers are difficult to identify in most of the cases, and the bowel detail is completely lost.

In breath-held T1-weighted images (Fig. 1b) the overall detail is clearly improved. Because of the freeze of respiratory motion, image blurring in the craniocaudal direction is largely eliminated. Nevertheless, some image unsharpness persists. The kidneys and liver frequently show a double contour. The large abdominal vessels including the peripheral segments are better displayed, but the visibility of the fine anatomy such as the perirenal fascias and the peritoneal layers suffer from the lower resolution and C/N. In addition, the organ contours are falsely accentuated by chemical shift artefacts (Fig. 1b).

Reformatted spiral CT scans acquired with a slice thickness and a table incrementation of 5 mm (Fig. 1c, d) provide better anatomical detail than regular SE images and detail similar to breath-held gradient echo scans. Reformatted CT images are characterized by a constant blurring in the craniocaudal direction but not in the lateral direction. Therefore, the upper and lower edges of organs are somewhat less well delineated. After intravenous contrast enhancement the vessels are well seen but enlarged compared with their actual size (Fig. 1f). The aorta can show a shaggy or sawtooth contour. Reformatted spiral CT images show the perirenal fascias and perirenal layers with greater detail than MRI (Fig. 2).

Because of the shorter acquisition time of spiral scanning needed to cover a large body region, the dose of the contrast agent and the injection made have to be adapted. Timing of the acquisition also has to be optimized to avoid incomplete enhancement of the organ studied (Fig. 3).

Discussion

As already mentioned in the "Introduction", the main limitation for the application of image reformatting in regular incremental body or chest CT is the impossibility of avoiding data gaps during the acquisition of the consecutive scans. Data gaps occur because of inconsistencies in the level of the consecutive breath-holds. Images reconstructed from this type of incomplete data set results in discontinuous reformatted images.

A second important factor for good image reformatting is to start with a stack of thin adjacent or overlapping slices. The slice thickness defines the resolution in the *z*-axis (perpendicular to the original slices). The larger the slice thickness, the coarser the image detail and the more irregular the organ contours. However, the acquisition of thin slices requires a longer total examination time, a higher tube load, and a greater patient irradiation dose. In addition, a long total acquisition time also prevents the optimal use of CT and the bolus technique, since only a small part of the total volume to be scanned will be acquired during the early vascular phase.

In comparison with regular incremental scanning, spiral CT has the following advantages. Data from a large body volume can be acquired during a single-breath-hold period. Spiral CT data are therefore truly 3D, with no data gaps. From these data, multiple contiguous or overlapping slices can be calculated [12]. Because the present study focussed on the diagnostic value of reformatted spiral CT in the abdomen, the sequence parameters were chosen so that a large volume could be covered during a single breath-hold, without compromising too much the resolution in the *z*-axis. During previous simulations and experiments, it was shown that a maximal slice thickness of 5 mm with a table incrementation speed between 5 and 10 mm/s was probably most appropriate if images could be calculated after a linear or 180° splice interpolation of the raw data [3, 14, 15].

With this interpolation algorithm, the effective slice thickness is only slightly thicker than the selected nominal slice thickness of 5 mm [16]. If overlapping slices with only 1-mm incrementation are used for image reformatting, the displayed organs will show only minimal contour irregularities.

Some image blurring in the *z*-axis persists as a consequence of the slice-thickness-related volume averaging. Multiplanar reformation from CT images is, on the contrary, only a limited number of pixels thick and shows almost no deterioration due to averaging (in the *x* or *y* direction).

Compared with reformatted spiral CTs, direct multiplanar MRI (2D or 3D) has the following theoretical advantages and drawbacks. In MRI, even large volumes can be acquired at once with or without breath-holding. However, the image quality of regular 2D SE sequences is affected by respiratory blurring and motion-induced ghosting. Respiratory motion can be frozen and almost eliminated by the application of breath-held fast SE or gradient-echo sequences, though with this approach compromises on signal to noise, contrast to noise, image matrix, and the type of reconstruction have to be made. Finally, for both regular SE and fast sequences, the slice thickness used induces and additional volume averaging artifact in the through plane direction. In comparison with MRI, spiral CT has the advantage that once the raw data have been acquired, images can be reformatted in any plane, whereas in MRI the image plane has to be defined before acquisition.

Our findings confirm previous clinical studies [17] on the feasibility of 2D reformatting of data acquired with spiral scanning. Though the number of cases examined in this study is still limited, the present results clearly demonstrate that in the abdomen, reformatted spiral CT scans can offer image detail and diagnostic information similar to that of direct multiplanar MRI.

References

1. Kalender WA, Seissler W, Vock P (1989) Single-breathhold spiral volumetric CT by continuous patient translation and scanner rotation. Radiology 173(P): 414
2. Kalender WA, Seissler W, Klotz E, Vock P (1990) Spiral volumetric CT with single-breathhold technique, continuous transport, and continuous scanner rotation. Radiology 176: 181–183
3. Rigauts H, Ooms D, Marchal G, Nuyts J, Suetens P (1991) Optimization of image quality in spiral scanning. Fourteenth annual course of the Society of Computed Body Tomography, Washington, April
4. Oudkerk M, Kalender W (1989) CT of hilar adenopathy with 1-second and subsecond scan times. Radiology 173(P): 452
5. Remy-Jardin M, Deffontaines C, Remy J (1991) Chest evaluation with use of spiral volumetric CT with the single-breathhold technique. Radiology 181(P): 273
6. Bautz W, Skalej M, Kalender W (1990) Diagnosis of pancreatic disease: clinical impact of spiral CT. Radiology 177(P): 154
7. Marchal G, Rigauts H, Baert AL (1991) Enhancement of the pancreas after single bolus injection combined with spiral scanning: a comparative study with conventional incremental scanning after biphasic contrast injection. European Congress of radiology, bi-annual meeting, Vienna, September
8. Dupuy DE, Costello P, Ecker CP (1991) Comparative study of spiral CT and conventional CT of the pancreas. Radiology 181(P): 350
9. Costello P, Dupuy DE, Ecker CP (1991) Spiral CT of the thorax with small volumes of contrast material: a comparative study. Radiology 181(P): 274
10. Bautz W, Strotzer M, Lenz M, Dittler HJ, Kalender WA (1991) Preoperative evaluation of the vessels of the upper abdomen with spiral CT: comparison with conventional CT and arterial DSA. Radiology 181(P): 274
11. Anno H, Kondo T, Katada K, Ida Y, Tsujioka K, Koga S (1991) Three-dimensional coronary angio-imaging with helical-scanning CT. Radiology 181(P): 336
12. Vock P, Jung H, Kalender W (1989) Single-breathhold spiral volumetric CT of the hepatobillary system. Radiology 173(P): 377
13. Costello P, Ecker CP, Tello RJ, Hartnell CG (1990) Spiral CT assessment of coronary artery bypass grafts. Radiology 181(P): 150
14. Rigauts H, Marchal G, Baert AL, Hupke R (1990) Initial experience with volume CT scanning. J Comput Assist Tomogr 14: 675–682
15. Rigauts H, Marchal G, Baert AL, Hupke R (1991) Spiral scanning and the influence of the reconstruction algorithm on image quality. European Congress of Radiology, bi-annual meeting, Vienna, September
16. Polacin A, Kalender WA, Marchal G (1992) Evaluation of slice sensitivity profiles and image noise in spiral CT with different data processing algorithms. Radiology (manuscript submitted)
17. Kuhlman JE, Ney DR, Fishman EK (1991) Two- and three-dimensional imaging of the in vivo lung: combining spiral CT with multiplanar and volumetric rendering techniques. Radiology 181(P): 274

Workshop

Chairmen: K. Lackner, C. D. Claussen, P. Vock, and M. Langer

Spiral CT: A New Technique for Better Evaluation of Upper Urinary Tract Filling Defects

M. Soucek, P. Vock, W. Kalender, and A. Stenzl

Introduction

Radiolucent filling defects of the upper urinary tract (UUT) are a relatively common finding in intravenous urography (IVU) and ureteropyelography (UPG). Despite further evaluation by additional imaging modalities such as sonography and conventional computed tomography (CT), a conclusive diagnosis cannot be made in some of these patients. Endoscopy combined with cytology and histology reveals further information regarding the nature of some of the lesions but is invasive, with a chance of complications, inconclusive with regard to invasiveness, and not economic [1, 2].

The purpose of this study was to determine the diagnostic value of spiral CT in the evaluation of radiolucent filling defects of the UUT and compare it with standard radiological methods.

Material and Methods

The study group comprised 20 patients seen during 1 year between April 1990 and April 1991. There were 12 men and 8 women, 33–80 years old (mean age 60 years). In all patients, one or several radiolucent filling defects were detected either on the IVU ($n = 18$) and/or UPG ($n = 19$). A lavage cytology was done in all patients with UPG. Further evaluation with sonography ($n = 19$), conventional CT ($n = 13$), and magnetic resonance imaging (MRI) ($n = 1$) did not result in a conclusive diagnosis. These patients therefore underwent a single-breath-hold volumetric CT commonly called a spiral CT examination. We used a Somatom Plus scanner (Siemens). The ranges of parameters for the technique employed were 10–24 s continuous scanning, 2–8 mm collimation, 2–8 mm/s table feed, 165 mA current, and 120 kV. If necessary, an intravenous bolus injection of 50–80 ml of contrast agent was given. Retrospective raw data interpolation produced images usually at intervals of 2–4 mm. Multidimensional reconstructions were obtained mainly in the sagittal, coronal, and paraxial planes. Occasionally, three-dimensional reconstructions were necessary. The conventional CT was usually performed by contiguous scanning using a 10 mm slice thickness at 210 mA and 120 kV. After each individual imaging modality a diagnosis was formulated. These preliminary diagnostic results were compared with the final diagnosis based on the outcome of spiral CT. In 18 out of 20 patients, the diagnosis was verified either by open surgery or endourological methods. In the remaining two patients, long-term clinical follow-up data combined with radiological control examinations were available.

Results

Malignant Tumors ($n = 10$)

The final diagnosis was based on the histological results of the surgical specimens in all patients. Surgery consisted of nephroureterectomy in seven patients and pyelotomy with local tumor excision and intraoperative nephroscopy in three.

The tumor was located in the pelvicalyceal system in nine patients and in the proximal ureter in one patient (Fig. 1). One of these tumors in the pelvicalyceal system was multifocal; all the others were solitary and measured 0.5–6.0 cm. The results of the lavage cytology were negative or questionable for malignancy in eight out of ten patients. The definite histological results of the surgical specimens are listed in Table 1.

Conventional CT scans depicted medium to large tumors. However, the exact site of location within the kidney could not be determined. Sonography even failed to visualize the tumor in eight out of ten patients. The presumptive diagnosis from spiral CT was correct in all these patients.

Nonopaque Calculi ($n = 6$)

In all six patients, the definitive diagnosis of ureteral ($n = 3$) or pyelocalyceal ($n = 3$) radiolucent calculi was established solely by spiral CT. The size of the stones varied between 0.2 and 2.5 cm (mean 0.8 cm). Only one patient underwent an additional

Table 1. Examination results of 20 patients with radiographic filling defects

Diagnosis by spiral CT	No. of patients	Operative/clinical results	No. of patients
Malignant tumor	10	TCC Pelvis	5
		TCC Calyx	2
		TCC Ureter	1
		SCC Pelvis	1
		Metastasis Renal/pelvis	1
Nonopaque UUT stone	6	PNL + URS	3
		URS	2
		ESWL	1
Blood clot	2	PNS	1
		URS	1
Benign tumor	2	No clinical and radiological change after 22–36 months	2

TCC, Transitional cell carcinoma; SCC, squamous cell carcinoma; PNL, percutaneous nephrolitholapaxy; PNS, percutaneous nephroscopy; URS, ureteroscopy; ESWL extracorporeal shock-wave lithotripsy; UUT, upper urinary tract.

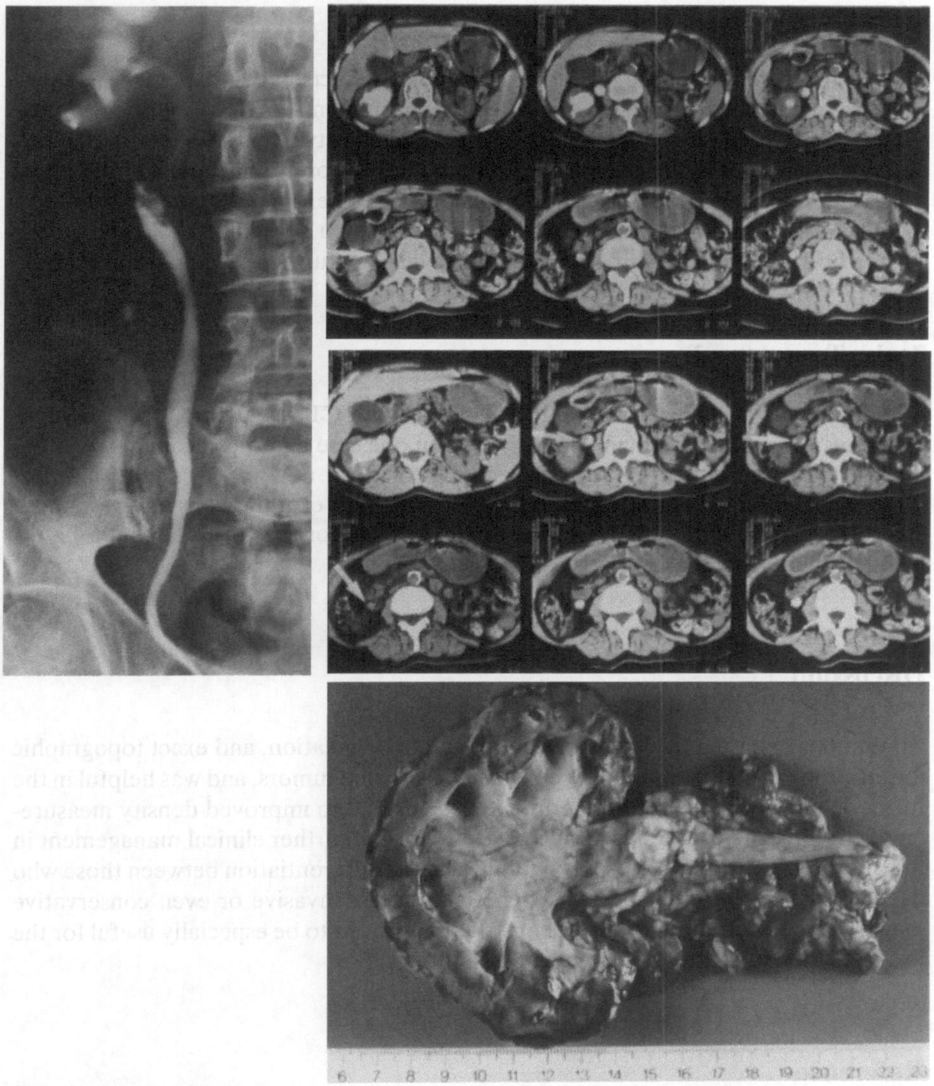

a b c d

Fig. 1. **a** A 72-year-old woman with an episode of painless macrohematuria and a radiolucent filling defect on a retrograde ureteropyelography. **b** On conventional CT, the tumor was missed. In retrospect, however, it can be suspected *(white arrow)*. **c** Spiral CT shows clearly a mass in the proximal ureter and delineates its full extent *(white arrows)*. **d** Surgery revealed an invasive transitional cell carcinoma (pT3b) of the proximal ureter

conventional CT scan, which missed a small midureter calculus. Sonography was negative or inconclusive for stone detection in five patients, because of either abnormal kidney location and/or interposition of fat, bone, or gas. Stone treatment was done in all patients (see Table 1).

Blood Clots ($n = 2$)

Blood clots were the reason for radiolucent filling defects in two patients. The diagnosis was made due to characteristic density measurements (60 HU) before and after contrast enhancement. With conventional CT the density measurements were more difficult because of large spacing with subsequently poorer delineation of the questionable lesion. Sonography was performed in one patient but did not contribute to the diagnosis. The blood clots were evacuated through a percutaneous nephrostomy tract in both patients. Nephroscopy did not reveal any further pathological findings.

Benign Tumors ($n = 2$)

In two patients a solitary filling defect seen on spiral CT was thought to be benign. On conventional CT, it remained undetected in one case and was inconclusive in the other one. These patients have been closely followed now for 22 and 36 months. There was no change of the lesions on repeat radiologic examinations nor were there any clinical signs of a progressive disease. It can therefore be assumed that a stationary lesion after such a long period is probably benign.

Discussion

Continuous scanning leads to a better detection, delineation, and exact topographic localization of small lesions [4, 5], e. g., small urothelial tumors, and was helpful in the further characterization of indeterminate lesions due to improved density measurements [3]. In conclusion, spiral CT was useful for the further clinical management in this selected group of patients by enabling a better differentiation between those who need open surgery and those who benefit from less invasive or even conservative management. Multidimensional reconstruction proved to be especially useful for the exact location and extent of complex UUT stones.

References

1. Bagley DH, Rivas D (1990) Upper urinary tract filling defects: flexible ureteroscopic diagnosis. J Urol 143: 196–200
2. Biester R, Gillenwater JY (1986) Complications following ureteroscopy. J Urol 136: 380–382
3. Parienty RA, Ducellier R, Pradel J, Lubrano JM, Coquille F, Richard F (1982) Diagnostic value of CT numbers in pelvocalyceal filling defects. Radiology 145: 743–747
4. Soucek M, Vock P, Daepp M, Kalender W (1990) Spiral CT: Eine neue Technik für Volumenaufnahmen, Teil II: Klinische Anwendungsmöglichkeiten. Röntgenpraxis 10
5. Vock P, Soucek M, Daepp M, Kalender W (1990) Lung spiral volumetric CT with single-breath-hold technique. Radiology 176: 864–867

CT Indications and Criteria for Asbestos-Related Findings of the Pleura and Parenchyma

K. G. Hering and S. Adomeit

The WHO defines pneumoconioses as changes in the lungs caused by the inhalation and deposition of dust-like particles. Asbestosis which leads to progressive, radiologically verifiable pulmonary fibrosis with functional impairment is often underestimated from a radiological viewpoint both medically and economically, although the various forms may have substantial implications.

Pleural reactions [3, 8, 13] which are most likely to be caused by exposure to asbestos are:

1. Hyaline plaques, with or without calcification (Fig. 1)
2. "Diffuse" pleural thickening, caused by:
   a) Confluent, flat plaques (Fig. 2)
   b) Expansion of the pulmonary fibrosis into the subpleural interstitium and with involvement of the visceral pleura (Fig. 2)
   c) Adhesive fibrothorax following pleuritis
3. Acute exudative pleuritis
4. Mesothelioma

The following early fibrotic changes of the parenchyma are found after exposure to asbestos, although they may also be seen following interstitial fibrosis of other origins:

1. Intra- and interlobular consolidated lines and isolated, micronodular structures, located subpleurally, centrilobular (Fig. 3)

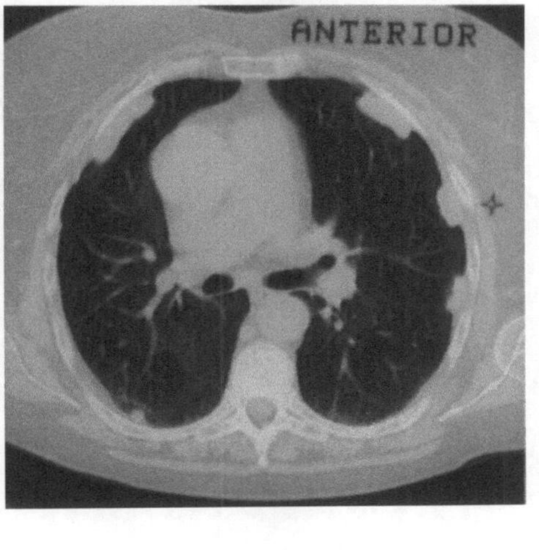

Fig. 1. Hyaline plaques, with and without calcification

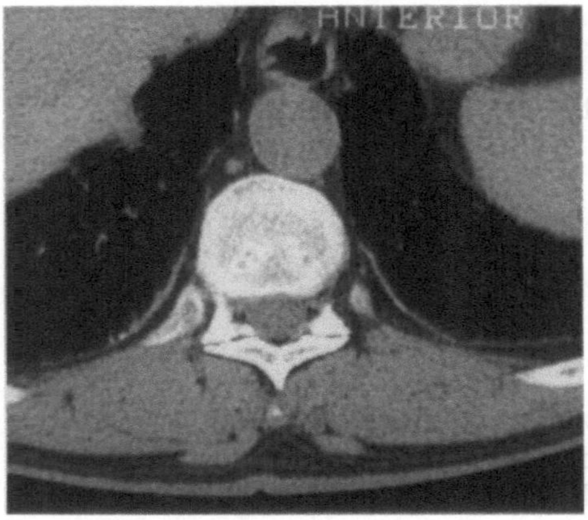

Fig. 2. Confluent, flat plaques and expansion of pulmonary fibrosis of the subpleural interstitium with involvement of the visceral pleura

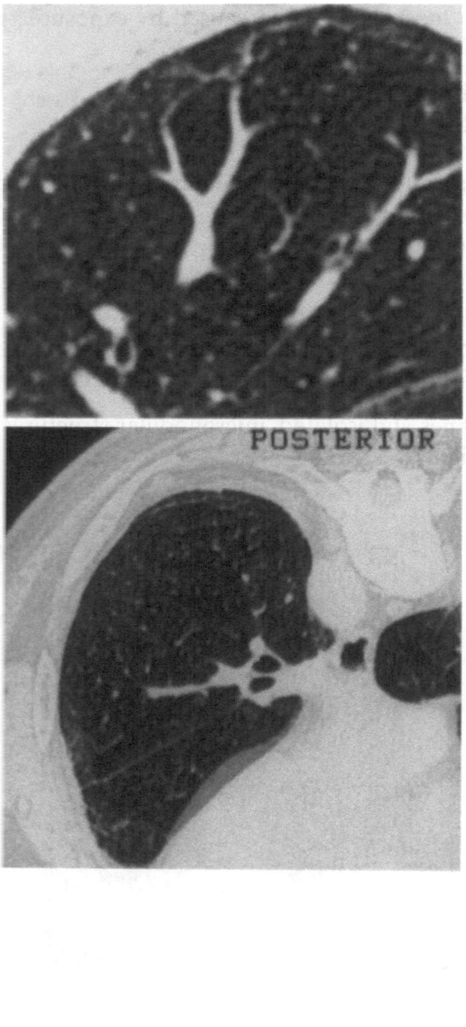

a

b

Fig. 3 a, b. Intra- and interlobular consolidated lines, isolated, micronodular structures, located subpleurally, centrilobular, and subpleural curvilinear lines in the parenchyma

2. Subpleural curvilinear lines in the parenchyma, about 1 cm from the pleura and parallel to the thoracic wall (Fig. 3)
3. Pleural-based nodular irregularities, sometimes wedge-shaped (Fig. 4)
4. Hazy patches of increased attenuation with a ground-glass appearance, located subpleurally; persistent even after a change in position, occasionally combined with cystic-like spaces (Fig. 5)

Both fibrosis due to asbestosis and malignomas induced by asbestos dust have a relatively long latency period lasting between 20 and more than 40 years from the initial, occupational exposure to asbestos to the characteristic clinical manifestation [4]. The frequency peak of these malignomas is therefore expected to be found between the years of 2010 and 2015, since the use of asbestos was highest around 1975 and has been decreasing constantly since then. Asbestos can now only be used with special permission or is encountered in activities of redevelopment.

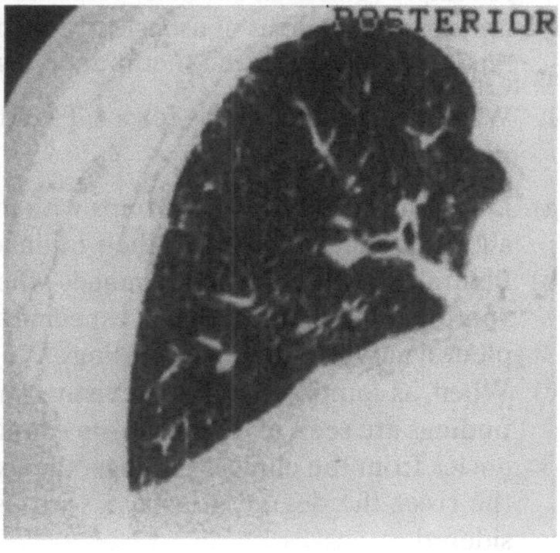

Fig. 4. Pleural-based nodular irregularities, sometimes wedge-shaped

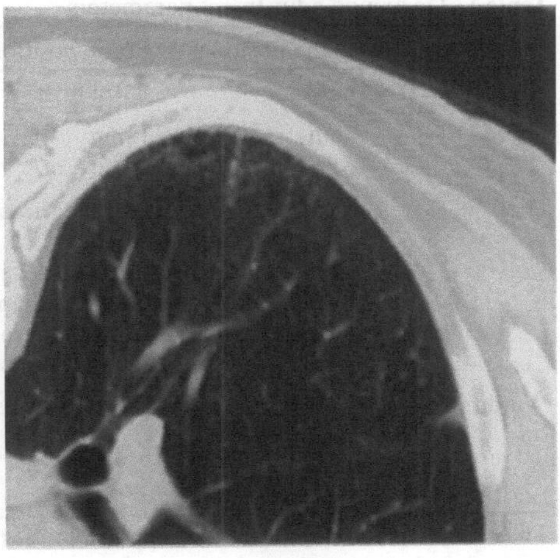

Fig. 5. Hazy patches of increased attenuation with a ground-glass-appearance, occasionally combined with cystic-like spaces

Aside from a detailed occupational history with consideration of past exposure, noninvasive radiological procedures play a central role in the diagnosis of this illness [6, 10, 11]. In addition to the conventional chest x-radiograph, the consequent application of computed tomography (CT) with the high resolution technique (HRCT) [12] permits an earlier and more exact evaluation of pathological pulmonary and pleural changes, since patients with sufficient asbestos exposure have a risk of developing a pulmonary carcinoma or a mesothelioma. It must be pointed out that a smoker who has been exposed to asbestos has a synergistic and multiplicative risk of suffering from bronchial carcinoma. The question of adequate compensation must also be decided in many cases.

Our experiences are based on > 400 CT evaluations as a medical expertise evaluation of persons who had been exposed to asbestos. By February 10, 1992, 140 of these insured persons had been examined with the Somatom Plus.

A regular application of CT/HRCT is expected to result in:
- An improvement in causality relationships
- An earlier diagnosis of asbestos-related malignancies
- An improvement of the therapeutic regimen

1. What are the indications for a CT study in the event of occupational pulmonary disease?

a) Differentiated follow-up groups with an increased exposure to asbestos dust and a long latency period from their initial exposure
b) Pleural and parenchymal changes whose etiology cannot be clarified with conventional techniques; this is especially true when there are hints for malignant pleural and/or pulmonary findings
c) When, as compared with the existing chest X-radiographs, relevant changes in the findings are seen in the follow-up examination, or in the event of distinct discrepancies from the clinical findings; the examination intervals should be adapted to the risks; the degree of asbestos exposure and the latency period must be considered

Table 1. Dortmund adjustment parameters

	Supine position	Prone position
Algorithm	High	Ultra high
Slice	5 mm 1 s, 255 mA	1 mm 1 s, 255 mA
Feed	15 mm	Apex, 2 slices Aortic arch Carina tracheae Dome of diaphragma Costodiaphragmatic sinus Plus 2 intermediate slices at regular intervals in the lower fields
Window	a) W = 450 C = 50 b) W = 1400 C = −500	W = 2000 C = −500

These adjustment parameters are applicable for the evaluation in case of a medical expertise evaluation. A reduced number of slices are performed for a medical screening examination, see Fig. 6.

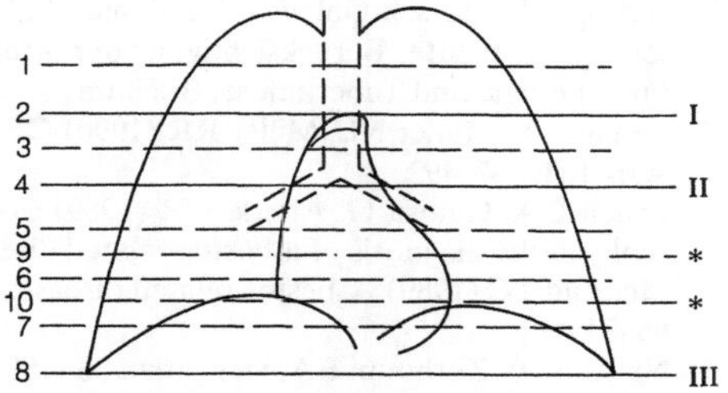

Fig. 6. Reduced number of 8–10 slices in the "screening" examination: Algorithm "high", 8 slices in the supine position, slice thickness 5 mm; if there is a decreased ventilation in the dorsal, basal parts, 2 additional slices (*) in the prone position, slice thickness 1 mm. Points of reference for repeated examinations are the aortic arch *(I)*, carina tracheae *(II)*, and the costodiaphragmatic sinus, the other slices should be distributed at regular intermittent intervals

2. How many slices should be made and with what examination parameters?

Many groups have rejected the general use of CT because of their considerations of radiation exposure and of discussions concerning the possible multiplicative carcinogenic effect of ionising radiation in a population already endangered by asbestos and smoking [7]. It is impossible to take sides in this debate at the moment. However, based on these considerations and on the papers from Leung et al. [8] and from the group of Aberle, Gamsu, Lynch et al. [1, 9], we have suggested a differentiated number of slices adapted to the clinical objective and to the risks [7] (Table 1).

"Diagnostic" CT of the chest does not permit a reduction in the number of slices. Specific clinical objectives can be differentiated using contrast medium administration in further slices or eventually even with additional HRCT slices in the supine and prone positions.

"Follow-up" examinations with a defined clinical objective can be performed with a reduced number of slices and a reduced slice thickness.

"Screening" examinations for the control of groups likely to be exposed occupationally must take into consideration that these individuals are actually still healthy, so that aside from the costs, the question of radiation exposure must also play a role.

References

1. Aberle DR, Gamsu G, Ray CS, Feuerstein IM (1988) Asbestos-related pleural and parenchymal fibrosis: detection with high-resolution CT. Radiology 166: 729–734
2. Akira M, Yokoyoma K, Yamamoto S, Higashihara T, Morinaga K, Kita N, Morimoto S, Ikezoe J, Kozuka T (1991) Early asbestosis: evaluation with high-resolution CT. Radiology 178: 409–416
3. Bohlig H, Calavrezos A (1987) Development, radiological zone patterns, and importance of diffuse pleural thickening to occupational exposure of asbestos. Br J Ind Med 44: 673–681
4. Coenen W, Schenk H (1990) Ermittlung von Risikogruppen bei Asbestexponierten. Die BG 718–726
5. Fiel SB, Friedman AC, Radecki PD (1989) Evaluation of pulmonary disease – clinical role of conventional and high-resolution CT. Radiol Rep 1: 188–205
6. Hering KG, Wiebe V (1990) Radiologische Diagnostik der Pneumokoniosen. Radiologe 30: 574–580

7. Hering KG, Borsch-Galetke E, Adomeit S, Peters T (1990) Rationaler Einsatz der Computertomographie unter Berücksichtigung der Strahlenexposition. Poster, 34 Kongreß der Dtsch Ges Pneumologie und Tuberkulose, Bochum
8. Leung AN, Müller NL, Miller RR (1990) CT in differential diagnosis of diffuse pleural disease. AJR 154: 487–492
9. Lynch DA, Gamsu G, Aberle DR (1989) Conventional and high resolution computed tomography in the diagnosis of asbestos-related diseases. Radiographics 9: 523–551
10. McLoud TC (1989) Asbestos related disease: the role of imaging techniques. Postgrad Radiol 9: 65–74
11. Naidich DP, Zerhouni EA, Siegelman SS (1991) Computed tomography and magnetic resonance of the thorax, 2nd ed. Raven, New York
12. Remy-Jardin M, Remy J, Deffontaines C, Duhamel A (1991) Assessment of diffuse infiltrative lung disease: comparison of conventional CT and high-resolution CT. Radiology 181: 157–162
13. Schwartz DA (1991) New developments in asbestos-induced pleural disease. Chest 99: 191–198

Three-Dimensional Printing from Somatom Plus CT Data

P. Brennan, H. Stucki, A. Ghezal, P. Stucki, W. A. Fuchs

Introduction

Stereolithography (three-dimensional, 3D printing) is a new technology in which plastic models are constructed from computed digital raw data. Its primary commercial use is in design model building for prototype construction. Its application in medicine is a natural extension of its commercial use.

Material and Methods

Fine slice, 2-mm, high-resolution CT was performed with the Somatom Plus. Then, 3-D reconstruction using a 256 or preferably a 512 matrix was performed. The raw data was transferred to the stereolithography workstation using a magnetic disc. Preprocessing is the next step in which 3-D mathematical reconstruction of the CT raw data takes place. In this operation, the object's outer boundaries are detected, thinned, and joined together.

The final preprocessing step consists of creating a wire frame model mathematically [1]. The stereolithography system (3D Systems) consists of a helium-cadium laser, an optical scanner, a photopolymer vat with elevator, and a controlling com-

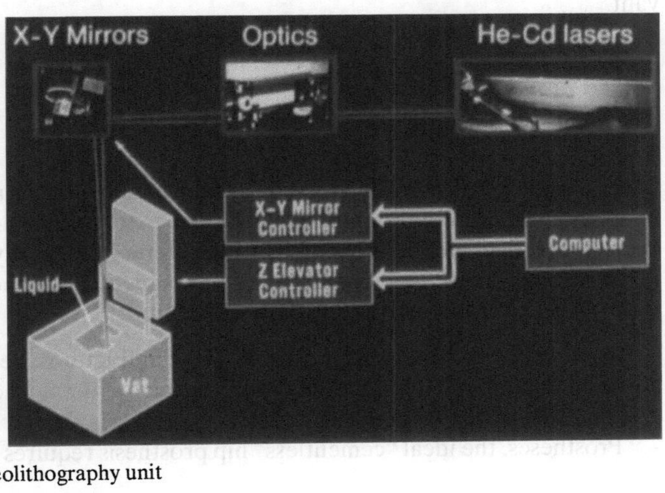

Fig. 1. Diagram of the stereolithography unit

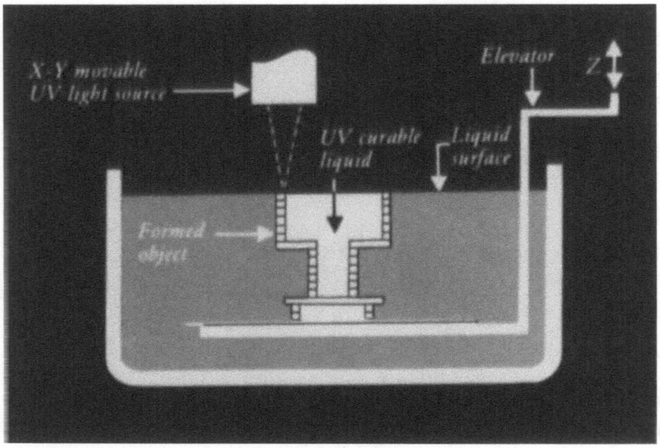

Fig. 2. Detail of vat with the photopolymer liquid

puter (Figs. 1,2). The photopolymer liquid(Cibatool SL) changes to solid resin on exposure to light and is particularly sensitive to ultraviolet (uv) light – this process is called curing. The ultraviolet laser generates a small intense spot of UV light which is precisely moved across the liquid surface by computed generated vectors. The slice is illuminated, and therefore solidified (curred) and is mechanically lowered into the vat allowing a new layer of liquid resin to flow over the object. This sequence is repeated slice by slice until the model is complete. The cured model is then removed and is strengthened by further exposure to UV light in a postcuring oven. A 3-D reconstruction of a knee (contiguous 2-mm slices, 256 matrix) and its stereolithographic plastic model are demonstrated (Fig. 3). The preprocessing steps are currently performed by computer manipulation, which delays the development of the model considerably. When performed automatically in the near future, models will be available in 12–18 h, making the process more clinically relevant.

Discussion

Several publications have discussed the clinical advantages and applications of 3-D imaging [2-5]. Stereolithography is a further extension of 3-D imaging. Computer-derived raw data can be transferred to the stereolithography unit by magnetic tape directly through workstations from CT or magnetic resonance units. The main purposes of 3-D printing of imaging data will be in:

- Trauma, for the operative planning of facial fractures, depressed zygomatic arch or mandibular fractures, spinal and especially sacral fractures, such as those of the tibial plateau and the calcaneus.
- Prostheses, the ideal "cementless" hip prosthesis requires a perfect fit of the pros-

Fig. 3. a A 3-D reconstruction of CT data of a knee with **(b, c)** corresponding 3-D printout

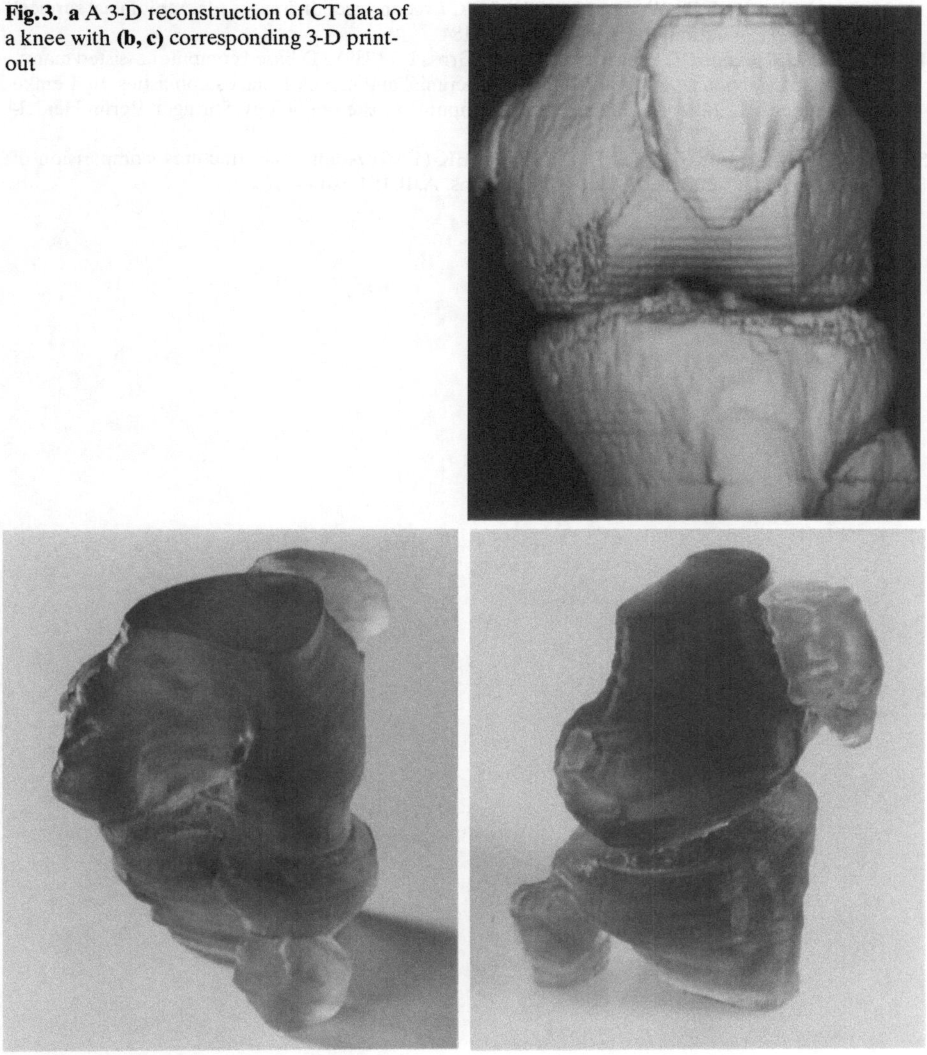

a

b

c

thesis into the distal intramedullary cavity, and individual prosthesis design based on the resin model will hopefully fulfill this goal. Prosthesis design will also play a role in oncology patients.

References

1. Ghezal A, Stucki P (1991) 3D-Copies of surface-reconstructed 3D-models mustererkennung. Springer, Berlin Heidelberg New York, pp 528-535
2. Fishman EK, Magid D, Ney DR, Chaney EL et al. (1991) Three dimensional imaging. Radiology 181: 321–337

3. Vannier MW, Marsh JL, Warren JO (1984) 3D CT reconstruction images for craniofacial surgical planning and evaluation. Radiology 150: 179–184
4. Schmitz HJ, Tolxdorff T, Honsbrok J, Fritz T, Gross U (1989) 3D based computer assisted manufacturing of individual alloplastic implants for cranial and maxillofacial osteoplasties. In: Lemke HU, Rhodes ML, Jaffe CC, Felix R (eds) Computer assisted radiology. Springer, Berlin Heidelberg New York, pp 390–395
5. Magid D, Michelson JD, Ney DR, Fishman EK (1990) Adult ankle fractures: comparision of plain films and interactive 2D and 3D CT scans. AJR 154: 1017–1023

A New Imaging Aid: Dental CT

R. Hupke and J. Ezrielev

Introduction

Recently, the requests for the preoperative modeling of custom subperiosteal implants as well as for the preoperative planning of endosseous dental implants have been strongly increasing. In the USA, approximately 300000 implantations are expected for the year 1992. Dental implant surgery, however, is still a delicate procedure which calls for exact planning [1–3]. In the past, preoperative radiographic evaluations typically included lateral radiographs of the skull, intraoral films, and panoramic views. More recently, the use of computed tomography (CT) has improved the quality of preoperative information, mostly utilizing direct coronal scans. This technique is very uncomfortable for the patient. Even more disadvantageous is that this procedure suffers frequently from artifacts caused by metallic fillings. Clearly, the results obtained by CT scanning needed improvement [4, 5]. It was the clear clinical need for the development of a new imaging aid: dental CT. This software package was driven first by the question of how can a CT scan provide a complete view of the mandible and be optimized for implant surgery and second by the need, to guide the oral surgeon to locate and avoid such vital parts of anatomy like the inferior alveolar nerve. The program offers the possibility of reconstructing out of the measured images panoramic views (PV) and synthetic transaxial images (STI) of the jaw. The first reconstruction offers the referring dentist the well-known panoramic image without superposition as in plain films. The STI add new information; they are defined to be locally perpendicular to the panoramic views. By this means, small transaxial images of the jaw are calculated, showing quantitatively the size of the wall thickness and the alveolar nerve.

Image Acquisition

Optimal positioning of the fixtures requires a detailed knowledge of the corss-sectional anatomy of the alveolar ridges of the edentulous region along the entire curvature of the bone. The most important requirement for successful implant surgery is the exact knowledge of the size of the wall thickness of the alveolar bone of the mandible and maxilla. For excellent images, it is necessary to spend some care in patient preparation. The patient must be comfortably placed in the supine position on the table, the head restrained in the headholder, and the mouth held open with a oral positioning aid to immobilize the jaw. The patient's jaw should be orientated in such a way that the alveolar ridge is perpendicular to the table, so that the scan plane will be parallel to that ridge. This is important to obtain a maximum geometric resolution with a minimum of axial slices. For superior results, a different patient positioning for the evaluation of the mandible and the maxilla are required. Only in a few cases are both parts of the jaw subject for evaluation. The correct positioning should be verified by a short lateral topogram.

In the next step, axial slices are acquired as usual, either with dynamic screening of spiral CT. We recommended 1-mm- or at most 2-mm-thick slices with a table feed not greater than the slice thickness. Because here only osseous structures are of interest, it will be sufficient to scan with a low-dose mode. Therefore, the time of measurement for the mandible (3 cm) varies from 30 s to roughly 3 min. A fixed protocol for the image reconstruction will help to minimize the set-up time for the evaluation software.

The Software: Dental CT

The Somatom Plus-S features the SMI 96 which is designed to hold the previously measured, transaxial images in a fast RAM storage. This allows the user to run the application software, in our case in dental package, immediately after finishing the measurement itself. First, all images available in this study are listed for individual selection. If images are to be loaded from a disk, it will take approximately 2 s per image for retrieval. If the images are still accessible in the SMI 96, the reference image is displayed immediately after invoking the program itself.

The very first use of the package is somewhat different from the following ones. The program prompts for an input of the actually used film size. The user has to measure the size of the CT image printed on the X-ray film. We recommend a 6-in-1 format for a laser camera, which results in an actual size of the CT image on the film of approximately 133 mm. The program runs through this procedure, and as long as there is no change in the camera, film size, and format this is a one time only procedure. By utilizing this information, all the resulting images of dental CT are scaled in such a way that 1 cm on the film corresponds with 1 cm in reality. The feature is greatly appreciated by the referring dentists, because it makes available the opportunity to compare directly an implant with the results on film.

In the next step, the definition of the reconstructions takes place. A transaxial image acts as the reference image. In the very first run, a parabolic curve with several handles appears as an overlay on this image. The user moves this curve by dragging these handles until the reference line for the panoramic reconstruction fits the individual jaw. The system responds to each user-interaction in real time. The resulting shape of the curve is stored for future applications. With fixed protocols for the measurement, it can be expected that the definition of the shape will not vary too much from patient to patient. However, different protocols may be utilized for the evaluation of mandible and maxilla, so it is possible to store two basic curves.

The orientation of the STI is then calculated and displayed on top of the definition of the PV in the reference image. The number as well as the width of the STIs can be selected between precalculated limits. The reason for not having here the absolute freedom of selecting these parameters is because the result on film is supposed to be life-size. After completing the definition phase, the program calculates, displays, and stores all PVs and STIs without any further user-interaction. Since the measured TA and the reconstructed PV and STI are two-dimensional, accurate measurements (distance, angle, profile, etc.) can be performed in any image. For example, dental CT permits the measurement of the bone depth on the maxillary sinus or the width of bone available for an implant.

Results

All comparative studies were performed by means of a dry skull phantom with a Somatom Plus with a spiral capability of 24 s. It was set up to define optimal measurement as well reconstruction parameters. As demonstrated in the lateral topogram in Fig. 1, the scan plane was chosen parallel to the alveolar ridge, and the graphics reflects the position and size of the transaxial images. A common zoom factor will be around 5; the field of view is about 10 cm with a pixel size of 0.2 mm. From this consideration, slice thicknesses of more than 2 mm are not recommended.

Resulting panoramic views of different combinations of slice thickness and table feed are shown in Fig. 2 for dynamic screening and in Fig. 3 for spiral CT. In every case, the scan time was 1 s, and the same dose, zoom, center, and standard kernel were used. It becomes clear that the scans performed with 1-mm slice and feed result in the best quality. There is no difference between the methods, even though spiral CT with 1-mm collimation has the drawback of not covering the whole mandible as seen in Fig. 3 on the top. With the version of the longer spiral (32 s), it is feasible to image the important part of the mandible and maxilla.

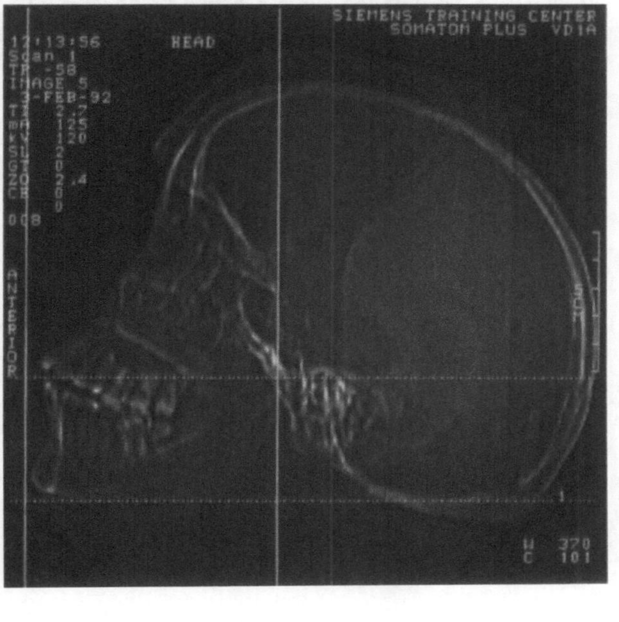

Fig. 1. Lateral topogram of a dry skull phantom; the graphics reflects the size of reconstructed images

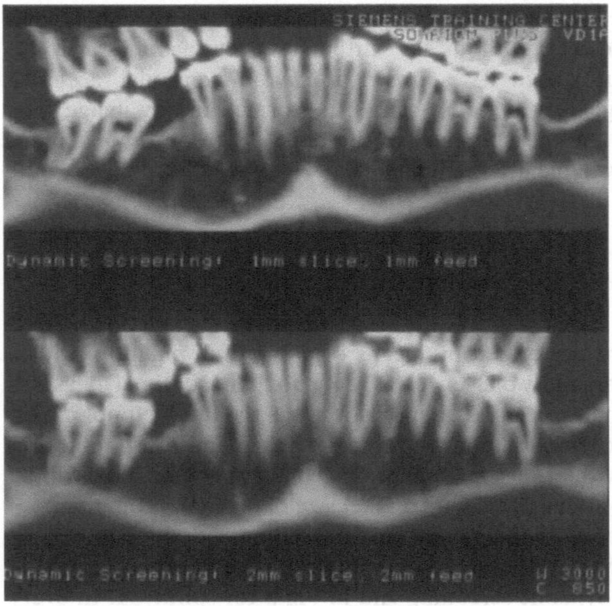

Fig. 2. Dynamic screening: comparison of two combinations of slice thickness/table feed: *top*, 1 mm/1 mm; *bottom*, 2 mm/2 mm

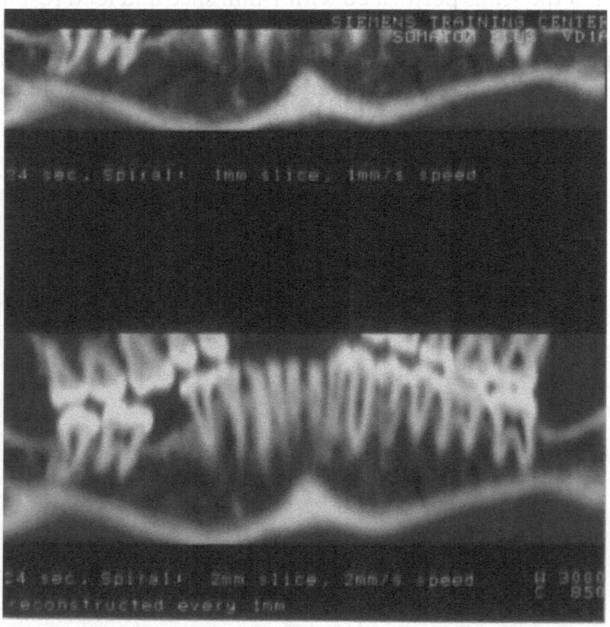

Fig. 3. Spiral CT: two combinations of slice thickness/table speed: *top*, 1 mm/1 mm; *bottom*, 2 mm/2 mm; in each case reconstruction offset is 1 mm

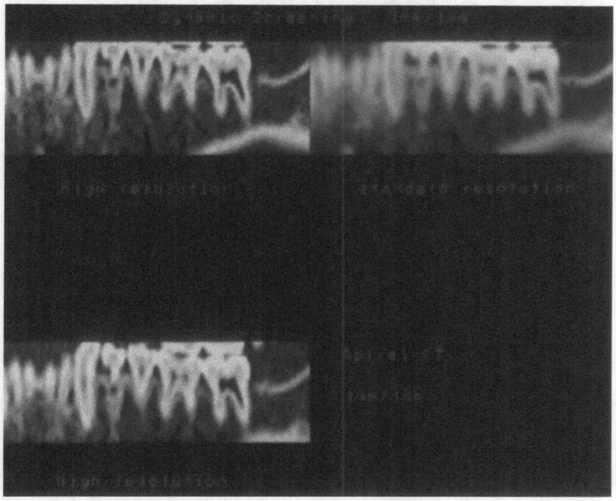

Fig. 4. The influence of different kernels on panoramic views: *top left*, high-resolution; *top right*, standard for dynamic screening; *bottom left*, high resolution spiral CT

The interesting result here is that the spiral with technique with 2-mm collimation and 2-mm table speed and reconstructed at every 1 mm gives nearly the same image quality as the dynamic screening. Similar statements are valid also for the STI. In the top part of Fig. 4, a comparison is presented between PV resulting from reconstructions of image stacks created with different convolution kernels. Top left shows a PV created with an edge enhancement kernel in contrast to a standard kernel in top right position. The spiral study on the bottom of Fig. 4 created with a high resolution kernel shows no disadvantages compared with the conventional scan. Since the measurement time is minimal, spiral CT should be applied whenever available. This will be greatly appreciated by the patients. According to these results, we recommend:

Scan time:	1 s	(spiral or dynamic screening)
Collimation:	1 mm	(1 mm table speed/feed)
Dose:	110 mA	(137 kV)
Algorithm:	AH_07041	(logical assignment # 9)
Zoom:	approx. 5	
Window/center:	approx. 3000/800	

For frequent and easy application, it is also suggested to create a separate scan mode containing these parameters. By utilizing this scan technique, a standard examination will take about 10 min (3 min for measurement and evaluation each, 3 min for filming, 1 min overhead).

Clinical Examples

In Figs. 5–8, we demonstrate the most important steps of the program. The first dental image screen consists of a regular transaxial image, displaying all usual patient information as well as scan protocol data. This image serves as the reference image for

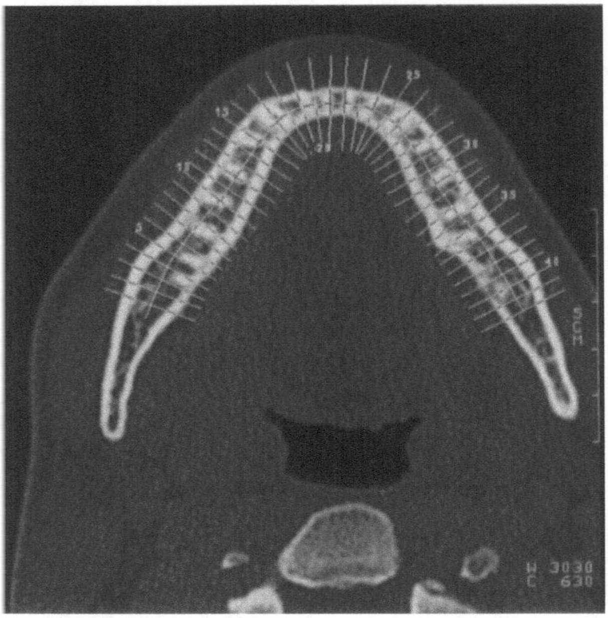

Fig. 5. Dental of the mandible: the graphic shows the orientation of the reconstructions

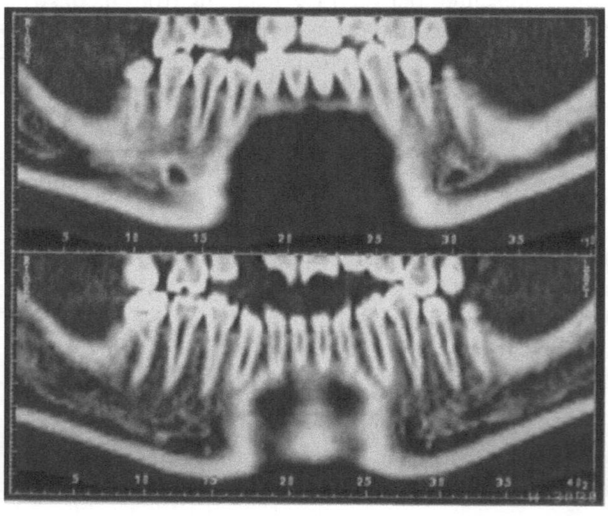

Fig. 6. Panoramic reconstructions of a mandible

the interactive definition of the dental reconstructions. An example is shown in Fig. 5: The definition for the PV is shown as a curved line running the length of the jaw. Locally perpendicular to this curved line and to the jaw are the location and orientation of each synthetic cross-sectional image. Every fifth tick mark is numbered for ease of counting. The length of these lines reflects the size of reconstructions. Two PVs of a mandible are presented in Fig. 6. Vertical markers indicate the position of the measured transaxial images. The horizontal tick marks refer to the positions of the

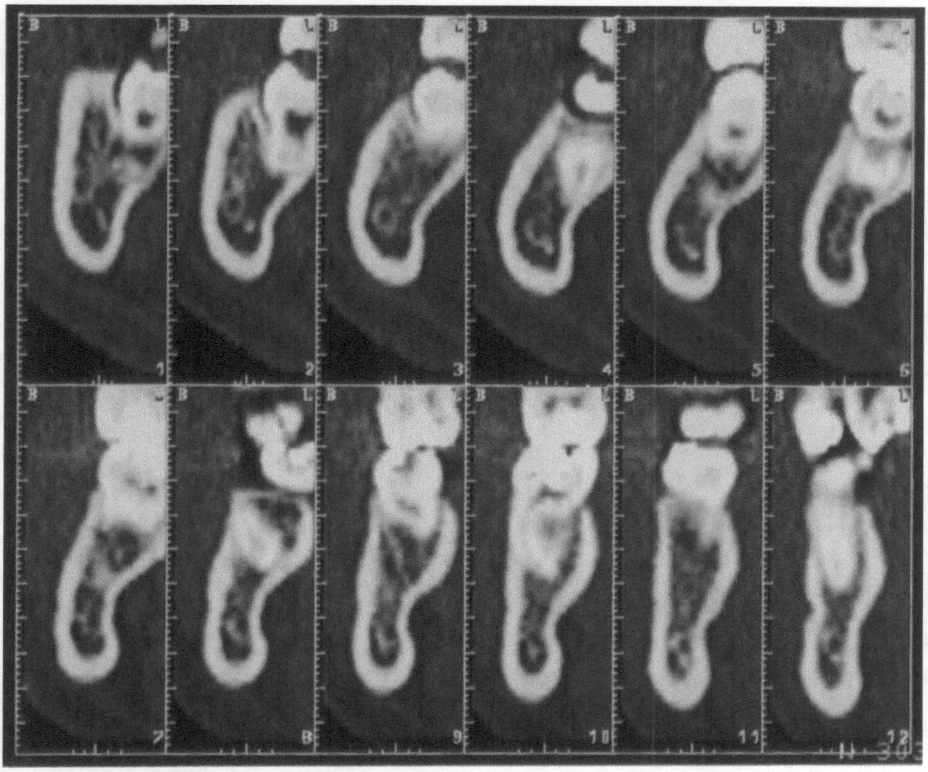

Fig. 7. Synthetic transaxial images of a mandible

STI. A standard labeling of orientation is displayed also. Up to five PVs are reconstructed; however, only one serves for reference purposes. The example in the lower right part of Fig. 6 demonstrates the alveolar nerve canal partially.

Dental CT produces two-dimensional synthetic cross-sectional images perpendicular to the long axis of the jaw and to both the panoramic and the transaxial scan planes. As demonstrated in Fig. 7, each of the small STIs is numbered as indicated in the reference image. The tick marks along the vertical edge of the STIs gives the location of the transaxial scans. The tick marks along the horizontal edge indicate the location of each PV produced by dental CT. The capital letter "B" symbolizes the buccal and the letter "L", the lingual orientations. The size and the number of displayed STIs in a presentation like that in Fig. 7 depend on the film size and the region of interest itself. Each of these small STIs manifests clearly the size and position of the alveolar nerve. The true cross-sectional images enable the dental surgeon to measure the wall thickness of the bone and the depth of the nerve. It even becomes possible to match real implant with the results on film to verify the selected size of the implant.

In Fig. 8, an example of the evaluation of a maxilla study is shown. The actions to achieve these results are similar to the examination of a mandible. The same type of labeling applies here also. Two important issues for clinically valuable results

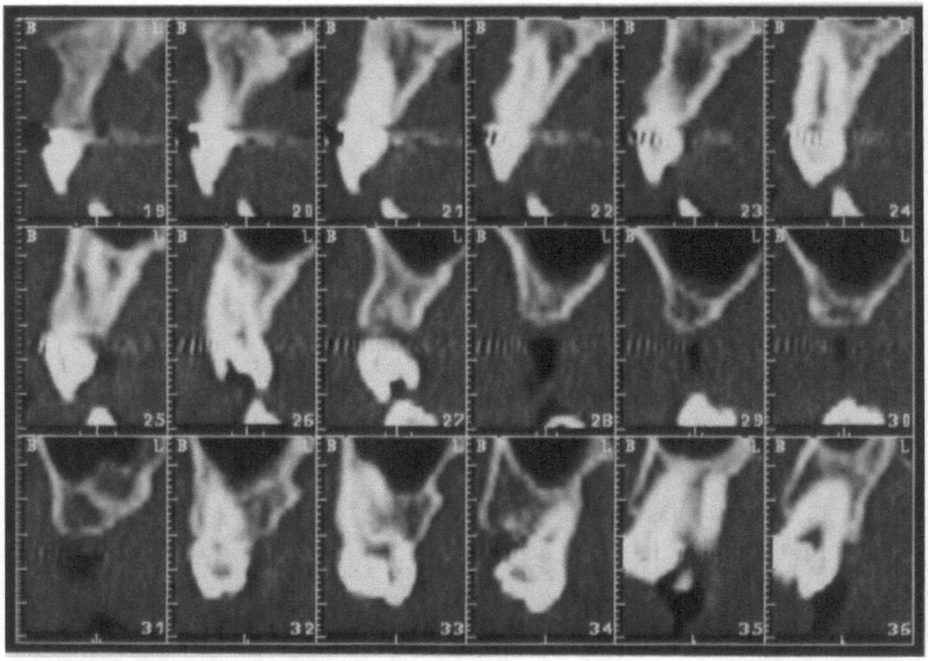

Fig. 8. Synthetic transaxial image of a maxilla

become obvious in these images. The bone of the maxilla is significantly thinner than that of the mandible. Therefore, it is here most important to scan with the smallest slice thickness possible and to select a high resolution mode. The second observation points to an imaging problem which is hard to overcome: metallic artifacts. This artifact often dramatically degrades the quality of transaxial images; however, secondary reconstructions like dental CT suffer less from this problem. To some extent, examinations which include metallic fillings may result in well-diagnosable dental images.

Conclusion

The special computer graphics technique realized in the software package dental CT provides cross-sectional reformats parallel and perpendicular to a curved line defined by the curvature of the mandibular or maxillary arches. These reformatted PVs and the STIs present the mandible and the maxilla to the oral surgeon for fast and easy evaluation of the patient's pathology. The capability of accurate measurements in these reformatted 2D images, even on X-radiography film, offers a safe and easy-to-use planning tool for oral surgeons and prosthodontists.

References

1. Schwarz MS, Stauts B (1987) Fixture placement. CDA J: 45–50
2. Branemark PI et al. (1977) Osseointegrated implants in the treatment of the edentulous jaw. Experience from a 10 year period. Scand J Plast Reconstr Surg [Suppl 16]
3. Jemt T (1986) Modified single and short-span restorations supported by osseointegrated fixtures in the partially edentulous jaw. J Prosthet Dent 55: 243–246
4. Rothman SL et al. (1988) CT in the preoperative assessment of the mandible and maxilla for endosseous implant surgery. Radiology 168: 171–175
5. Gotec TS (1986) CAD-CAM multiplanar imaging for subperiosteal implants. Dent Clin North Am 30: 85–95

A Prospective View of the Importance of Three-Dimensional CT in the Diagnosis of Brain Tumors Based on Clinical Experience

A. Dickschas

Introduction

Surface-oriented three-dimensional (3D) reconstructions with computed tomography (CT) were initially conceived for the display of the skin surface and that of bony structures. It is based on the spatial differentiation of tissue areas with high contrast. Thus, soft-tissue differentiation was primarily not intended. This was first mase possible using a trick: The application of contrast medium into the circulatory system results in a sufficiently high contrast of the vessels to the marginal tissue and thereby also of the highly vascularized soft tissue structures. The neuroradiologist therefore has the posibility of including this new CT imaging method for the specific diagnosis of tumors.

No reliable figures are available concerning the frequency of brain tumors in the population. Nevertheless, the high mortality of brain and spinal tumors is estimated to affect between 20000 and 25000 inhabitants here. It is therefore a matter of priority for physicians in the neurological fields to provide excellent preoperative images of the tumor so that surgery can be performed as soon as possible. The 3D reconstruction of axial CT is a diagnostic aid which will be especially important for preoperative planning and radiation therapy.

Patients and Methods

The present paper introduces four case histories of patients with brain tumors displayed synoptically with imaging of the masses being performed with the 3D CT technique.

They were four of the five tumor-afflicted patients on our station at the time of this examination. The types of tumor were therefore purely random: two meningiomas, one neurinoma, a prolactinoma of the pituitary gland, and a suprasellar, well-encapsulated, cystic tumor which was most likely a craniopharyngioma. Four of the brain tumors revealed such substantial contrast medium enhancement that a 3D reconstruction appeared useful. No appreciable contrast medium enhancement was found in the case of the cystic, encapsulated tumor. Because the contrast was insufficient here to differentiate the tumor surface from the marginal tissue, no 3D reconstruction was attempted.

The examinations were performed on a Somatom Plus-S (Siemens, Erlangen, FRG). The surface-oriented procedure together with the use of the high-speed processor of the system served to generate the 3D images. For this imaging method, the surface of the structure displayed with CT is reconstructed from a series of many slices. A binary contour matrix is thereby recalculated slice-by-slice.

In the course of our study, we initially used a series of 2-mm slices and later used two overlapping series with 2- and 3-mm slices.

Contrast medium was administered as is common for conventional CT. The rigid temporal coordination required by the high-speed processor of the angio-CT was not necessary here, since the contrast medium enhancement persisted sufficiently long and was extensive.

All of the examinations presented here were performed using standard software and without an editing program.

Case Studies

Case one was a female patient with a paraparesis of the legs, more evident on the right, and increasing disorientation. Two juxtapositional tumors were diagnosed in the preliminary examination with CT. In spite of the high image quality of the thin, overlapping axial slices, a clear relationship of the complex structure could not be provided even with the 2D imaging of the Somatom Plus-S. It appeared to be two portions of the same tumor connected by a thin parenchymal bridge (Fig. 1 a).

Only the 3D reconstruction shows that it is a complex, solitary tumor formation with uninterrupted continuity. The piniform meningioma extending from the parasagittal sinus cauded into the cranium reveals no appreaciable change in caliber at the margin of the calcified and soft tissue portions (Fig. 1 b, c).

Figure 1 d, e shows an isolated display of the calcified region of the tumor on a 3D reconstruction of the axial, precontrast CT.

Figure 1 f demonstrates how the inclusion of further reconstructed slices provide a better recognition of the complex tumor formation than do the axial projections alone. The step-by-step increase in information by gradually including further slices supports the expectation that a synoptical view of the tumor with "all" slice levels provides the best possible information concerning its form and expansion.

Our second case is a female patient who was referred to our station for neurological clarification of a continuous metopodynia and cephalodynia, with an increasing loss of vision in the right eye. The examination with CT revealed a 2 × 3 cm contrast medium-enhanced mass in the region of the right temporal pole and without perifocal edema. The 3D reconstruction of the axial slices displayed an easily differentiable, circular tumor in the middle right cranial fossa, with contact to the sphenoid process and with a relatively smooth surface. The form and localization thereby support the diagnosis of a meningioma of the mediolateral sphenoid process. The tumor extends cranially from the basal dura mater and has already reached the basal region of the trunk of the right middle cerebral artery which it has partially surrounded. The furrow in the relief of the tumor surface is seen clearly after subtracting the blood vessel (Fig. 2). It is clear what importance this information can have for the operating surgeon.

The case described here clearly displays the spatial structure of the tumor with the adjacent, intraoperatively relevant anatomical structures which can be visualized

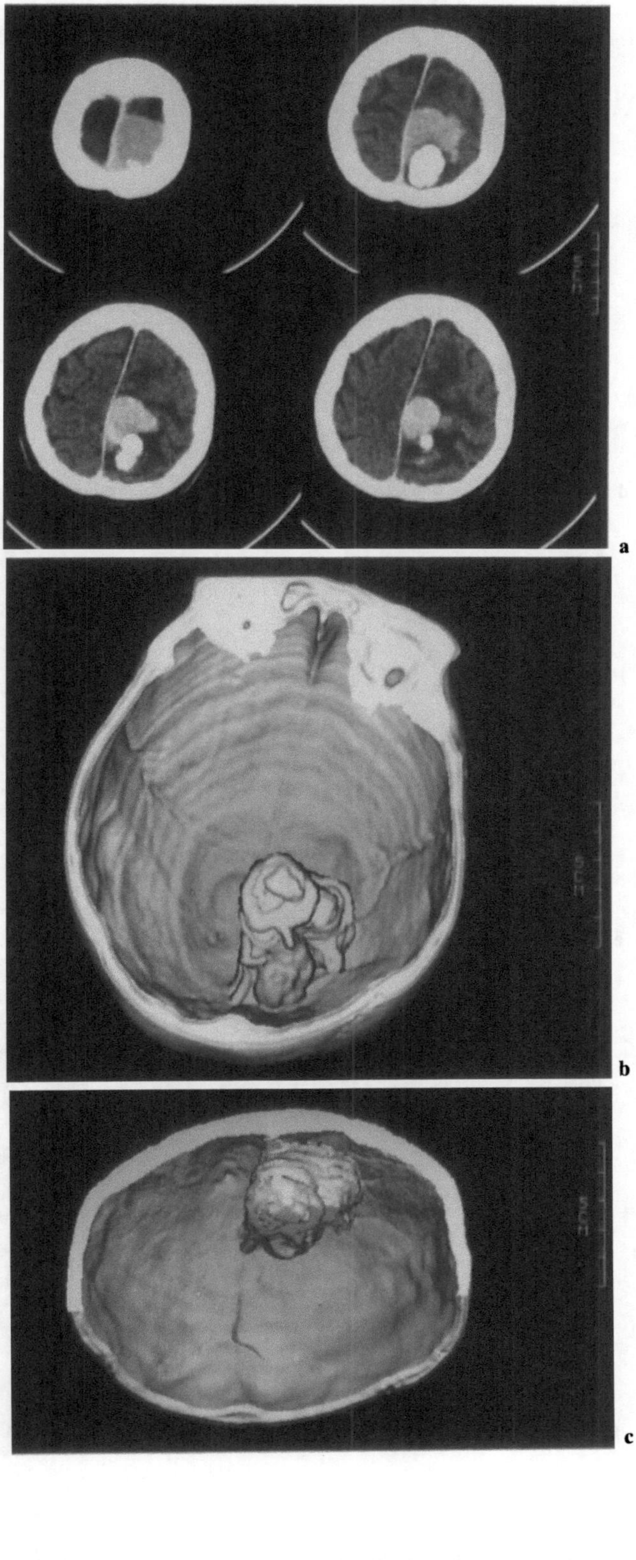

Fig. 1 a–c

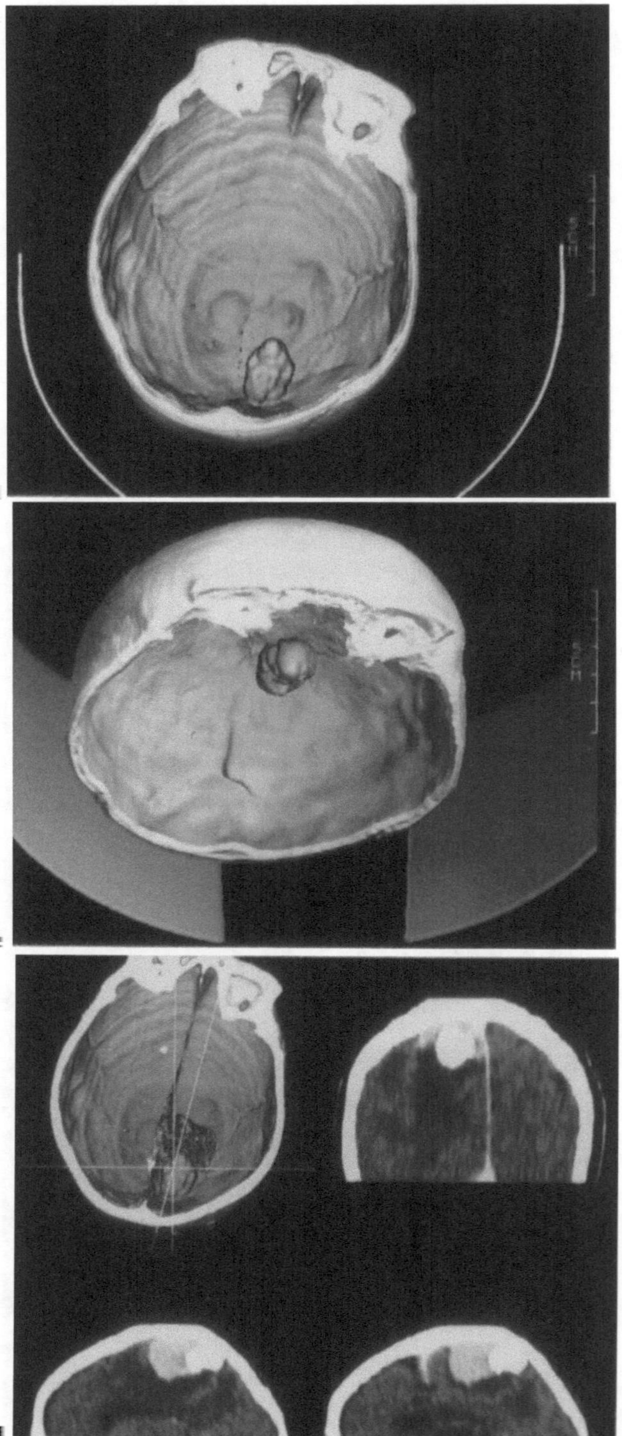

d

e

f

Fig. 1d–f

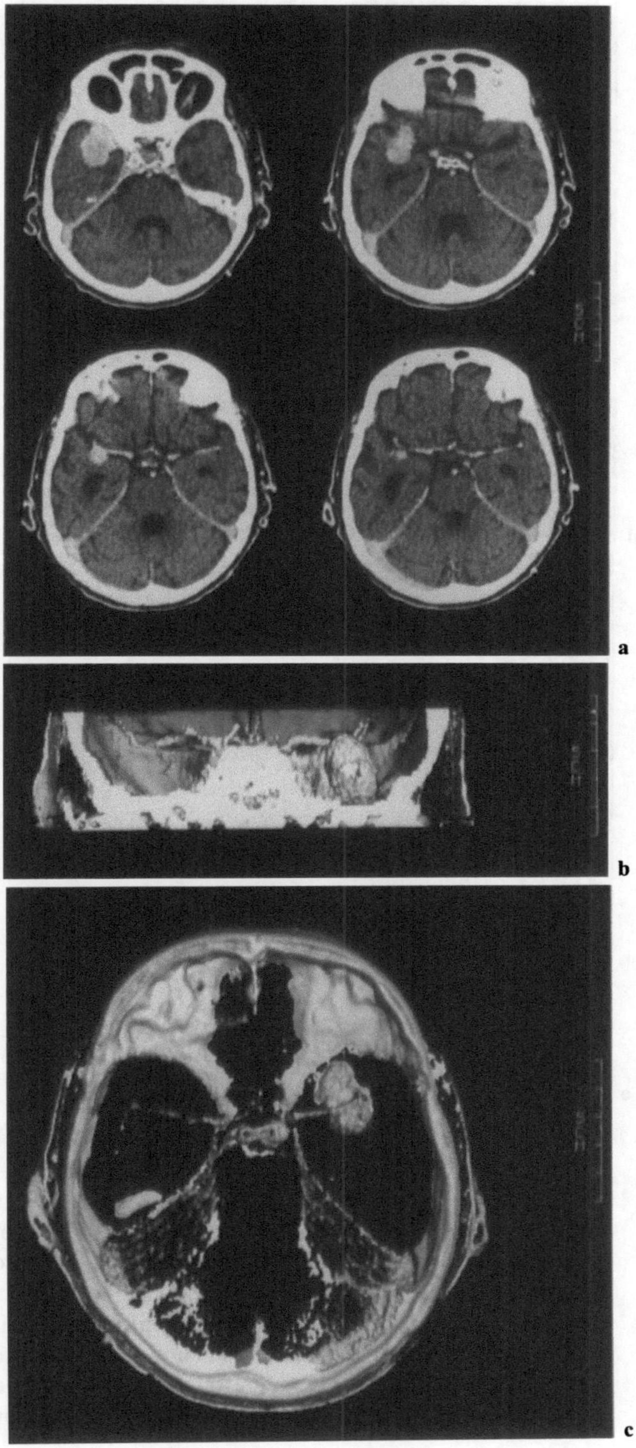

Fig. 2 a–c

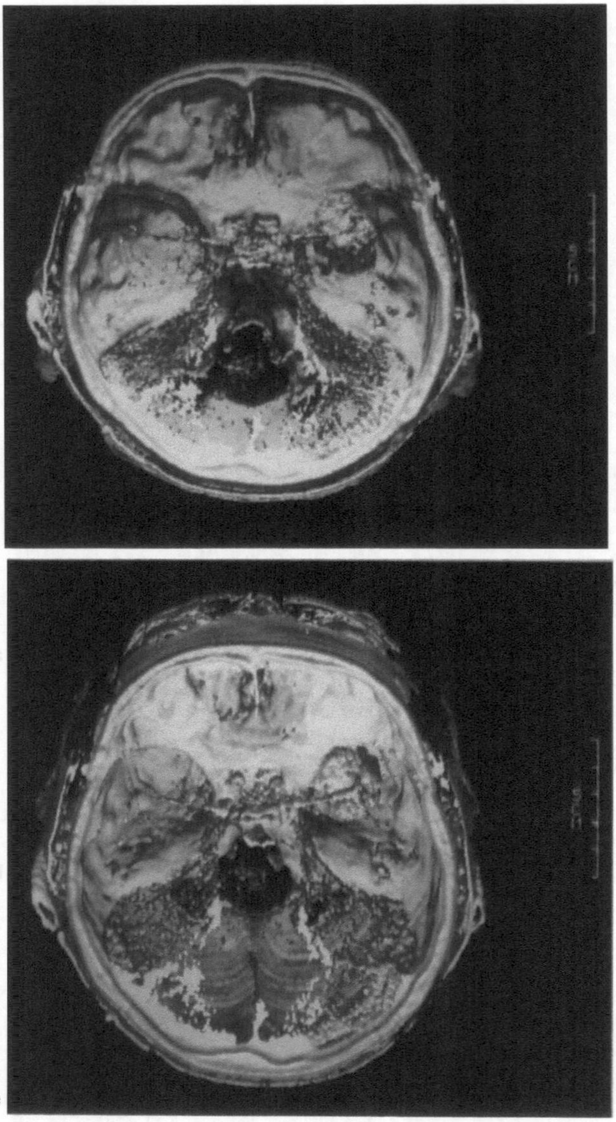

d

e

Fig. 2d, e

hyperdensely enough with CT. It also displays the exact spatial position of the tumor with the "scenery" of the cranial fossae as well as such other freely selectable spatial parameters as the crista galli, falx, tentorium, etc. A reconstruction of the tentorium permits the local classification of processes in the region of the occipital bone or the posterior cranial fossa as being either supratentorial or infratentorial.

On the other hand, this case also shows that an optimal increase in information results from the combined evaluation of axial slices and of the 3D reconstructions: the identification of the meningioma was established from the characteristically lacking edema, which could only be seen on the 2D CT, and the characteristic surface composition of the mass which, in contrast, was to be seen with 3D CT.

Case three is a male patient who was admitted for a left-sided hearing loss and increasing ataxic gait. A circular tumor with moderate contrast medium enhancement was found in the left cerebellopontine angle at the level of the porus acusticus internus with CT. Reduced contrast medium enhancement is seen in an area with regressive alterations. The localization, form, structure, and contrast medium behavior are most likely indicative of a neurinoma of the acoustic nerve (Fig. 3 a).

The 3D CT image also reveals a circular tumor which is adherent to the petrosal bone at the level of the porus acusticus internus, although easily differentiable from

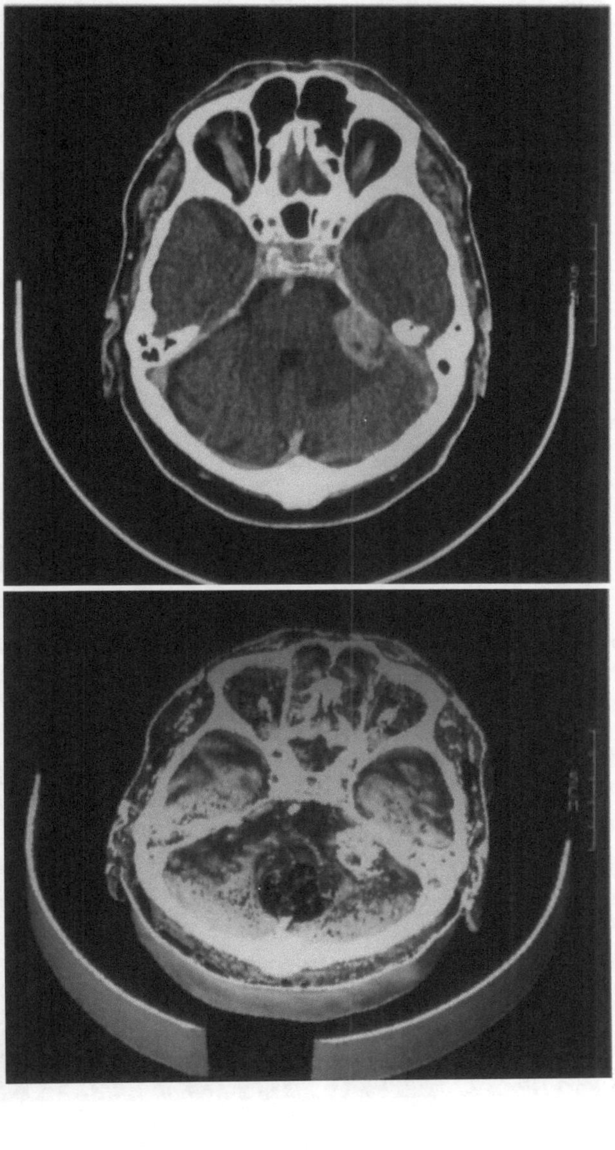

a

b

Fig. 3 a, b

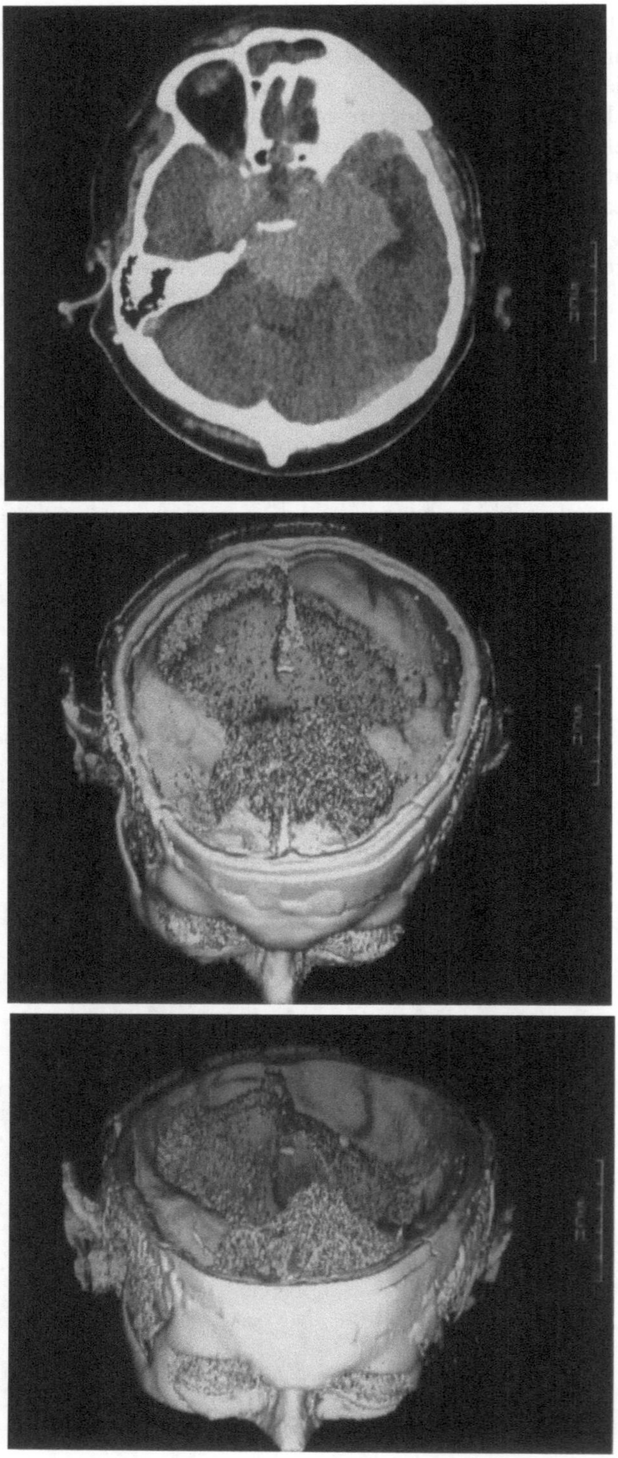

a
b
c

Fig. 4a–c

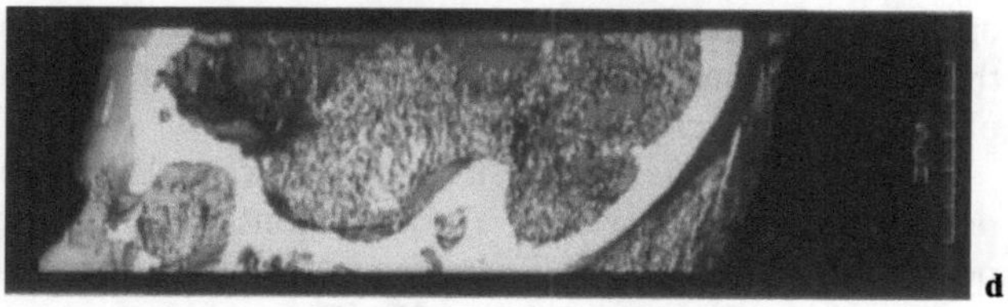

Fig. 4 d

the surrounding tissue. Erosion of the bone and a broadening meatus acusticus are seen in Fig. 3b).

Binding of the contrast medium also decreases in areas where vascularization is reduced such as in cystic necrotic decomposition, thereby lacking the mandatory contrast for 3D imaging. The lateral pole of the tumor can no longer be reconstructed fully: An indication of the limitations of this technique!

Case four describes the findings in a male patient in whom a pituitary tumor was resected 7 months ago. Histological findings were indicative of a prolactinoma. A bilateral amaurosis and substantial changes in behavior were seen clinically. Hormone analysis again revealed a high elevation in the prolactin level.

The precontrast CT scan revealed a congested temporal horn left, whereas the right temporal horn and the parasellar cistern were wasted away fully. The tumor region could only be seen with CT after contrast medium administration. The extensive pituitary adenoma extending into the intrasellar, parasellar, and retrosellar regions compressed the parasellar cisternae and only revealed moderate contrast uptake and a homogeneous enhancement (Fig. 4a). The 3D reconstruction reveals a tumor recurrence which extends from the subfrontal to the clivus, lies broadly and parasellar along the base of the brain, and has a domed configuration. The parasellar and interpeduncular cisternae are filled, and the middle cerebral arteries are surrounded bilaterally, although they are not fully blocked (Fig. 4b–d).

Results and Discussion

Based upon experience gained from examinations of five patients with brain tumors, we have attempted to make an analysis of the operational possibilities and the meaningfulness of 3D CT in the diagnostic clarification of brain tumors.

The first requirement for performing 3D imaging of a tumor is a high degree of contrast with the surrounding tissue either through adequate contrast medium enhancement or abundant calcifications. In our study, it was impossible to perform 3D imaging on one patient. Highly homogeneous contrast medium enhancement is seen especially in tumors which are solid and therefore easily operable, meningiomas, neurinomas, adenomas of the pituitary, and solid angioblastomas as well as medulloblastomas, the most frequent tumor in children, nodular glioblastomas, and chorioepitheliomas.

Thus, 3D CT is especially useful for surgeons and radiation therapists. For the latter, the technique is able to provide metric data concerning the tumor and its surroundings for measurements, intervals, and angles. Neurosurgeons usually make preoperative plans based on two-dimensional CT scans before they are able to confirm their expectations during the operation, which must than be performed with the aid of our physiological 3D vision and recognition.

The 3D CT offers a plastic image of complex tumor structures which is comparable with our 3D vision. The "relationship" of irregular structures which might possibly be lost with 2D CT can be visualized with this technique. As indicated by the study, we are of the opinion that 3D CT provides a more complete image of brain tumors than is possible with 2D imaging. Aside from the information available in the underlying axial slices, 3D reconstructions can, of course, provide no more information than that found in the raw data.

Since transaxial imaging has become a standard examination technique, we have meanwhile become accustomed to seeing images in the axial mode. In general diagnosis, however, it has usually been accepted that "the importance of axial slices is intensified by the addition of coronary slices." This is true even when the coronary slice is reconstructed from axial slice data. Consequently, each slice which we include provides additional information, until the greatest possible formation is finally attained by computing a conglomeration of all cumulative slices. Here, this information is concerned with both the form and expansion of the tumor.

It is our opinion that the image with 3D CT inevitably offers more extensive information than the 2D images in one (generally the axial plane) or two slices.

Our case studies reveal that a reconstruction of typical cranial/intracranial structures, with the exception of large-caliber cerebral blood vessels, the tentorium, and the falx, enables a more secure localization of the mass as well as important information concerning the relationship of the tumor to adjacent cerebral arteries and sinuses.

The disadvantage to 3D CT is its dependency on high contrast already mentioned above. The solitary application of this new variant for the diagnosis of brain tumors is therefore not sensible. However, in combination with 2D CT, which also permits soft tissue differentiation, it can be seen to be a useful addition to neuroradiological diagnostics. The 2D CT scan not only visualizes a larger part of the tumors which cannot be displayed with 3D reconstruction but also reveals such secondary changes in brain tissue brought about by tumors as perifocal edema, for instance. The combined application of both techniques (2D and 3D reconstructions) provides optimal information concerning the localization and specific diagnosis of brain tumors and requires an extremely short examination time as well.

References

1. Hodler J, Kuoni W, Rodriguez M (1990) Three-dimensional Imaging: advances in CT. Springer, Berlin Heidelberg New York
2. Imhof K, Die dreidimensionale Darstellung von CT-Bildern: Methode und Möglichkeiten. Elektomedica 57 (4)
3. Lange S, et al. (1988) Zerebrale und spinale Computertomographie. S. Karger, Basel
4. Mummenthaler M (1989) Neurologie. Georg Thieme, Stuttgart
5. Poeck K (1977) Neurologie. Springer, Berlin Heidelberg New York
6. Sager WD, Ladurner G (1979) Computertomographie. Georg Thieme, Stuttgart
7. Scheid W (1980) Lehrbuch der Neurologie. Georg Thieme, Stuttgart

Subject Index

D

FSC
www.fsc.org
MIX
Papier aus verantwortungsvollen Quellen
Paper from responsible sources
FSC® C105338

If you have any concerns about our products,
you can contact us on
ProductSafety@springernature.com

In case Publisher is established outside the EU,
the EU authorized representative is:
Springer Nature Customer Service Center GmbH
Europaplatz 3, 69115 Heidelberg, Germany

Printed by Libri Plureos GmbH
in Hamburg, Germany